CONTENTS

Quality of Life in Child and Adolescent Illness

Concepts, Methods and Findings

Edited by

Hans M. Koot
Erasmus University Rotterdam, The Netherlands
and
Jan L. Wallander
University of Alabama, Birmingham, USA

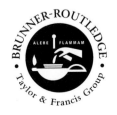

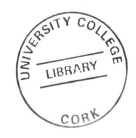

First published 2001 by Brunner-Routledge
27 Church Road, Hove, East Sussex, BN3 2FA

Simultaneously published in the USA and Canada
by Taylor & Francis Inc,
29 West 35th Street, New York NY 10001

Brunner-Routledge is an imprint of the Taylor & Francis Group

© 2001 Brunner-Routledge

Cover design by Richard Massing
Printed and bound in Great Britain by Biddles Ltd, Guildford and
King's Lynn

British Library Cataloguing in Publication Data
A catalogue record for this book is available from the British Library

Library of Congress Cataloging-in-Publication Data
A catalogue record for this book is available from the Library of
Congress

ISBNs 1-58391-233-9 (hbk)
      1-58391-234-7 (pbk)

TABLES AND ILLUSTRATIONS

The end of the last century has seen a wide-spread interest in the quality of people's lives. For many in the developed countries living standards have risen to unknown heights and technical possibilities seem unlimited. At the same time the efficacy and effectiveness of both private and public services and expenditures are seriously questioned. The main issue regards their contribution to a life of quality for their recipients. Program and service evaluation have never attracted this much attention. In the last few decades this has promoted the development of a vast amount of quality of life (QL) studies on adult persons, most notably in the arenas of public health and intellectual disabilities. More recently these activities have started to include children and adolescents as well.

Major progress in the diagnosis and treatment of a number of severe and chronic diseases in childhood has drastically increased the rate of survivors. Along with this progress in medical therapy the psychological and social task of children and adolescents and their families has become one of adapting to and coping with frequently uncertain survival, impact of chronic disease, and the costs of treatment. In recent years, this has led to efforts to assess the impact of disease on the QL in children and adolescents with physical conditions from the viewpoint of pediatrics, psychology, and public health and social policy administration. Similarly, QL studies involving people with intellectual disability have started to include youths as well.

Developments in the field of QL research reflect larger societal trends concerning the individual, the importance of subjective views in evaluating life, and the recognition that material, social, or medical indicators alone do not define QL. People react differently to the same circumstances, and they evaluate conditions based on their unique expectations, values, and previous experiences. A balanced definition of QL emphasizes "the combination of objectively and subjectively indicated well-being in multiple domains of life considered salient in one's culture and time, while adhering to universal standards of human rights" (Wallander, this volume) as core features of QL. However, the study of QL in children and adolescents has only just begun and is hampered by a myriad of theoretical and operational problems. Despite this, the QL studies with young people constitute a rapidly expanding, challenging, and exciting field of research.

Given the wide-spread interest in the study of QL in young people and its growing body of research, we felt there was a need for a book that provides an overview of conceptual and methodological issues concerning QL measurements amongst children and youths, of the impact of chronic conditions and their treatment and care on the QL of children, and of the results of recent efforts to develop QL instruments for this age group. We thought such a book should be both introductory to the field, and should contain in-depth contributions by leading researchers in this emerging field. To reach a balanced overview three main areas are addressed: (1) the conceptual basis of different approaches to QL assessment; (2) the impact of the most prevalent and disabling chronic conditions on the QL of children and adolescents; and (3) detailed overviews of efforts and methodological issues in the development of appropriate QL measures for this age group and their characteristics.

The first part of this book contains an introductory chapter by Koot that outlines the concepts, methods, and issues related to the study of QL in children and adolescents.

In the second part, Wallander's chapter expands this outline by a much needed in-depth discussion of theoretical and developmental issues in QL studies. Spieth reviews and evaluates generic measures currently available for the assessment of QL of children and adolescents. The generic measure is acknowledged by virtually all authors in this volume to be an indispensible instrument for the study of QL. Next, the chapter by Kaplan introduces the health care policy perspective and a number of innovative, thought provoking applications of it.

The third part includes three chapters on QL and chronic conditions as a general class. Ireys' chapter discusses methodologic and conceptual issues related to defining and classifying childhood chronic conditions and describes a number of consequences resulting from decisions made about these issues. The patient group perspective, discussed by Ravens-Sieberer and Bullinger, seems to be a promising approach for the evaluation of the QL implications of specific treatments in pediatrics. Hanson, in her chapter on QL in families of youths with chronic conditions, presents a framework for understanding the deep impact of having a child or adolescent with a chronic condition in the family.

The fourth part constitutes a major part of the book, covering QL in children and adolescents suffering from a number of the most common chronic childhood conditions. The aim of this section is to give an overview of the consequences of having the disease or handicap that constitutes a risk for the child's or adolescent's QL, either directly or through its treatment. Each chapter first describes the disease in functional terms. Then, a literature-based description is given of the impact of the disease and its treatment on QL in relation to the different domains of QL. Each chapter provides information on child and adolescent QL measures that have been applied to or specifically developed for this condition, including their strenghts and limitations. The chapters concern abdominal disorders (by Bouman), asthma (by French), cancer (by Eiser), cardiovascular disease (by Delamater and Pearse), cystic fibrosis (by Thompson and Karlish), headaches (by Langeveld and Passchier), insulin-dependent diabetes mellitus (by Johnson and Perwien), and intellectual disabilities (by Wallander and Turrentine). The reader will notice that many of the issues and findings discussed in these condition-specific chapters are not very condition-specific, and that several of them add considerable to the general childhood QL literature due to remarkable conceptual or methodological contributions.

In their concluding chapter, Koot and Wallander give an overview and integration of the issues that have been raised in the previous chapters, and identify a number of promising alleys for future research and applications.

This book is intended for psychologists; pediatricians; pediatric nurses; child psychiatrists; other medical specialists; public health professionals and administrators; researchers; and others and who are interested in the QL of children and adolescents with an acute or chronic disease or handicap and those who need intensive treatment or chronic care. We hope it will be suitable as a text for courses, seminars, or in-service training programs that aim at the development of knowledge on psychosocial issues in pediatrics, child psychology, child psychiatry, and services for the handicapped at the graduate level and above. In addition, it should be informative for working professionals. Although the focus is on the child with a chronic condition, we expect that the content of the book will have implications for studies on children and adolescents at large, including those from the general population and those with special needs due to adverse personal or environmental circumstances, or receiving other services or treatment such as those with intellectual or sensorimotor impairments or disabilities, learning problems, or psychiatric disorders.

Hans M. Koot
Jan L. Wallander

Nico H. Bouman, Department of Child and Adolescent Psychiatry, Sophia Children's Hospital, Rotterdam, The Netherlands

Monika Bullinger, Department of Medical Psychology, University Hospital Eppendorf, University of Hamburg, Hamburg, Germany

Alan M. Delamater, Mailman Center, School of Medicine, University of Miami, Miami, Florida, USA

Christine Eiser, Department of Psychology, University of Exeter, Exeter, United Kingdom

Davina J. French, Department of Psychology, University of Western Australia, Nedlands, Western Australia

Cindy L. Hanson, University of Central Florida, Orlando, Florida, USA

Henry T. Ireys, Departments of Maternal and Child Health and Pediatrics, Johns Hopkins University School of Hygiene and Public Health, Baltimore, Maryland, USA

Suzanne Bennett Johnson, Center for Pediatric Psychology Research, University of Florida, Gainesville, Florida, USA

Robert M. Kaplan, Family and Preventive Medicine, University of California, San Diego, California, USA

Lisa Karlish, Division of Medical Psychology, Duke University Medical Center, Durham, North Carolina, USA

Hans M. Koot, Department of Child and Adolescent Psychiatry, Erasmus University Rotterdam, Rotterdam, The Netherlands

Johannes H. Langeveld, Rogaland Psychiatric Hospital, Stavanger, Norway

Jan Passchier, Institute of Medical Psychology and Psychotherapy, Erasmus University Rotterdam, Rotterdam, The Netherlands

Lee Ann Pearse, University of Miami School of Medicine, Miami, Florida, USA

Amy R. Perwien, Center for Pediatric Psychology Research, University of Florida, Gainesville, Florida, USA

Ulrike Ravens-Sieberer, Department of Medical Psychology, University Hospital Eppendorf, University of Hamburg, Germany

Leslie E. Spieth, Harvard Medical School, Children's Hospital, Boston, Massachusetts, USA

Robert J. Thompson, Jr., Division of Medical Psychology, Duke University Medical Center, Durham, USA

Luanne Turrentine, Civitan International Research Center, University of Alabama, Birmingham, Alabama, USA

Jan L. Wallander, Civitan International Research Center, University of Alabama, Birmingham, Alabama, USA

INTRODUCTION

Chapter 1

THE STUDY OF QUALITY OF LIFE: CONCEPTS AND METHODS

Hans M. Koot

The last century has seen a marked change in how we view children and adolescents and how we have come to put a value on each and every one's life. Whether you are a child or adult, it is not merely enough to *have* life, rather, society strives to *enhance the quality of life* (QL) of all its citizens through programs such as health care, education, housing, and resource planning. One example of this change in emphasis from maintaining life to enhancing QL is seen in the major progress in the diagnosis and treatment of a number of severe and chronic diseases in childhood, which has drastically increased the rate of survivors (Newachek & Taylor, 1992). Along with this progress in medical treatment the psychological and social task of children and adolescents and their families has become one of adapting to and coping with various problems such as frequently uncertain survival, impact of chronic disease, and the costs of treatment. In recent years, this has led to efforts to assess the impact of disease on QL in children and adolescents from the viewpoint of pediatrics, psychology, and public health administration (Spieth & Harris, 1996). The time seems right to review concepts and methods of research that are relevant for the study of quality of life in children and youth. Although several such reviews exist, they are focused on specific populations (e.g., Eiser, 1997; Eiser & Jenney, 1995; Mulhern, et al., 1989) or included in books essentially covering quality of life in adults (e.g., Landgraf & Abetz, 1996; Rosenbaum, Cadman, & Kirpilani, 1990; Rosenbaum & Saigal, 1996). This chapter gives an introductory overview of aims, concepts, and methods related to the study of quality of life with children and adolescents.

CONCEPTS

Once we start thinking about QL, the concept itself becomes intriguing. We can imagine visiting someone who lies in the hospital for some serious disease. A very likely question would be: "How are you?" If not merely pronounced for reasons of politeness these three words seem to contain the essence of the question of QL. This may be illustrated by the following example.

A few years ago, my eleven year old niece was hospitalized because she had recurrent headaches and increasing difficulty walking. Because she was born with spina bifida and was living with a shunt that had been replaced already several times, her family was very worried about her present state and future development. When a diagnosis still had not been established after a week, I visited her in the hospital and asked her: "How are you?" Fifteen minutes later we appeared to have talked in a very natural way about the possible origin of her recurrent difficulties, how ill she felt, what kind of diagnostic investigations she had gone through, and how stressful these were to her. She conveyed to me some of her pain, distress and anxiety. We talked over what she could and could not do in the hospital, how she tried to cope with the situation, and the additional stress she was confronted with because she had to share the room with several profoundly handicapped younger children. But she also mentioned the support she got from the daily visits by her parents, her good relationship with the nursing staff, and the postcards and letters she received from her family and friends.

This anecdotal account conveys many aspects of QL. However, public health administrators, clinicians, and researchers need a more formal definition of quality of life.

DEFINITION OF QUALITY OF LIFE

In this book the major emphasis is on aspects of quality of life that may be influenced by having a chronic condition. Studies in the young field of QL research with children and adolescents have borrowed frequently from health-related quality of life research in adults, and the applied definitions proposed for that purpose. Therefore, most definitions identify QL as a multidimensional construct incorporating primarily the patient's (and his/her caregiver's) evaluation of his/her life with respect to the domains of somatic sensation, physical and cognitive functioning, psychological well-being, and social interaction (cf. Schipper, Clinch, & Olweny, 1996).

However, large discrepancies exist across operational definitions of QL and in the identification of specific domains of QL (e.g., Gill & Feinstein, 1994; Hughes, Hwang, Kim, Eisenman, & Killian, 1995). Conceptually, QL encompasses all domains of a person's life. Since the beginning, researchers have agreed that QL is a multidimensional concept tapping functional impairments, handicaps, and living conditions of the individual. However, the diversity of QL criteria and outcome measures has been described as "almost researcher specific"

(Borthwick-Duffy, 1989). For example, Hughes et al. (1995) reviewed quality of life studies of persons with disabilities and identified 44 different definitions that could be aggregated into 15 dimensions of quality of life. In 87 of the reviewed empirical studies 1,243 different operationalizations of these dimensions could be identified. As a consequence, most researchers abandon the idea of defining QL as an entity, but instead are satisfied to use QL as a working construct or organizing concept, and restrict the domains under consideration to about 4 to 8 depending on the purpose to which it is applied (e.g., Schalock, 1996; Schipper et al., 1996; Spilker, 1996).

Since QL in principle regards all domains of life for all people, only practical or philosophical reasons can be forwarded to limit the set of domains to cover any specific application. From the patient's perspective at least the domains of physical, psychological, and social functioning should be included since each may be affected by acute or chronic conditions. It certainly cannot be limited to merely physical or medical considerations. Another consideration is to define relevant domains from the perspective of care for a certain group. For example, Stark and Faulkner (1996) reasoned that for individuals with disabilities QL domains can be identified that are valid across the life-span and in which different levels of support are needed, including health care, living environment, family, social/emotional relationships, education, work, and leisure. Across the life-span and across domains, the level of support needed may vary from intermittent or limited, through to extensive and pervasive.

In another, more philosophical account Laplège and Hunt (1997) argued that the existential framework of QL with its emphasis on human freedom, patient preferences and subjective importance would make it undesirable for medicine to keep it as an object of scientific enquiry for the benefit of medical decision making or health policy. They suggested that in the health field QL could be more clearly defined as an outcome variable and measured more validly if it were replaced with the notion of "subjective health status," limiting its definition to the patient's view of his/her physical and psychological symptoms.

An important distinction can be made between health-related quality of life and overall quality of life. There seems to be general agreement that health-related QL is "a multidimensional concept that includes the broad areas of functional status, psychologic and social well-being, health perceptions, and disease- and treatment-related symptoms" (Aaronson et al., 1991, p. 840). It therefore advocates a medical and health-care perspective on QL. Overall quality of life expands upon this and incorporates non-medical-related aspects of a person's life such as influence of jobs, family, friends, and other living circumstances.

Another important conceptual differentiation regarding QL is between the subjective and objective perspectives. Some researchers argue that the assessment of QL is essentially subjective and that the patient should be the primary source of information regarding his/her quality of life. The target individual then is regarded the primary source of information of the quality of his or her life. However, others state that QL refers to both subjective and objective evaluations (cf. Spieth & Harris, 1996). In this view it is crucial to have an objective description of the individual and his/her circumstances in order to identify life conditions that are associated with subjective well-being and may be amenable to change through service and policy. Most health-related quality of life research has included both of these levels in their studies. More recently, a third level is being emphasized; the importance attached by the individual to his/her life conditions and his/her valuation of these (e.g. Felce & Perry, 1995; 1997). Although still quite limited, the issue of subjective importance is now starting to be addressed in child and adolescent QL research (e.g., Cummins, 1997; Juniper, Guyatt, Feeny, Ferry, Griffith, & Townsend, 1996b).

Despite the large variation in definitions and the numerous obstacles to be overcome, there are many common issues in the conceptualizing and defining of QL. These commonalities lead us to submit the following definition of the QL of children and adolescents with chronic conditions: *Quality of life is the combination of objectively and subjectively indicated well-being in multiple domains of life considered salient in one's culture and time, while adhering to universal standards of human rights.* We propose to take this definition as a guideline for the present volume. The derivation of the definition and what domains should be included will be explained in Chapter 2.

IMPORTANCE OF QUALITY OF LIFE AS AN OUTCOME MEASURE

In 1947 the World Health Organisation defined health as a state of complete physical, mental and social well-being. Aspects of disease to be distinguished include pathology, morbidity, functional impairment, and associated handicap (Verbrugge & Jette, 1994). In the past, most studies of disease outcome only regarded the first two aspects. However, during the last few decades it became clear that the association between morbidity and health as defined above is seriously limited. Morbidity and functional impairment are only partially related to life satisfaction. For example, Guyatt, Juniper, Feeny, and Griffith (1997a) found only small correlations between respiratory flow in child and adolescent asthma patients and their self-rated QL. By contrast, regarding long-term outcome, general life satisfaction appears to have significantly better predictive power than morbidity parameters, at least in adults. Further, there is a notable discrepancy between the assessed efficacy and the patient-perceived effectiveness of many treatments. Thus, even for treatments with proven efficacy, decisions on whether or not to treat may depend on the gain in subjective QL (see Kaplan, 1990, for an elaboration of these points).

Another issue is that until quite recently, outcome from medical care and policy was mainly assessed through physician's report. However, physicians seem to underestimate patients' quality of life and over-estimate patients' feelings of anxiety, depression, and distress (see Sprangers & Aaronson, 1992, for an overview). Equally, they seem to have limited sensitivity to the psychological burden caused by the condition and its treatment. Due to these and other factors, agreement between proxies and patients is notoriously poor (Sprangers & Aaronson, 1992). Finally, an important impetus to the development of QL measures for children and adolescents, is that the numerous instruments needed to tap important outcomes as reported in, for example, the *Journal of Pediatric Psychology* or the *Journal of Developmental and Behavioral Pediatrics* might be efficiently summarized in concise QL instruments covering the same domains for effective use in and comparison across outcome studies and clinical trials. For example, it is much more convenient to apply one standardized and normed QL measure that comprises all relevant domains presented in a similar format than to have separate instruments for different domains, such as, physical, emotional and social functioning, that were originally developed for goals other than assessing outcomes of medical care. This aspect is especially evident in studies involving different age groups or longitudinal follow-up, since developmental differences may reduce the utility of outcome developed for a specific age range.

APPROACHES TO QUALITY OF LIFE ASSESSMENT

Aside from the several conceptual issues in applying QL notions to children and adolescents, there are several salient methodological questions to clarify. The most basic questions for the assessment of QL, whether for clinical or research purposes, are: "What should I

TABLE 1.1 PERSPECTIVES, INSTRUMENTS, AND VALUATION OF QUALITY OF LIFE ASSESSMENTS

PERSPECTIVES	INSTRUMENTS	VALUATION
SOCIETAL	→ GLOBAL	
HEALTH CARE POLICY	→ GENERIC	→ REPRESENTATIVE SAMPLE FROM THE GENERAL PUBLIC
PATIENT GROUP	→ DISEASE SPECIFIC	→ SIMILAR GROUPS OF PATIENTS IN RANDOMIZED CLINICAL TRIALS
INDIVIDUAL PATIENT	→ PATIENT SPECIFIC	→ INDIVIDUAL PATIENT / PROXY

ask?", "Whom (or where) should I ask?", "When should I ask?", and "How should I ask?" Generally, the answers to these questions should to a considerable extent be determined by the answer to the question: "What do I intend to do with the answer?" That is, for the best choice among alternative assessment procedures, the *purpose* of the assessment is of primary importance.

As indicated above, a person's health and its outcomes can be measured at a number of levels, the most prominent being mortality, morbidity, functional status and handicaps, and economic values. The assessment of QL can be ordered around at least four different *perspectives*, which typically lead to the choice of a specific *type of assessment*, and the potential to *weigh* or *valuate* the outcome to inform health-related decision-making (Table 1.1; also see Essink-Bot, 1995).

Perspectives

The four perspectives can be ordered along a dimension of application from macro to micro. The *societal* perspective concerns decisions on the distribution of public resources over areas such as education, housing, public transportation, and health care. It is closely tied to national priorities. From the *health care policy* perspective, decisions may be taken on the distribution of health care funds based on priorities set by knowledge of costs and effects of different interventions (e.g., from preventive strategies in the prenatal period to life extension at the end of life). The *patient group* perspective regards decisions on alternative treatments for circumscribed groups of patients (e.g., bone marrow transplant vs. radiation for cancer). These decisions are of immediate relevance from the *individual patient* perspective, which relates to the choice of the best treatment for the individual patient by him or herself and the physician. The level of decision-making, as represented by the different perspectives, guides the choice of the type of instrument that is most approriate for the assessment of quality of life at that level.

Instrumentation

At the *individual patient level*, decision-makers, that is the patient and the physician, are most interested in patient-specific instruments that assess the impact of disease and treatment on that patient's quality of life from his/her own perspective (e.g., by assessing the impact on domains of life that are of particular importance for this patient). At the *patient group level* the instrument must enable the assessment of the group under study in comparison with a control group. Therefore it is most important to include domains of functioning and experience that are relevant to the patients in the study group (e.g., continence-related impairments in patients with inflammatory bowel disease), that is to have a disease- and treatment-specific instrument available. By contrast, at the *health care policy level*, the impact of different diseases and interventions on outcome should be compared, which requires generic and comprehensive instruments. Finally, from the *societal perspective* data on the distribution of public resources should be obtained from population-based studies. The valuation of the information obtained at any of these levels of assessment becomes important to reach decisions on the allocation of resources or interventions.

Valuation

From the *individual patient* perspective the best decision is the one that most precisely reflects the individual patients' values without being in conflict with the values held by the physician. From the *patient group* perspective values attached to different outcomes by representatives of the patient group involved may be used to decide on alternative treatment strategies within a disease category. Values to be used in decisions made at the *health care policy* level should reflect the societal viewpoint and be obtained from a representative general population sample. In this sense, health care policy and *societal* priorities are closely connected.

The perspective that is taken in any situation will depend on a combination of factors. In practice we have to consider at least the following alternatives: Do we want to assess QL for clinical use or for public health purposes? Do we want to focus on health status, broadly construed, or on distress related to physical, psychological, and social functioning? Do we want to monitor treatment or assess outcomes? Do we want to study populations, groups, or individuals? Of course, these options are not necessarily mutually exclusive. In fact, most people who want to study QL may have several purposes in mind at the same time.

METHODS

Recent reviews of child and adolescent psychopathology (e.g., Verhulst & Koot, 1995) show convincingly that seemingly straightforward clinical notions and definitions of child and adolescent dysfunction are extremely resistant to adequate operationalization. Similar to the field of child and adolescent psychopathology, the development of child and adolescent QL measures is hampered by the lack of a gold standard, dependence on informants other than the child/adolescent, and the need to account for developmental differences. At the same time, scientific standards of reliability and validity should be met and normative standards included. From a practical point of view, users prefer a QL instrument that is long enough to yield robust data on the topic, and at the same time short enough to be practical, that is easy to administer, easy to score, and easy to interpret.

Thus, desiderata for a QL measure for children and adolescents are that it:

- operationalizes an accepted QL definition;
- includes both objective and subjective measures;
- includes domains broadly encompassing QL;
- has parallel forms for the patient, child and other informants;
- weighs satisfaction on domains of perceived importance to the child/adolescent;
- has satisfactory psychometric characteristics (internal structure, internal consistency, test-retest reliability, convergent and divergent validity, discriminative validity, sensitivity to change);
- has norms for the general population and/or specific patient groups.

Not surprisingly, and as will become evident in the following chapters, the task of developing adequate QL instruments for use with children and adolescents is far from accomplished. This charge will be revisited and elaborated in the concluding chapter.

MEASURING QUALITY OF LIFE IN CHILDREN AND ADOLESCENTS

In the last two decades numerous instruments have been developed to obtain information on QL in children and adolescents. These instruments can appropriately be distinguished into *generic* instruments, that are applicable to children and adolescents from the general population and to a range of different conditions, and *disease-specific* instruments. Among generic interviews and questionnaires, a distinction can be made between instruments used for epidemiologic survey work, utility measures, health profiles, and functional status and multi-dimensional instruments to assess clinical outcomes (Spieth, Chapter 3, this volume). Although the number and content of the items and scales show enormous variation, most instruments tap physical as well as psychological and social aspects of the child's functioning. Of the measures reviewed by Spieth most are to be rated by parents (n = 11), although quite recently questionnaires are developed for adolescents (n = 6) and children themselves (n = 4). A wealth of instruments have been developed for specific conditions, including asthma, cancer, diabetes, epilepsy, headaches, inflammatory bowel disease, juvenile rheumatoid arthritis, neuromuscular disorders, otitis media, rhinoconjunctivitis, and short stature. It is obvious that work on disease-specific measures that first mainly focused on cancer and asthma is now rapidly expanding. In addition, some of the generic instruments have modules designed for specific disease groups. For example, the HAY (Bruil, Maes, le Coq, & Boeke, 1997; le Coq et al., 2000) has specific modules for asthma, diabetes mellitus, epilepsy, and juvenile chronic arthritis. Recently, emphasis is put on the derivation of item content from adolescents and children themselves, for example through focus-group discussions with affected children and adolescents to develop items that are more relevant to the specific population (e.g., Griffiths, Nicholas, Smith, Munk, Durno, & Sherman, 1999).

Children are dependent on the support of their parents for the first 15–20 years, at least, of their lives and family functioning is regarded one of the strongest influences on child adjustment to chronic illness. Conversely, parents of children with serious or chronic diseases may themselves be at risk for psychological problems to the extent that they can no longer be an effective source of protection and development for the child (e.g., Varni & Setoguchi, 1992). Effects of chronic childhood illness on the family, including parents and siblings have recently received increasing attention (see Hanson, Chapter 7, this volume). In addition, a number of standardized instruments have been developed to assess this impact, including the Impact on Family Scale (Stein & Reissman, 1980), Parents of Children with Disabilities Inventory (Noojin & Wallander, 1996), Handicap-Related Problems for Parents

Inventory (Wallander & Marullo, 1997), Paediatric Asthma Caregiver's Quality of Life Questionnaire (Juniper, Guyatt, Feeny, Ferrie, Griffith, & Townsend, 1996a), and Life Situation Scale for Parents (Enskar et al., 1997). In addition, some generic QL instruments (e.g., the Child Health Questionnaire; Landgraf, Abetz, & Ware, 1996) have a parent impact scale.

There is a number of measurement issues that are especially relevant for the assessment of QL in children and adolescents. Some of these regard general psychometric aspects such as reliability and validity (see Spieth, Chapter 3, this volume), others regard aspects more specific to this age range, including developmental considerations and the issue of proxy reports. These latter represent major challenges for the development of QL measures for children and adolescents.

DEVELOPMENTAL CONSIDERATIONS

What can I ask? How should I ask? Can I ask the child him/herself? What are important areas of functioning at different ages? These are all questions that are affected by the child's development. First, developmental tasks vary by age. Examples of universal developmental tasks are: getting acquainted with peers at the age of 4 or 5 years; performing school-related tasks at school age; gaining a position among your peers and developing romantic relationships as an adolescent, and transitioning towards autonomy by late adolescence (e.g. Sroufe, 1979). Having a chronic condition may affect the process and outcome of dealing with these tasks considerably (e.g., Eiser, 1993). Also, how can tasks that are applicable to certain developmental periods, but not others, be addressed in any given assessment?

Second, developmental changes in attention span, perception of time, language level, and understanding of health, illness and QL related concepts, should all be accounted for in the assessment of children. Quite different demands are placed on the respondent in different instruments. For example, Juniper, Guyatt, Feeny, Griffith, and Ferrie (1997) studied the minimum age and reading skills required to complete four different formats for QL and health utility measures: the 7-point rating of the Paediatric Asthma Quality of Life Questionaire (Juniper et al., 1996b); the Feeling Thermometer that asks to indicate feelings about one's own health state on a thermometer ranging from 0 to 100 with clearly defined end points; the Health Utilities Index (Feeny et al., 1995; Torrance et al., 1995), that progressively ascertains the level of impairment on 10 attributes; and the Standard Gamble procedure (Torrance, 1986), in which patients are asked whether they would prefer the certainty of remaining in their current health state or would prefer to take a gamble with a treatment which will result in either perfect health or death. While the first three procedures could be reliably completed through reading or interview by children ages 7 and up, the latter was only reliable for children with above grade 6 (about 11–12 years of age) reading and comprehension skills.

Third, the importance that children attach to different areas of concern may vary both with age and disease or handicap. For example, especially during adolescence patients may be more concerned with reactions to their adherence behaviors than with proper adherence to treatment prescriptions (e.g. French et al., 1994; La Greca & Schuman, 1995). As another example, the visibility of the condition may play a different role at different periods of development.

It might be suggested that developmental increases in competence, broadening of areas of functioning, and age-specific changes in the relative importance of different domains of functioning, all argue for the development of age-specific QL measures or at least age-specific modules in QL measures. Taking this issue seriously, French, Christie, and Sowden (1994) designed three different versions of the Child Asthma Questionnaires. Form A for ages four to seven (14 items) uses picture items ('Smiley' faces expressing emotions) to ask about feelings, but not about frequency or duration of disease-related problems. Form B for ages 8 to 11 (23 items) uses more advanced pictures and includes items about the frequencies of activities and symptoms; Form C for ages 12 to 16 years (41 items) requires numerical responses to questions about feelings and frequencies. Also the level of independence of completion varies with age. The form for younger children is completed by child and parent together, the form for the intermediate age group is completed by the child with the help of an adult, if needed, and Form C requires individual completion stressing confidentiality. Another example along these lines is Cummins (1997) pre-testing approach to match response scale to respondent's ability (see Wallander & Turrentine, Chapter 15, this volume). Although these approaches partially solve the issue by producing formats that are reliable for each separate age group, its main drawbacks are difficulty in comparing data for children of different age groups, and using these different formats in longitudinal studies that cross the age borders.

DEVELOPING QUALITY OF LIFE MEASURES FOR CHILDREN AND ADOLESCENTS

The development of QL instruments for children should pass through all common and well-known phases of instrument development (e.g., Bullinger, Power, Aaronson, Cella, & Anderson, 1996; Guyatt, Naylor, Juniper, Heyland, Jaeschke, & Cook, 1997b). From a psychometric point of view, these include: the choice of the intended function or functions of the measurement; careful selection of the initial item pool; construction of scales by exploratory and confirmatory factor analyses; assessment of reliability; and assessment of discriminative validity, divergent and convergent construct validity, and sensitivity to change (see Spieth, Chapter 3, this volume). Not many of the current efforts in QL measurement in children have gone through all these phases, but even if they would, many often thorny conceptual and practical issues remain. To name a few: Should we try to develop instruments that are useful from all perspectives mentioned earlier, i.e., society, health care policy, treatment evaluation, and the individual? How should we construct psychometrically sound measures with sufficient practical value? For example, striving for high internal consistencies without content-related considerations may compromise applicability of these scales in the real world. Should we try to assess discriminative validity if there is no gold standard available for comparison? Are all QL instruments appropriate for the assessment of the outcome of all interventions or should we only use disease- or treatment-specific measures for that purpose? How should we deal with weighting of objective, subjective, and importance scores? What is our methodological answer to response shift, i.e. the tendency of respondents to change rating standards across time?

PROXY REPORTS

Informant variance is a continual problem when ratings from different informants on the same subject are obtained, as is typically required for children. Low agreement between informants appears to be the rule rather than an exception. For example, Achenbach, McConaughy, and Howell (1987) performed a meta-analytic study on 269 samples found in 119 studies on consistency between informants' reports of behavioral and emotional problems in subjects aged from 1.5 to 19 years. The mean correlation between pairs of informants who played similar roles to the child, such as pairs of parents, pairs of teachers, and pairs of mental health workers was .60. However, the mean correlation between informants playing different roles in relation to the child was only .28, and between children's self-reports and the other informants' reports only .22. Thus, informants who see the child in the same situation show higher agreement than informants seeing the child in different situations.

Agreement between informants may also differ by sex, age, and type of problem. Verhulst and Van der Ende (1992) reported on the agreement between parents' reports and adolescents' self-reports of problem behaviors in 883 11–19-year-olds from the general population. Adolescents reported many more problems than their parents reported about them. Discrepancies were larger for externalizing than for internalizing problems, and became larger with age. Discrepancies were largest for older girls on internalizing problems.

Lack of agreement between informants may be attributable to several sources including situation specificity of behavior; lack of knowledge on the part of the informant; the relationship between the child and the informant; value differences; denial, social desirable answers, or exaggeration; and the informant's own biases, personality, and personal problems (Achenbach, 1991). As yet we do not know the best way to integrate information from different informants in a standardized way.

The general phenomenon of moderate cross-informant agreement is an issue in all situations involving proxy reports, such as when we try to get a picture of the QL of a pediatric patient from different informants, such as the patient, the clinician, or family members. Sprangers and Aaronson (1992) performed a review of the literature on this topic in adult patients and identified a number of clear trends. In general, while health providers and significant others, such as family members and close companions appear to evaluate the patients' QL with a comparable degree of accuracy, they tend to underestimate it compared to the patient's own report. In addition, health care providers tend to underrate the patients' pain intensity. Further, evidence shows that proxy ratings are more accurate when the information sought is concrete and observable, and tend to be more accurate when the proxy lives in close proximity to the patient. However, they can also be biased by the caregiving function of the rater.

This latter issue may be even more of importance when parents are rating their child's QL. Parents of chronically ill children have an increased risk for symptoms of maladjustment (e.g., anxiety, depression) than parents of well children (e.g., Wallander & Varni, 1998), and these tend to influence their ratings of childhood adjustment (Boyle & Pickles,

1997). However, parental (especially maternal) ratings also contain substantive portions of variance (up to 50%) attributable to the child's condition (Rowe & Kandel, 1997).

Despite the less than optimal agreement to be expected among child and proxy on QL, proxy reports cannot be discarded. First, they are indispensable when a person is too young, ill, or handicapped to reliably report on his/her own condition. Second, although not highly correlated to the patient's own reports, proxy reports may contain both reliable and valid information. For example, both parent and teacher ratings of behavioral and emotional problems are valid indicators of later child outcomes (Koot & Verhulst, 1992; Verhulst, Koot, & Van der Ende, 1994), over and above the information obtained from youngsters themselves (Heijmens Visser, Van der Ende, Koot, & Verhulst, 1999). However, in most cases proxy reports of objective, easily observable aspects of QL are probably significantly more valid than proxy reports on the patient's subjective well-being.

CONCLUSIONS

In conclusion, we can be fairly sure that QL measurement in children will have to address numerous issues that until now have not been fully answered in QL assessment with adults. Nonetheless, it would be wise to draw on the experience of two decades of QL research with adults. For example, in 1990 a working group on QL research in oncology (Aaronson et al., 1991) reviewed the state of the art and future priorities in QL research regarding the conceptualization of QL, the focus and content of QL investigations, best research design and implementation strategies, and ways to transfer knowledge gained from QL research to clinical practice and medical decision making. Conclusions from this review should be taken seriously by any investigator of childhood QL. Furthermore, based on a critical review of available adult QL measures, Gill and Feinstein (1994) concluded many of the published instruments for adults seem to lack clinical appropriateness, have poor conceptualizations of QL, and do not sufficiently incorporate patients' values and preferences. That is, these instruments measure various aspects of health status instead of QL. They recommend the use of global ratings of both overall quality of life and of health-related quality of life; the rating of severity or magnitude of problems, but also of the importance of problems to the patient; and the possibility for patients to add important factors not included in the instrument. Again, these recommendations apply to the developing field of QL research with children and adolescents. However, it would be unforgivable to not also apply the basic findings of developmental psychology and developmental psychopathology, and the growing body of knowledge of pediatric psychology research. In doing so, we may turn the relatively immature position of QL assessment with children and adolescents into an advantage.

References

Aaronson, N.K., Meyerowitz, B.E., Bard, M. et al. (1991). Quality of life research in oncology: Past achievements and future priorities. *Cancer*, *67*, 839–843.

Achenbach, T.M. (1991). *Integrative guide for the 1991 CBCL/4-18, YSR, and TRF profiles.* Burlington, VT: University of Vermont Department of Psychiatry.

Achenbach, T.M., McConaughy, S.H., & Howell, C.T. (1987). Child/adolescent behavioral and emotional problems: Implications for cross-informant correlations. *Psychological Bulletin*, *101*, 213–232.

Boyle, M.H., & Pickles, A. (1997). Influence of maternal depressive symptoms in ratings of childhood behavior. *Journal of Abnormal Child Psychology*, *25*, 399–412.

Bruil, J., Maes, S., le Coq, E., & Boeke, A. (April, 1997). *Assessing the quality of life among children with chronic illness: The development of a questionnaire.* Paper presented at the Sixth Florida Conference on Child Health Psychology, Gainesville, FL.

Bullinger, M., Power, M., Aaronson, N.K., Cella, D.F., & Anderson, R.T. (1996). Creating and evaluating cross-cultural instruments. In B. Spilker (Ed.), *Quality of life and pharmacoeconomics in clinical trials* (2nd ed.) (pp. 659–668). Philadelphia: Lippincott-Raven.

Cummins, R.A. (1997). *Comprehensive Quality of Life Scale — Student (Grades 7–12): ComQoL-S5.* (5th ed.). Melbourne: School of Psychology, Deakin University.

Eiser, C. (1993). *Growing up with a chronic disease: The impact on children and their families.* London: Jessica Kingsley.

Eiser, C., & Jenney, M.E. (1995). Measuring symptomatic benefit and quality of life in pediatric oncology. *British Journal of Cancer*, *73*, 1313–1316.

Eiser, C. (1997). Children's quality of life measures. *Archives of Disease in Childhood*, *77*, 350–354.

Enskar, K., Carlsson, M., von Essen, L., Kreuger, A., & Harmin, E. (1997). Development of a tool to measure the life situation of parents of children with cancer. *Quality of Life Research*, *6*, 248–256.

Essink-Bot, M.L. (1995). Health status as a measure of outcome of disease and treatment. Erasmus University Rotterdam. Doctoral dissertation.

Feeny, D.H., Furlong, W., Boyle, M., & Torrance, G.W. (1995). Multi-attribute health status classification systems: Health utilities index. *Pharmacoeconomics*, *7*, 490–502.

Felce, D., & Perry, J. (1995). Quality of life: Its definition and measurement. *Research in Developmental Disabilities*, *16*, 51–74.

Felce, D., & Perry, J. (1997). Quality of life: The scope of the term and its breath of measurement. In R.I. Brown (Ed.), *Quality of life in people with disabilities* (pp. 56–71). Cheltenham: Stanley Thornes.

French, D.J., Christie, M.J., & Sowden, A.J. (1994). The reproducibility of the Childhood Asthma Questionnaires: Measures of quality of life for children with asthma aged 4–16 years. *Quality of Life Research*, *3*, 215–224.

Gill, T.M., & Feinstein, A.R. (1994). A critical appraisal of the quality of quality-of-life measurements. *JAMA*, *272*, 619–626.

Griffiths, A.M., Nicholas, D., Smith, C., Munk, M., Stephens, D., Durno, C., & Sherman, P.M. (1999). Development of a quality-of-life index for pediatric inflammatory bowel disease: Dealing with differences related to age and IBD type. *Journal of Pediatric Gastroenterology and Nutrition*, *28*, S46-52.

Guyatt, G.H., Juniper, E.F., Feeny, D.H., & Griffith, L.E. (1997a). Children and adult perceptions of childhood asthma. *Pediatrics*, *99*, 165–168.

Guyatt, G.H., Naylor, C.D., Juniper, E., Heyland, D.K., Jaeschke, R., & Cook, D.J. (1997b). User's guide to the medical literature: XII. How to use articles about health-related quality of life. *JAMA*, *277*, 1232–1237.

Heijmens Visser, J., Van der Ende, J., Koot, H.M., & Verhulst, F.C. (2000). Predictors of psychopathology in young adults referred to mental health services in childhood or adolescence. *Britsih Journal of Psychiatry, 177,* 59–65.

Hughes, C., Hwang, B., Kim, J.H., Eisenman, L.T., & Killian, D.J. (1995). Quality of life in applied research: A review and analysis of empirical measures. *American Journal of Mental Retardation, 99,* 623–641.

Juniper, E.F., Guyatt, G.H., Feeny, D.H., Ferrie, D.H., Griffith, L.E., & Townsend, M. (1996a). Measuring quality of life in the parents of children with asthma. *Quality of Life Research, 5,* 27–34.

Juniper, E.F., Guyatt, G.H., Feeny, D.H., Ferrie, D.H., Griffith, L.E., & Townsend, M. (1996b). Measuring quality of life in children with asthma. *Quality of Life Research, 5,* 35–46.

Juniper, E.F., Guyatt, G.H., Feeny, D.H., Griffith, L.E., & Ferrie, P.J. (1997). Minimum skills required by children to complete health-related quality of life instruments for asthma: Comparison of measurement properties. *European Respiratory Journal, 10,* 2285–2294.

Kaplan, R.M. (1990). Behavior as the central outcome in health care. *American Psychologist, 45,* 1211–1220.

Koot, H.M., & Verhulst, F.C. (1992). Prediction of children's referral to mental health and special education services from earlier adjustment. *Journal of Child Psychology and Psychiatry, 33,* 717–729.

La Greca, A.M., & Schuman, W. (1995). Adherence to prescribed medical regimens. In M.C. Roberts (Ed.), *Handbook of pediatric psychology* (2nd ed.) (pp. 55–83). New York: Guilford.

Landgraf, J.M., & Abetz, L.N. (1996). Measuring health outcomes in pediatric populations: Issues in psychometrics and application. In B. Spilker (Ed.), *Quality of life and pharmacoeconomics in clinical trials* (2nd ed.) (pp. 793–802). Philadelphia: Lippincott-Raven.

Landgraf, J.M., Abetz, L., & Ware, J.E. (1996). *The CHQ user's manual.* Boston, MA: The Health Institute, New England Medical Center.

Laplège, A., & Hunt, S. (1997). The problem of quality of life in medicine. *JAMA, 278,* 47–50.

le Coq, E.M., Colland, V.T., Boeke, A.J., Boeke, P., Bezemer, D.P., & van Eijk, J.T., (2000). Reproducibility, construct validity, and responsiveness of the "How Are You?" (HAY), a self-report quality of life questionnaire for children with asthma. *Journal of Asthma, 37,* 43–58.

Mulhern, R.K., Horowitz, M.E., Ochs, J., Friedman, A.G., Armstrong, F.D., Copeland, D., & Kun, L.E. (1989). Assessment of quality of life among pediatric patients with cancer. *Psychological Assessment, 1,* 130–138.

Newachek, P.W., & Taylor, W.R. (1992). Childhood chronic illness: Prevalence, severity, and impact. *American Journal of Public Health, 82,* 364–371.

Noojin, A.B., & Wallander, J.L. (1996). Development and evaluation of a measure of concerns related to raising a child with a physical disability. *Journal of Pediatric Psychology, 21,* 483–498.

Rosenbaum, P., Cadman, D., & Kirpilani, H. (1990). Pediatrics: Assessing quality of life. In B. Spilker (Ed.), *Quality of life assessments in clinical trials* (pp. 205–215). New York: Raven Press.

Rosenbaum, L.P., & Saigal, S. (1996). Measuring health-related quality of life in pediatric populations: Conceptual issues. In B. Spilker (Ed.), *Quality of life and pharmacoeconomics in clinical trials* (2nd ed.) (pp. 785–791). Philadelphia: Lippincott-Raven.

Rowe, D.C., & Kandel, D. (1997). In the eye of the beholder? Parental ratings of externalizing and internalizing symptoms. *Journal of Abnormal Child Psychology, 25,* 265–275.

Schalock, R.L. (1996). Reconsidering the conceptualization and measurement of quality of life. In R.L. Schalock (Ed.), *Quality of life, Volume I: Conceptualization and measurement* (pp. 23–32). Washington: American Association on Mental Retardation.

Schipper, H., Clinch, J.J., & Olweny, C.C. (1996). Quality of life studies: Definitions and conceptual issues. In B. Spilker (Ed.), *Quality of life and pharmacoeconomics in clinical trials* (2nd ed.) (pp. 11–23). Philadelphia: Lippincott-Raven.

Spieth, L.E., & Harris, C.V. (1996). Assessment of health-related quality of life in children and adolescents: An integrative review. *Journal of Pediatric Psychology, 21,* 175–193.

Spilker, B. (1996). Introduction. In B. Spilker (Ed.), *Quality of life and pharmacoeconomics in clinical trials* (2nd ed.) (pp. 1–10). Philadelphia: Lippincott-Raven.

Sprangers, M.A., & Aaronson, N.K. (1992). The role of health care providers and significant others in evaluating the quality of life of patients with chronic disease. *Journal of Clinical Epidemiology, 45*, 743–760.

Sroufe, L.A. (1979). The coherence of individual development. *American Psychologist, 34*, 834–841.

Stark, J., & Faulkner, E. (1996). Quality of life across the life span. In R.L. Schalock (Ed.), *Quality of life, Volume 1: Conceptualization and measurement* (pp. 23–32). Washington: American Association on Mental Retardation.

Stein, R.E.K., & Reissman, C.K. (1980). The development of an impact-on-family scale: Preliminary findings. *Medical Care, 18*, 465–472.

Torrance, G.W. (1986). Measurement of health state utilities for economic appraisal: A review. *Journal of Health Economics, 5*, 1–30.

Torrance, G.W., Furlon, W., Feeny, D.H., & Boyle, M. (1996). Multi-attribute preference functions: Health utilities index. *Pharmacoeconomics, 6*, 503–520.

Varni, J., & Setoguchi, Y. (1992). Effects of parental adjustment on the adaptation of children with congenital and acquired limb deficiencies. *Journal of Developmental and Behavioral Pediatrics, 14*, 13–20.

Verbrugge, L.M., & Jette, A.M. (1994). The disablement process. *Social Science & Medicine, 38*, 1–14.

Verhulst, F.C., & Koot, H.M. (Eds.) (1995). *The epidemiology of child and adolescent psychopathology*. Oxford: Oxford University Press.

Verhulst, F.C., Koot, H.M., & Van Der Ende, J. (1994). Differential predictive value of parents' and teachers' reports of children's problem behaviors: A longitudinal study. *Journal of Abnormal Child Psychology, 22*, 531–546.

Verhulst, F.C., & Van der Ende, J. (1992). Agreement between parents' reports and adolescents' self-reports of problem behavior. *Journal of Child Psychology and Psychiatry, 33*, 1011–1023.

Wallander, J.L., & Marullo, D.S. (1997). Handicap-related problems in mothers of children with physical impairments. *Research in Developmental Disabilities, 18*, 151–165.

Wallander, J.L., & Varni, J.W. (1998). Effects of pediatric chronic physical disorders on child and family adjustment. *Journal of Child Psychology and Psychiatry, 39*, 29–46.

MODELS AND PERSPECTIVES

Chapter 2

THEORETICAL AND DEVELOPMENTAL ISSUES IN QUALITY OF LIFE FOR CHILDREN AND ADOLESCENTS

Jan L. Wallander

The premise of this chapter is that the evolution of the Quality of Life (QL) notion for use in understanding outcomes in children/adolescents will benefit from attention to two sets of issues. First, there are issues related to the fact that QL is a theoretical notion, and secondly that children/adolescents are developing beings whose characteristics vary widely both between and within individuals over time. Thus far, QL has had insufficient development as a theoretical construct and developmental issues have been under-recognized for children/adolescents. Consequently, I will discuss a selection of the numerous issues related to these two facts.

I will begin with a discussion of some basic principles of psychological or behavioral measurement. The role of theory in the development of any construct will be reviewed and the recognized principles of construct validation as applicable to QL will be discussed. Following this, I will consider the previous work on QL for people for whom developmental issues are at the forefront; namely, the considerable body of work on defining and using QL for people with developmental disabilities. This literature should have implications for children/adolescents in general. More specifically, I will discuss approaches to defining and establishing the content of QL for people with developmental issues and then review the methodological challenges addressed by these endeavors. I will conclude this chapter by making some recommendations.

CONCEPTUALIZATION OF QUALITY OF LIFE AS A CONSTRUCT
QUALITY OF LIFE IS A CONSTRUCT

QL is a hypothetical construct. Like all hypothetical constructs, QL has no physical or temporal basis. It cannot be seen; instead it is an organizing concept that exists to guide its users (Foster & Cone, 1995; Silva, 1993). In other words, as a construct, QL "is not a visual image, nor is it external to the mind; it is analogous to a piece in a game in which thought plays" (Caws, 1959, p. 16). Hypothetical constructs, including QL, enjoy no universal agreement as to their definition.

Rather they are inferred from consistent differences in their measures and based on relations of those measures with measures of other constructs.

That said, constructs are also thought to be more than their measures. That is, constructs are distinct from their operationalizations. Even when QL is operationalized by a measure, that measure is not synonymous with QL. The user of the QL measurement can view it merely as an indicator of an underlying characteristic. Often referred to as a latent trait, or a process. This reciprocity between constructs and measures was enunciated by Kant as: "[Constructs] without factual content are empty; sense data without [constructs] are blind" (cited in Mackay, 1977, p. 84).

Furthermore, constructs are unobserved variables hypothesized to explain the covariance between observed or measured variables. The observed variables are presumed to be tangible but imperfect indices of the underlying construct. For example, the Vocabulary and Block Design subscales of the WISC-III, a measurement of cognitive processing speed, and grades in school could be taken as indices of intelligence, but clearly, they are imperfect as indicators of intelligence.

Because of these assumptions about what scores on measures represent, a construct can never be fully operationalized by its measurements. There is always a figurative distance present between that which we are truly interested in (e.g., QL), and its measurements. This creates challenges. A given measurement can be used to reflect different constructs and the same construct can be manifested by different measurements. For example, while the rating by a child of his satisfaction with support from peers can be used as one indicator of the child's QL, it can also be used to measure negative affectivity, environmental insularity, and perceived social support, among other constructs. Conversely, QL can be measured by, for example, material resources, ratings of psychological well-being, and frequency of physical symptoms, in addition to the child's rating of satisfaction with support from peers.

PSYCHOLOGICAL MEASUREMENT PRINCIPLES

Psychological assessment, as a scientific and professional endeavor, has been developed in part to make it possible to study hypothetical constructs, such as QL. Based on theories and procedures that have evolved over a period of about 100 years, psychological assessment refers to the systematic measurement of a person's behavior. It incorporates measurement principles, strategies and the inferences and clinical judgments derived from the obtained measures. Psychological assessment includes many methods, such as direct observations, physiological recordings, and self-report questionnaires, and many different assessment instruments. In this terminology, a specific assessment instrument refers to a specified method for acquiring data about behavior.

Among other things, psychological assessment principles include a set of guidelines for evaluating and communicating about the quality of a measurement instrument. It is my contention that these guidelines are applicable to QL measurement instruments. Indeed, these principles form the framework for much of the discussion that follows in the chapters reviewing QL measurement for different conditions. The most important measurement qualities are how consistently an instrument measures something, or its reliability, and how well it measures the hypothetical construct it is purported to measure, or its validity.

Most efforts at developing and evaluating QL instruments have attended fairly well to the reliability issue. In my opinion, however, the development of the QL construct and evaluation of the construct validity of any given QL instrument have generally not received sufficient attention. Admittedly, QL is a thorny construct that challenges our ability to define it, embed it in a theoretical framework, and operationalize it. However, we need to improve in these endeavors. To this end, it should be helpful to consider guidelines for construct development and validation.

CONSTRUCT VALIDITY

Construct validity refers to the extent to which an instrument can provide a good representation of a construct. Construct validity is at the core of psychological assessment, as elaborated, for example, in the *Standards for Educational and Psychological Testing* (American Psychological Association, 1999). According to the Standards, construct validity is one of the most important forms of validity (beside content validity and criterion-related validity). Construct validity is built on evidence that a test measures the construct it claims to measure, for example, that a quality of life measure indeed measures quality of life. Yet, a widespread misunderstanding remains regarding precisely what construct validity is and what establishing construct validity entails.

The process of establishing construct validity represents a key element in differentiating behavioral measurement as a science from other, nonscientific approaches to the analysis of human behavior (Clark & Watson, 1995). Cronbach and Meehl (1955) argued that elaborating the construct validity of a measure necessarily involves at least three steps:

- articulating a set of theoretical concepts and their interpretations;
- developing ways to measure the hypothetical constructs proposed by the theory;
- testing empirically the hypothesized relations among constructs and their observable manifestations that follow from the above.

This means that without an articulated theory, which Cronbach and Meehl termed "the nomological net," there can be no construct validity. Thus, to develop a construct, the theory undergirding it must first be elaborated. However, very few efforts at developing the QL concept for children/adolescents and the instruments existing to measure QL in children/adolescents have followed this dictum.

THE ROLE OF THEORY IN CONSTRUCT DEVELOPMENT

I have elaborated the role of theory in the study of behavioral issues in health and medicine in children/adolescents elsewhere (Wallander, 1992). These ideas will be briefly summarized here. As a premise, scientific inquiry is not really a search after the truth, nor is it a search after laws of nature, waiting to be discovered. "A scientific law is not part of nature. It is only a way of comprehending nature" (Thurstone, 1947, p. 5). That is, what is considered true from one conceptual framework for a given purpose, and under given conditions, may not be deemed true from another conceptual framework for a different purpose and under different circumstances.

"We never encounter 'facts' " (Nietzsche, 1968, p. 264). Rather, what we see — the facts — is largely determined by what we are looking for, by our beliefs, expectations, orientations, and *by our theories*. This is the most basic argument for needing explicit theories in our scientific work. We have to make our theories about QL explicit as we engage in science to understand it and use it so that others may know what guided our interpretations of the facts. "Theory is an invention aimed at organizing and explaining specific aspects of the environment" (Pedhazur & Schmelkin, 1991, p. 180). De Groot (1969) emphasizes a major characteristic of scientific theory:

"Theory means . . . a system of logically interrelated, specifically noncontradictory statements, ideas, and concepts relating to an area of reality, formulated in such a way that *testable hypotheses can be derived from them*" [italics added] (p. 40).

Consequently, theory provides a frame of reference; it provides the researcher with a "selective point of view." Without theory, science loses much potential for providing an organized, integrative answer to a question. Lynd (1939) made this point in graphic language: without theory, science would be "the ditty bag of an idiot, filled with bits of pebbles, straws, feathers, and other random hoardings" (p. 138). The literature on QL in children and adolescents can appear random, with many differences appearing among its various users and procedures without a clear understanding of why. Differences will, and probably should, continue; but we would be helped if the premise of each different approach to QL were made explicit.

By providing an orientation for what to look for, theory also helps determine which constructs are and are not relevant. Additionally, theory will guide the type of research design, analyses, and interpretations of results to consider. It must also be acknowledged that being a way of seeing, a theory is also a way of not seeing. This is a potential drawback. Theory can bias or even blind the scientist. For example, the researcher may not "see" evidence that is contrary to his or her theory. Or explanations for "seeing" contradictory results may be explained as due to deficiencies in the design or execution of the study. Individual vigilance and scholarly debate can guard against such problems.

A theory contains constructs and explicates relations among constructs, be they antecedent consequences or concomitant ones. Theoretical definitions of constructs entail the use of terms that may also require definitions. Pedhazur and Schmelkin (1991) suggest that a definition should (a) not be too broad or narrow, (b) not contain vague, ambiguous, obscure, or figurative language, (c) not be circular, and (d) state the essence of things named. A major impediment to cumulative knowledge regarding QL in children/adolescents is the "loose" state of theoretical definitions in this area. In many instances, researchers do speak of different things, although they call them by the *same name.* In other instances, researchers do speak of the same thing, although they call it by different names. Health, QL, health-related QL, life satisfaction, and well-being are terms that some times have meant different things and some times the same thing. Again, making the underlying theory, and therefore definitions, clear would reduce this problem.

Theoretical constructs derive their meaning from relations with other constructs in a theoretical context. To test hypotheses derived from theory, however, it is necessary to relate constructs to observed phenomena. This relating is accomplished by means of empirical definitions of the construct. Although all constructs have to be theoretically defined, they do not always require empirical definitions. Constructs not empirically defined are related to observable phenomena through their relations with other constructs that have been empirically defined.

The theoretical conception of a construct is a paramount guide to the type of measures that may be considered. Ignoring this can lead to proliferation of empirical definitions in lieu of theoretical ones. The oft-repeated statement that "Intelligence is what intelligence tests measures" may exemplify the degeneration of the idea that a construct is synonymous with a specific set of operations. As Bridgman (1945) pointed out, "the assertion as it stands begs the question. The question-begging word is the humble 'what' " (p. 249). We have to guard against defining QL in terms of what is measured by instruments named "QL." Using explicit theories is imperative to this end.

CONSTRUCT VALIDATION OF MEASURES OF QUALITY OF LIFE

Developing a construct and validating a measure of that construct is based on a theoretical explication of that construct. However, this only serves as a starting point. Construct validity cannot be inferred from a single set of observations rather a series of investigations is required to even begin the process of confirming a construct. Nonetheless, Cronbach and Meehl's (1955) dictum that "one does not validate a test, but only a principle for making inferences" (p. 297) is often ignored as instrument developers address lightly — sometimes in a single sentence — the establishment of the construct validity of an instrument.

There are numerous discussions of and arguments for how best to conduct theoretically based measurement construction. The following material is based on Clark and Watson's (1995) and Loevinger's (1957) expositions. Accordingly, for purposes of measurement development, (a) substantive, (b) structural, and (c) external components of construct validity must be addressed.

SUBSTANTIVE VALIDITY

The substantive validity addressing theoretical context, definition, and content, is largely developed through a series of cognitive activities of the scientist following a set of initial steps:

Conceptualization

Instruments can be developed to assess constructs at many levels of abstraction, from narrow, to broader, and on to general levels. Consequently, a key issue to be resolved initially when developing a measure of QL is the scope or generality of the target construct. Nevertheless, even narrow-band measures should be embedded in a theoretical framework. A critical first step thus is to develop a precise and detailed conception of QL and its theoretical context. Writing a brief, formal description of the construct is very useful in crystallizing the conceptual model. Addressing these theoretical issues prior to the actual process of instrument construction increases the likelihood that the resulting instrument will make a substantial contribution.

Literature review

To articulate the basic construct as clearly and thoroughly as possible, it is necessary to review the relevant literature to see how others have approached the same problem. This needs to include attempts to conceptualize and assess both the same construct and closely related constructs. For example regarding QL, concepts such as life satisfaction, general well-being, and health would need to be considered. Subsequently, the review should be broadened to encompass what may appear to be less immediately related constructs, to articulate the conceptual boundaries of the target construct. For example, QL might need to be differentiated from functional status. In other words, a good theory articulates not only what a construct is, but also what it is not. This process will also identify predicted convergent and differential patterns of relations with other constructs (Smith & McCarthy, 1995), which will be used in later empirical validation.

Creation of an item pool

The fundamental goal in creating an item pool is to sample systematically all content that is potentially relevant to the target construct. Loevinger (1959) articulated this principle: "The items of the pool should be chosen so as to sample all possible contents which might comprise the putative [construct] according to all known alternative theories of the [construct]" (p. 659). The initial item pool therefore should (a) be broader and more comprehensive than one's own theoretical view of the target construct and (b) include content that ultimately will be shown to be tangential or even unrelated to the core construct. In other words, one should err on the side of over-inclusiveness in the initial stages.

Good instrument construction is inevitably an iterative process involving several periods of item writing, followed in each case by conceptual and psychometric analysis. There are many recommendations available regarding principles of item writing and item format (e.g., Comrey, 1988; Kline, 1986), which are beyond the scope of this chapter.

While the theoretical and operational premises are set through the above largely cognitive activities, the connection between the instrument and the construct is established through several sequential behavioral activities:

Test construction

The choice of stategy for item selection is as important as the compilation of the initial item pool. Item selection strategy should be matched to the goal of the instrument development and the theoretical conceptualization of the construct. In this regard, Loevinger (1957) described three main models: (a) quantitative models that differentiate individuals with respect to the target construct, (b) class models that seek to categorize individuals into qualitatively different groups, and (c) more complex dynamic models. QL, at least implicitly, is typically viewed according to some quantitative model, that is it is seen as existing on a continuum.

There are three main item selection strategies in use for quantitative model constructs: (a) criterion-based — primarily concerned with extra-instrument or external manifestations; (b) internal consistency — concerned with inter-item structure; and (c) item-response theory — focused on the latent trait. However, exclusive reliance on a single method is neither required nor necessarily desirable. Because these strategies are detailed in many psychological measurement monographs or books (e.g., Clark & Watson, 1995; Cronbach, 1990), they will not be discussed here.

Initial data collection

It is important to administer the initial item pool together with additional items or instruments to permit examination of the boundaries of the target construct. This process is often missed in QL instrument development. It is also important to complete this step with respondents for whom the instrument is intended. This can be challenging when patient groups are the intended population, given their finite and often small size in any given location.

Psychometric evaluation

There are many different considerations to attend to in evaluating the technical quality of the instrument being developed. These are also elaborated in many texts and monographs (e.g., Cronbach, 1990; Spector, 1992). Clark and Watson (1995) highlight the need to inspect item distributions, unidimensional item consistencies, and multidimensional item structures. Unfortunately, their application and standards are too often seen as absolute (e.g., Cronbach's alpha must be above .75 to be acceptable). Rather, each application must be considered in light of the theoretical context of the construct, theoretical definition of the construct, and intended purpose of the instrument used to measure the construct. For example, maximizing internal consistency almost invariably produces a scale that is quite narrow in content; if the scale is narrower than the target construct, its validity is compromised. Many constructs are not homogeneous and therefore instruments measuring those constructs should not evidence homogeneity. More often the goal of instrument development is to maximize validity rather than reliability, which typically puts a limit on the internal consistency of the items.

EXTERNAL VALIDITY

External validity procedures are dependent upon clearly explicated theory and construct definitions. Once established, these will identify appropriate construct validity tests. External validation is an ongoing process; construct validity is not really proven at any given point or after that certain *a priori* standards are met. An instrument merely accumulates more or less support for its validity in measuring the target construct.

The basic approach to testing construct validity externally is to delineate hypotheses based on the theory undergirding the construct. In other words, if the instrument in question is used to operationalize the construct, will it behave as predicted by that theory? Various investigations can be set up to test such hypotheses. Common variants and simplistic examples applicable to QL in children and adolescents are:

- comparison of scores between groups that should differ (e.g., QL scores should differ between children in an acute stage of an illness and healthy children);
- comparison of scores within a group that should differ over time (e.g., QL scores for a group of children with acute lymphoblastic leukemia should differ at different stages of the disease process, from initial diagnosis, to acute treatment, return to school, and complete remission);
- inspection of associations with scores on different instruments of the same or highly similar construct (e.g., scores on a newly developed QL measure should correlate highly with those on an existing, well accepted QL measure);
- inspection of differential relationships with scores of measures of both similar and quite independent constructs (e.g., scores on a newly developed QL measure should have higher correlations with a measure of symptom severity than with a measure of intelligence);
- comparison of instrument scores between or within groups that should differ due to experimental manipulations, such as an intervention (e.g., QL scores of children that receive a less intrusive medical intervention should differ from those receiving a highly aggressive medical intervention); and
- inspection of relationships with scores representing processes that are components or consequences of the construct (e.g., children with high scores on a new QL measure should have higher scores on established measures of mental health, social support, and physical health status compared to those with low scores).

QUALITY OF LIFE AND CHILD DEVELOPMENT

Developmental issues in QL have not received sufficient attention despite the obvious fact that children and adolescents are continuously and quite rapidly developing beings. This means that QL may need to be approached differently in children at different ages or in the same child over time. This fact raises a number of questions, for example: Can the same definition of QL be used across child development? Should QL address different content across child development? Can the same measurement methodology be used across child development? If the answer is "no" to any of these questions, then how can we best handle those developmental issues?

A potentially useful approach to illuminating developmental issues in defining and measuring QL for children and adolescents is to consider the work that has been done with another population for whom development is also a highly salient issue. To this end, we propose there are developmental similarities between adults with developmental disability, especially in terms of intellectual functioning, and children and adolescents with chronic conditions without intellectual disability. Consider that intellectual disability (ID) is defined as a deficit in *development*, primarily in cognitive and social capacities (e.g., Hodapp & Dykens, 1996). Likewise, childhood by definition is a stage of immature development. Hence, just as adults with ID are compromised in their development compared to adults without ID, so are all children and adolescents compared to adults in the population (despite following a typical developmental path).

This results in some similarities of relevance to QL. For example, these two groups both present with issues in comprehension, introspection, life experience, choice, diversity in supports, and living in environments primarily of others' construction. For these and other reasons, these two groups may also present with similar conceptual and methodological challenges for the QL notion. A discussion of how some of those issues have been dealt with in developing the QL notion for people with ID therefore should aid in stimulating advances in QL applications to children and adolescents with chronic conditions.

The concept QL has been applied with people with ID (or mental retardation and other developmental disabilities) for quite some time. This is evidenced in the numerous volumes published on QL in people with ID (e.g., Brown, 1997; Goode, 1994; Renwick, Brown, & Nagler, 1996; Schalock, 1996, 1997), as well as many journal articles (see Hughes, Hwang, Kim, Eisenman, & Killian, 1995, for a content analysis of this literature). A number of issues have been addressed in this literature. For example, Raphael (1996) identified several that have caught much attention:

- sociological versus psychological perspectives
- positivist, idealist, and realist approaches
- value-based versus value-free approaches
- social policy versus basic research orientations
- system versus individual data collection
- naturalistic versus positivist methodologies
- quantitative versus qualitative methods
- objective versus subjective measurements
- self-reports versus reports by others
- traditional versus participatory approaches

It is evident that discussions about QL for people with ID have included a broad range of issues ranging from philosophical, to conceptual and methodological ones. Our discussion herein will have to be limited to a selection of conceptual and methodological issues where developmental themes are especially salient.

CONCEPTUAL ISSUES
DEFINITIONS OF QUALITY OF LIFE

The literature on QL of people with ID is replete with definitions. In one review, Cummins (1995) found over 100. This plethora led Schalock (1996) to propose that QL should not be considered "an entity that one has or does not have to some degree, [but] should be viewed as an organizing concept. [As such, QL] can be used for a number of purposes" (p. 123). Therefore, it would be reasonable to expect variations in definitions depending on the purpose to which they are applied. This notwithstanding, there are many commonalties in conceptualizing and defining QL evidenced in these many offerings (cf. Borthwick-Duffy, 1997; Cummins, 1997, Felce & Perry, 1995; Schalock, 1996).

Recognizing these similarities, I submit that *QL can be defined as the combination of objectively and subjectively indicated well-being in multiple domains of life considered salient in one's culture and time, while adhering to universal standards of human rights.*

The tension between culturally and universally held standards for a life of quality is challenging to resolve. This definition attempts to do so — but not without difficulties, it must be recognized — by emphasizing that there may be cultural differences in life styles and values that need to be taken into account when defining the quality of life in that culture. Making the definition culturally relevant can in fact make it universally applicable, although standards would vary across cultures. However, some cultures stipulate quite limited rights for some groups, for example for females compared to those accorded males. This definition holds that some standards for a life of quality are unalterable by culture.

Furthermore, this definition is not unique to young people with ID, but is applicable to all people. That is, I agree with Cummins (1995) that, regardless of the specific definition chosen, "[i]t is imperative that all definitions of [QL] be referenced to the general population both in their conception and operational measures" (p. 14). Consequently, QL must be defined universally and certainly similarly for persons with or without disability, whether they are young or old. Otherwise society will hold different standards for different groups of people.

As it is, minority groups, defined as having little or no power in society and including people with ID and children and adolescents in general, may experience a lower average standard of living than the general population. There is a great danger of defining QL for such people in terms that seem appropriate for minority groups, but would be unacceptable to the majority group which hold the power in society. Of course, we run this same risk when we make a condition-specific definition of QL for young people with a chronic condition (e.g., diabetes). Thus, this theoretical definition of QL primarily recognizes development by advocating that, at this level, the definition must be developmentally universal.

PERSPECTIVES ON QUALITY OF LIFE

Our definition of QL also includes both objective and subjective perspectives, consistent with advances in the conceptualization of QL in people with ID. Historically, four perspectives have characterized theories about what indicates QL (Borthwick-Duffy, 1992; Felce & Perry, 1995). They focus on:

A. the *objective quality of the conditions* in which the person lives;
B. the person's *subjective satisfaction* with life conditions;
C. some *combination* of the objective, life-condition and subjective, satisfaction perspectives (e.g., additive or multiplicative combinations);
D. some combination of the objective and subjective perspectives when specific domains of QL are weighted by the *person's values*, aspirations, and expectations.

Regarding the last perspective (D), it is argued that a person's values should moderate the role of life conditions and personal satisfaction in establishing that person's QL. For example, if the condition of one's residence is not a priority, where and how one lives should have a lower weighting in establishing one's QL than would higher valued domains of one's life.

The distinction between objective and subjective perspectives on QL, whether adopted strictly (A and B above) or in some combination (C and D above), has important implications. Emphasizing *objectively measurable life conditions* experienced by a person (e.g., income, residence, work status, symptoms, illness days, functional achievements, social contacts) follows from the premise that a person only has the right to a life and equality of opportunity, not the right to satisfaction with that life (Felce & Perry, 1995). Few advocates for people with ID, youth with a chronic conditions, or children/adolescents in general would find that philosophy acceptable.

Moreover, the appropriateness of using a normative basis (as is inherent in the objective perspective) to establish a person's QL can be challenged. For example, if we observe that a person cannot do something that is normative (e.g., an adolescent with a gross motor impairment may not be able to walk as far as an able-bodied adolescent can), we cannot use this fact to extrapolate that the former necessarily has a poorer QL. As Leplege and Hunt stated (1997, p. 48): "To imply that physically disabled or elderly persons have a poorer [QL] than younger or able-bodied individuals is a reinforcement of stereotypes that underlie discriminatory practices." I strongly feel this point applies to all vulnerable groups, whether defined by a physical or intellectual disability, as well as for children and adolescents in general.

Satisfaction with life has therefore become one important criterion of individual QL. Equating QL solely with personal satisfaction, however, has its own issues. Edgerton (1990) points to the independence often found between a person's life conditions and their subjective well-being as a problem. For example, people living in substandard environments have been found to report a QL equal to that of people in what could objectively be considered better environments. Similarly, people with significant physical impairments have been found to report a health-related QL similar to people of excellent health and show improvements over time without objective changes in their physical condition (Bury, 1991). Finally, reports of well-being have repeatedly been found to be better explained by internal, stable dispositions than external conditions (e.g., Costa, McCrae, & Zonderman, 1987; Edgerton, Bollinger, & Harr, 1984; Flynn, 1989). These findings raise the possibility that subjective QL is primarily a personality characteristic and not much influenced by conditions.

One reason offered for the apparent lack of differentiation of subjective QL is that making a judgment on satisfaction is a *comparative activity* (Felce & Perry, 1995). Therefore, satisfaction depends on one's frame of reference, which is affected by one's experience and judgment both of what is typical and possible for one's situation. This applies to all people, but raises particular issues for young people and people with ID because they inhabit worlds of other people's construction (e.g., parents, teachers, service providers). People in these groups lack independence and experience constrained opportunities and autonomy. This raises significant concerns about what the life satisfaction expressed by people with limited control over and experience in life means. At this extreme, then, it is impossible to conclude that one's lifestyle necessarily reflects one's choice. Satisfaction with that lifestyle, therefore, cannot by itself be an adequate measure of QL (Felce & Perry, 1997).

Recognizing this, about 80% of all QL definitions for people with ID have applied a *combination of objective and subjective perspectives* (Cummins, 1997). While this approach is recommended also for children and adolescents in general, it is unclear how exactly to do this. The different perspectives would likely need to be applied differently at different developmental levels. Presumably, there would need to be a relatively stronger emphasis on objective standards of QL the younger or the less developmentally mature the target person is. At some point down the developmental continuum, only objective standards of QL would be considered. Conversely, with increased development, the subjective perspective on QL needs to be brought in, not to substitute, but to be put in parallel with the objective perspective. Thus, Perspectives C or D above would be applied. Empirical knowledge to guide these decisions, however, is much needed.

CONTENT OF QUALITY OF LIFE

There is considerable agreement across various definitions that QL refers to a concept that is *multidimensional*. Different approaches, however, have been followed to delineate what are the important dimensions. Hughes, Hwang, Kim, Eisenman, and Killian (1995) completed a structured content analysis of empirical measures of QL for people with ID referenced in the peer-reviewed literature. Others have proposed schemes derived from more informal analysis (e.g., Cummins, 1997; Felce & Perry, 1997; Schalock, 1996) or theoretical-philosophical considerations (e.g., Woodhill et al., 1994). Nonetheless, between five and 15 dimensions typically emerge from these efforts, often with hierarchical elements.

An illustrative sample of such schemes is presented in Table 2.1. As can be seen, there is considerable overlap among content systems, the differences being due mainly to whether and how much to subdivide life into domains and subdomains. Felce and Perry's (1997) delineation

TABLE 2.1 EXAMPLES OF DIMENSIONAL STRUCTURES OF QUALITY OF LIFE THAT HAVE BEEN APPLIED TO PEOPLE WITH INTELLECTUAL DISABILITY

AGER & EGLINTON (1989)	HOME
	LEISURE
	RELATIONSHIPS
	FREEDOM
	OPPORTUNITIES
BROWN & BAYER (1992)	HOME LIVING
	ACTIVITIES
	HEALTH
	SOCIAL LIFE
	FAMILY LIFE
	SELF-IMAGE
	LEISURE
	EMPLOYMENT
	LEGAL ASPECTS
	DESIRED SUPPORT
	LIFE SATISFACTION
CUMMINS (1997)	MATERIAL WELL-BEING
	HEALTH
	PRODUCTIVITY
	INTIMACY
	EMOTIONAL WELL-BEING
	SAFETY
	COMMUNITY
FELCE & PERRY (1995)	MATERIAL WELL-BEING
	FINANCE/INCOME
	HOUSING QUALITY
	TRANSPORT
	PHYSICAL WELL-BEING
	HEALTH
	FITNESS
	MOBILITY
	PERSONAL SAFETY
	SOCIAL WELL-BEING
	PERSONAL RELATIONSHIPS
	COMMUNITY INVOLVEMENT
	EMOTIONAL WELL-BEING
	POSITIVE AFFECT
	STATUS/RESPECT
	MENTAL HEALTH/STRESS
	FULFILLMENT
	FAITH/BELIEF
	SELF-ESTEEM
	PRODUCTIVE WELL-BEING
	COMPETENCE
	PRODUCTIVITY/CONTRIBUTION
HUGHES ET AL. (1995)	SOCIAL RELATIONSHIPS AND INTERACTION
	PSYCHOLOGICAL WELL-BEING AND PERSONAL SATISFACTION
	EMPLOYMENT
	SELF-DETERMINATION, AUTONOMY, AND PERSONAL CHOICE
	RECREATION AND LEISURE
	PERSONAL COMPETENCE, COMMUNITY ADJUSTMENT, AND INDEPENDENT LIVING SKILLS
	RESIDENTIAL ENVIRONMENT

TABLE 2.1   EXAMPLES OF DIMENSIONAL STRUCTURES OF QUALITY OF LIFE THAT HAVE BEEN APPLIED TO PEOPLE WITH INTELLECTUAL DISABILITY (*CONTINUED*)

	COMMUNITY INTEGRATION
	NORMALIZATION
	SUPPORT SERVICES RECEIVED
	INDIVIDUAL AND SOCIAL DEMOGRAPHIC INDICATORS
	PERSONAL DEVELOPMENT AND FULFILLMENT
	SOCIAL ACCEPTANCE, SOCIAL STATUS, AND ECOLOGICAL FIT
	PHYSICAL AND MATERIAL WELL-BEING
	CIVIC RESPONSIBILITY
OUELLETTE-KUNTZ & MCCREARY (1995)	HEALTH SERVICES
	FAMILY/GUARDIANSHIP
	INCOME MAINTENANCE
	EDUCATION/TRAINING/EMPLOYMENT
	HOUSING AND SAFETY
	TRANSPORTATION
	SOCIAL AND RECREATION
	RELIGION-CULTURE
	CASE MANAGEMENT
	AESTHETICS
	ADVOCACY
	COUNSELING
ROSEN, SIMON, & MCKINSEY (1995)	ACCOMMODATION
	EMPLOYMENT
	FRIENDS/FAMILY
	NEIGHBORHOOD
	FREEDOM
SCHALOCK (1996)	EMOTIONAL WELL-BEING
	INTERPERSONAL RELATIONS
	MATERIAL WELL-BEING
	PERSONAL DEVELOPMENT
	PHYSICAL WELL-BEING
	SELF-DETERMINATION
	SOCIAL INCLUSION
	RIGHTS
SCHALOCK & KEITH (1993)	EMPOWERMENT/INDEPENDENCE
	COMPETENCE/PRODUCTIVITY
	SATISFACTION
	SOCIAL BELONGING/COMMUNITY INTEGRATION
WOODILL ET AL. (1994)	BEING
	PHYSICAL
	PSYCHOLOGICAL
	SPIRITUAL
	BELONGING
	PHYSICAL
	SOCIAL
	COMMUNITY
	BECOMING
	PRACTICAL ACTIVITIES
	LEISURE ACTIVITIES
	PERSONAL GROWTH ACTIVITIES

appears to strike a useful balance between parsimony and comprehensive coverage, considering QL as manifested grossly in terms of material, physical, social, emotional, and productive well-being. Each major QL domain is then further divided, as can be seen in Table 2.1 (see also Wallander, Chapter 15, Figure 15.1 in this volume).

Some of the advantages of this model of QL include: It is a general model, delineating life as opposed to health or functional ability. It is comprehensive and on the face of it covers all important domains of life. It is quite consistent with various other approaches (see Table 2.1). It is hierarchical, such that for different purposes, one can use it to divide life into global or narrow domains. It also appears applicable across development, as will be elaborated below.

QUALITY OF LIFE CONTENT ACROSS DEVELOPMENT

The question remains, however, how do these content schemes apply to young people? Unfortunately, few have discussed these issues. Borthwick-Duffy (1996) argued that QL for people across the life span, with or without ID, should be conceptualized in terms of similar overall constructs. At the same time, each stage of the life span brings some unique considerations that may affect specific measured indicators.

As an example, although Felce and Perry's (1997) dimensions of QL (see Table 2.1) were developed originally for adults with ID, they appear applicable to young people at the most general level. Even "Productive Well-being" is applicable to children and adolescents. This dimension includes competence and productivity/contribution, as well as choice/control and independence. Considering the educational context, rather than the work context, would make this domain highly relevant for young people as well. Furthermore, these are important capacities on which young people vary, as do older people, both within one person across development and between people at the same stage of development.

Two modifications, however, may need to be made when applying to youth models of QL that have initially been proposed for adults. One is recognizing the different contexts in which children live, such as being a child in a family and going to school. Second, developmental considerations must be taken into account in selecting what specific aspects of a QL dimension to address. For example, Material Well-being in Felce and Perry's (1997) model may be less dependent on finance/income and transport in younger children than they would in adults. However, these would become important for adolescents. Likewise for the domain of Emotional Well-being, where sexuality, faith/belief, and fulfillment, for example, would emerge as important in adolescence, but may have little bearing on describing QL for younger children.

The emergence of different sub-dimensions of the major domains of QL in relation to cognitive and pubertal development needs investigation. One approach would be to expect the respondent to identify what domains are important to them (Cummins, 1997), as discussed under Perspective D above. However, it is likely that this would not be possible below some point in development. Nonetheless, the major domains of QL may be developmentally universal, but the sub-domains may vary (and certainly, the indicators will likely vary, as will be discussed).

METHODOLOGICAL ISSUES

Numerous methodological issues have been discussed in the application of the QL concept to people with ID and many have relevance to young people with and without chronic conditions. This chapter will only discuss issues around using self-report with developing beings and the possible need to make adaptations in measures dependent on the abilities of the respondent.

QUALITY OF SELF-REPORT

As discussed above, the individual's perspective on well-being is important in measuring QL in people with ID. However, this conceptual stance becomes challenged when operationalized into a measurement method. As Felce and Perry (1997) observed, "...gaining ratings of satisfaction from people with poor receptive and expressive language is associated with special problems of inconsistent reliability and uncertain validity" (p. 65). This concern should also hold for typical-developing, but still developmentally immature young people. Unfortunately, there is considerable empirical support for this problem regarding adults with ID.

For example, Sigelman, Schoenrock, Winer and colleagues (1981) demonstrated that it was not possible to gain responses to even simple questions from some adults with severe ID and most with profound ID. Moreover, inconsistency, inaccuracy, and the tendency to acquiesce and choose the last in a list of response choices offered were other problems they observed in a series of empirical studies. While these problems tended to increase with greater severity of ID, they were also found in some people with only mild or moderate ID. Moreover, these problems were somewhat magnified in young people with ID.

By implication, these studies raise some concerns about self-ratings of QL from young people *without* ID as well because their cognitive abilities are still developing. However, similar methodologically oriented studies need to be conducted on typical-developing youngsters to confirm whether this is the case and if so to identify more specifically which problems occur and when. There is a great need for these types of methodological studies to be conducted on child respondents.

ADAPTATIONS IN MEASUREMENT

Different strategies have been suggested to address the problem of self-reports from people with developmental challenges. Schalock, Keith, and Hoffman (1990) suggest obtaining proxy ratings from other knowledgeable sources, such as a parent, teacher, or other caregiver. More specifically, they suggest that two proxies should be used when a self-rating cannot be obtained with confidence. Others do not encourage that a third party can generally represent well the views of a given individual (Cummins, 1992). Koot (Chapter 1 in this volume) further discusses challenges in using proxies.

In contrast, Cummins (1997) suggests that the ability of people to respond to the demands of the measurement methodology should be assessed as a preliminary step before accepting responses to that method. He developed a testing protocol to determine the extent to which a respondent is able to use Likert response scales as part of his QL measure for people with ID (reviewed by Wallander & Turrentine, Chapter 15, in this volume). This testing is done in three stages. The first involves arranging wooden cubes of unequal sizes in an ordered progression. The second requires the transposition of relative block sizes to a Likert scale marked from "largest" to "smallest". The third requires the respondent to indicate an appropriate response on a Likert scale of importance using items of known importance to the client.

The results of this pre-testing then inform which response scale needs to be used for that respondent. For example, if a respondent is only able to manage the choice between two levels, then he or she will be provided with a version where choices are presented as binary. If he or she can differentiate three or five levels of responses, then the appropriate version of the instrument would have three or five response choices, respectively.

This type of pretesting is recommended for the assessment of any population with apparent or suspected cognitive limitations. This would obviously include children without ID who are at a cognitive developmental stage that may not support their responding to Likert scales. There are some indications that the youngest age at which self-report data may be obtained with acceptable reliability is about age four (Harter & Pike, 1985), for example by using pictorial response scales. However, empirical research is much needed to indicate what age ranges are generally challenged in providing self-report that can be used in scientific measurement.

While it is a step in the right direction, pretesting for the appropriate response scale still leaves unaddressed the difficulty of the conceptual comprehension of item content. Some QL instrument developers have written items in different ways to recognize abilities at different ages. As one example of how to handle this concern about young people's ability to handle items and response scales with differing complexity, French, Christie, and Sowden (1994) developed three age-specific forms to assess QL in children with asthma (see also Chapter 9 in this volume). Eiser (see Chapter 10 in this volume) also developed different forms to assess QL of children with cancer at different levels of developmental maturity. Additional empirical work is clearly needed into the important issue of how we merge our conceptual premises regarding QL with methodological realities in assessing developing beings. We believe the necessary empirical basis can be developed to address this challenge. Others are less optimistic. Edgerton (1990), for example, proposes that the only viable means of assessing the quality of an individual's life who cannot adequately report on that him/herself is to have prolonged contact with that person over time, to become a natural part of his/her life as a participant observer. He feels that scales and inventories, whether completed by the target or a proxy, cannot adequately meet the needs for which QL assessment is intended to fill. Before accepting this approach, however, we need to collect the empirical data to inform us about these issues.

SUMMARY AND RECOMMENDATIONS

The ideas put forth in this chapter will be summarized as a series of recommendations:

- QL needs to be further developed as a construct.
- To this end, theories about QL need to be elaborated.

- Both the developments of the QL construct and measurement procedures for operationalizing this construct need to be guided by principles of psychological assessment.
- QL needs to be defined for each use.
- The definition should be equally applicable to non-specific populations as well as people with specific characteristics, such as a chronic illness or being young, to ensure that the same standards for a life of quality are applied and that normative comparisons are available for special groups.
- QL addresses status in multiple important domains of life, including health and functioning, but certainly extends beyond these.
- What those dimensions exactly are remains in debate, but this seems largely an issue of semantics and where on a continuum from molar to molecular divisions one stands. While different uses will require different dimensional frameworks, there is considerable comparability among existing models of QL content.
- Felce and Perry's (1997) organization strikes a nice balance among comprehensiveness, applicability across the life span, parsimony, and utility.
- Because there are advantages and disadvantages with emphasizing either objective or subjective perspectives on QL — and clearly, neither is sufficient by itself — both are needed.
- When and how to join these perspectives or use them as two equally important, but independent perspectives, require further research in children and adolescents.
- The two sources of self-report and significant others' (e.g., parent or teacher) report need to be used to measure QL in young people.
- Further research is needed, however, to determine at what point in development self-report can be reliably used in this population.
- Cummins' (1997) pre-testing approach is recommended to address the concern about the optimal complexity of response scales for individuals at different points in development.
- Psychometric standards of reliability, validity, and sensitivity need to be considered in using QL measures. While some QL advocates have eschewed traditional psychometric standards as not being consistent with measuring QL (e.g., Brown & Bayer, 1992; Woodhill et al., 1994), this must enter into the consideration.
- A decision-making model should be used to deal with the dilemma in joining such considerations for psychometric standards with those of utility (Hubert & Wallander, 1988). This means that psychometric

standards are not the exclusive concern, nor are they sufficient standards for using a measure. However, they are necessary initial standards, beyond which must be considered measurement goals and context. Measures must be practical given these goals and context.

- Measuring QL in young people poses many challenges, such as the risk for acquiescence, tendency toward socially desirable responding, lack of effective communication, and the need to use proxies in some cases. These concerns need considerable empirical attention.

References

Ager, A., & Eglinton, L. (1989). *Working paper 4: Life experiences of clients of services for people with learning difficulties: Summary of findings from studies using the life experiences checklist.* Mental Handicap Research Group, Department of Psychology, University of Leicester.

American Psychological Association. (1999). *Standards for educational and psychological testing.* Washington, DC: Author.

Borthwick-Duffy, S.A. (1992). Quality of life and quality of care in mental retardation. In L. Rowitz (Ed.), *Mental retardation in the year 2000* (pp. 52–66). Berlin: Springer-Verlag.

Borthwick-Duffy, S.A. (1996). Evaluation and measurement of quality of life: Special considerations for persons with mental retardation. In R.L. Schalock (Ed.), *Quality of life* (Vol. I, pp. 105–119). Washington, DC: American Association on Mental Retardation.

Bridgman, P.W. (1945). Some general principles of operational analysis. *Psychological Review, 52,* 246–249.

Brown, R.I., & Bayer, M.B. (1992). *Rehabilitation questionnaire and manual: A personal guide to the individual's quality of life.* Toronto: Captus University Publications.

Bury, M. (1991). The sociology of chronic illness. *Social Health Illness, 13,* 451–468.

Caws, P. (1959). Definition and measurement in physics. In C.W. Churchman, & P. Ratoosh (Eds.), *Measurement: Definitions and theories* (pp. 3–17). New York: Wiley.

Clark, L.A., & Watson, D. (1995). Constructing validity: Basic issues in objective scale development. *Psychological Assessment, 7,* 309–319.

Comrey, A.L. (1988). Factor-analytic methods of scale development in personality and clinical psychology. *Journal of Consulting and Clinical Psychology, 56,* 754–761.

Costa, P.T., Jr., McCrae, R.R., & Zonderman, A.B. (1987). Environmental and dispositional influences on wellbeing: Longitudinal follow-up of an American national sample. *British Journal of Psychology, 78,* 299–306.

Cronbach, L.J. (1990). *Essentials of psychological testing* (Fifth ed.). New York: Harper & Row, Publishers.

Cronbach, L.J., & Meehl, P.E. (1955). Construct validity in psychological test. *Psychological Bulletin, 52,* 281–302.

Cummins, R.A. (1992). *Comprehensive Quality of Life Scale: Intellectual disability.* Melbourne, Australia: Deakin University.

Cummins, R.A. (1995). *Directory of instruments to measure quality of life and cognate areas.* Melbourne, Australia: Deakin University.

Cummins, R.A. (1997). Assessing quality of life. In R.I. Brown (Ed.), *Quality of life for people with disabilities* (2nd ed., pp. 116–150). London: Stanley Thornes (Publishers) Ltd.

Edgerton, R.B. (1990). Quality of life from a longitudinal research perspective. In R.L. Schalock (Ed.), *Quality of life: Perspectives and issues* (pp. 149–160). Washington, DC: American Association on Mental Retardation.

Edgerton, R.B., Bollinger, M., & Herr, B. (1984). The cloak of competence: After two decades. *American Journal of Mental Deficiency, 88,* 345–351.

Felce, D., & Perry, J. (1995). Quality of life: Its definition and measurement. *Research in Developmental Disabilities, 16,* 51–74.

Felce, D., & Perry, J. (1997). Quality of life: The scope of the term and its breadth of measurement. In R.I. Brown (Ed.), *Quality of life for people with disabilities* (2nd ed., pp. 56–71). London: Stanley Thornes (Publishers) Ltd.

Flynn, M. (1989). *Independent living for adults with a mental handicap: A place of my own.* London: Cassel.

Foster, S.L., & Cone, J.D. (1995). Validity issues in clinical assessment. *Psychological Assessment, 7,* 248–260.

French, D.J., Christie, M.J., & Snowden, A.J. (1994). The reproducibility of the Childhood Asthma Questionnaires: Measures of quality of life for children with asthma aged 4–16 years. *Quality of Life Research, 3,* 215–224.

Goode, D.A. (1994). *Quality of life for persons with disabilities: International perspectives and issues.* Boston: Brookline Books.

Harter, S., & Pike, R. (1985). The pictorial scale of perceived competence and social acceptance for young children. *Child Development, 55,* 1969–1982.

Hubert, N.C., & Wallander, J.L. (1988). Instrument selection. In T.D. Wachs, & R. Sheehan (Eds.), *Assessment of young developmentally disabled children* (pp. 43–60). New York: Plenum.

Hughes, C., Hwang, R., Kim, J.H., Eisenman, L.T., & Killian, D.J. (1995). Quality of life in applied research: A review and analysis of empirical measures. *American Journal on Mental Retardation, 99,* 623–641.

Kline, P. (1986). *A handbook of test construction: Introduction to psychometric design.* New York: Methuen.

Leplege, A., & Hunt, S. (1997). The problem of quality of life in medicine. *JAMA, 278,* 47–50.

Loevinger, J. (1957). Objective tests as instruments of psychological theory. *Psychological Reports, 3,* 635–694.

Lynd, R.S. (1939). *Knowledge for what? The place for social science in American culture.* Princeton, NJ: Princeton University Press.

Mackay, A.L. (1977). *The harvest of quiet eye: A selection of scientific quotations.* Bristol, UK: Institute of Physics.

Nietzsche, F. (1968). *The will to power.* W. Kaufman, & R.J. Hollingdale (Trans). New York: Vintage.

Ouellette-Kuntz, H., & McCreary, B.D. (1995). Quality of life assessment for persons with severe developmental disabilities. In R. Renwick, I. Brown, & M. Nagler (Eds.), *Quality of life in health promotion and rehabilitation: Conceptual approaches, issues, and applications* (pp. 268–278). Thousand Oaks, CA: Sage Publications.

Pedhazur, E.J., & Schmelkin, L.P. (1991). *Measurement, design, and analysis: An integrated approach.* Hillsdale, NJ: Erlbaum.

Raphael, D. (1996). Defining quality of life: Eleven debates concerning its measurement. In R. Renwick, I. Brown, & M. Nagler (Eds.), *Quality of Life in Health Promotion and Rehabilitation: Conceptual approaches, issues, and applications* (pp. 146–165). Thousand Oaks, CA: Sage Publications.

Renwick, R., Brown, I., & Nagler, M. (1996). *Quality of life in health promotion and rehabilitation: Conceptual approaches, issues, and applications.* Thousand Oaks, CA: Sage Publications.

Rosen, M., Simon, E.W., & McKinsey, L. (1995). Subjective measure of quality of life. *Mental Retardation, 33,* 31–34.

Schalock, R.L. (1996). *Quality of Life Volume 1: Conceptualization and measurement.* Washington, DC: American Association on Mental Retardation.

Schalock, R.L. (1997). *Quality of life Volume II: Application to persons with disabilities.* Washington, DC: American Association on Mental Retardation.

Schalock, R.L., & Keith, K.D. (1993). *Quality of life questionnaire.* Worthington, OH: IDS.

Schalock, R.L., Keith, K.D., & Hoffman, K. (1990). *Quality of life questionnaire: Standardization manual.* Hastings, NE: Mid-Nebraska Mental Retardation Services.

Sigelman, C.K., Schoenrock, C.J., Winer, J.L., Spanhel, C.L., Hromas, S.G., Martin, P.W., Budd, C., & Bensberg, G.J. (1981). Issues in interviewing mentally retarded persons: An empirical study. In R.H. Bruininks, C.E. Meyers, B.B. Sigford, & K.C. Lakin (Eds.), *Deinstitutionalization and community adjustment of mentally retarded persons* (pp. 114–129). Washington, DC: American Association on Mental Deficiency.

Silva, F. (1993). *Psychometric foundations of behavioral assessment.* Newbury Park, CA: Sage.

Smith G.T., & McCarthy, D.M. (1995). Methodological considerations in the refinement of clinical assessment instruments. *Psychological Assessment, 7,* 300–308.

Spector, P.E. (1992). *Summated Rating Scale Construction: An Introduction.* Sage University Paper Series on Quantitative Applications in the Social Sciences, 07-082. Newbury Park, CA: Sage Publications.

Thurstone, L.L. (1947). *Multiple-factor analysis*. Chicago: Chicago University Press.

Wallander, J.L. (1992). Theory-driven research in pediatric psychology: A little bit on why and how. *Journal of Pediatric Psychology, 17*, 521–535.

Woodill, G., Renwick, R., Brown, I., & Raphael, D. (1994). Being, belonging, becoming: An approach to the quality of life of persons with developmental disabilities. In D. Goode (Ed.), *Quality of life for persons with disabilities: International perspectives and issues* (pp. 57–74). Cambridge, MA: Brookline.

Chapter 3

GENERIC HEALTH-RELATED QUALITY OF LIFE MEASURES FOR CHILDREN AND ADOLESCENTS

Leslie E. Spieth

Health-related quality of life (QL) measures are categorized as either generic or specific. *Generic* QL measures are designed to assess all areas of functioning deemed to be directly affected by an illness and its treatment, whereas specific measures assess QL within the context of a specified disease, function, or age group. The two types of QL measures are thus contrasted in terms of the type of assessment data they yield. Generic QL measures are *broad-based* or *wide-band* instruments that broadly assess the different domains of childhood functioning that may be affected by an illness and/or its treatment (Richards & Hemstreet, 1994; Temkin et al., 1989). The core domains typically included in a generic QL measure are disease state, and physical, psychological, and social functioning, as outlined in the World Health Organization definition (WHO, 1948). Disease-specific measures are designed to be *high fidelity* instruments that assess primarily those symptoms associated with a particular disease and treatment effects. Although the relative merits of generic and disease-specific QL measures have been summarized and debated (Patrick & Deyo, 1989), neither assessment approach is inherently superior as each accords investigators unique information. Nor are the two approaches mutually exclusive, but rather may be used in a complementary fashion.

In this chapter the historical development of the several approaches to QL assessment is outlined and a taxonomy for organizing the different types of generic QL measures is introduced. The psychometric criteria used to evaluate QL measures are reviewed briefly and these criteria are applied in an evaluation of the generic QL measures currently available for children and adolescents.[1] Finally, considerations and guidelines for selecting a generic QL measure for clinical practice or research are provided.

HISTORICAL DEVELOPMENT OF GENERIC MEASURES

Generic measures have been developed within the context of three primary approaches to the assessment of health-related QL: (1) health care policy (macro level), (2) clinical research trials (intermediate level), and (3) clinical practice (micro level). Each approach has used QL outcomes to address a particular concern, and the measures that have emerged from the different approaches reflect very different objectives and definitions of QL.

Health-related QL assessment was first conducted within the context of population-based surveys. The goal of these surveys was to establish prevalence rates of childhood illnesses and associated limitations in the general population. These surveys (two of which are reviewed in this chapter) are very brief and unidimensional in the sense that they primarily evaluate functional limitations (e.g., school days missed). Thus, these surveys do not evaluate the multiple dimensions of QL as it is currently conceptualized.

In the 1970s, health care policy-makers became concerned with measuring the impact of the health care system on the health of the general population and used QL outcomes to guide health care funding allocations. QL assessment at the policy level has been based on two primary conceptual models: (1) the utility concept and (2) health status measurement. The utility approach is derived from theories of economic decision-making and has been applied to the health care field as a means of directing the allocation of health care funds. Similarly, the goal of health status measurement has been to assess the impact of health care policies on the health of the general population. Both of these approaches are, by definition, conducted at the level of the general population, or the macro level.

By contrast, clinical researchers have been mostly concerned with comparing the relative efficacy of treatment modalities. This work has been done primarily within the area of Phase III oncology clinical trials to assess the relative benefits of chemotherapeutic regimens and alternate treatment modalities. Such assessments are typically conducted at multiple sites at a national level to facilitate comparisons of QL outcome data from groups of cancer patients randomly assigned to different treatment arms. An extension of this approach has been to compare QL outcomes in other illness populations (e.g., cystic fibrosis patients, organ transplant patients) to either identify specific patient populations that may be at relatively higher risk for long-term dysfunction, and/or to determine whether QL differs across illness groups. The objectives of such investigations require relatively large subject samples and are conducted at an intermediate level of investigation.

Most recently, health care professionals have become increasingly interested in obtaining QL ratings from individual patients with a variety of acute and chronic illnesses. The goal of the individual assessment approach is to inform clinical decision-making by evaluating physical and psychosocial changes in individual patients secondary to medical and psychological interventions. QL data also has the potential to provide a means for clinicians to demonstrate the efficacy of psychological treatment protocols in this era of increased accountability to third party payors. Individual QL assessments can also help to: (1) identify unexpected health problems, (2) monitor disease progression or response to treatment, and (3) enhance provider–patient communication (MacKeigan & Pathak, 1992). This approach to QL assessment is conducted at the micro level.

Given the widely divergent goals of each of these three approaches to QL assessment, it is not surprising that the instruments developed to meet the needs of each approach are very different. Consequently, the term generic QL measures is commonly used to categorize a group of heterogeneous measures. To clarify these differences and facilitate the selection of an appropriate generic measure for a planned investigation, a taxonomy of generic measures is introduced here. The taxonomy includes four categories: (1) epidemiologic health surveys, (2) utility measures, (3) health profiles, and (4) clinical outcome measures. The fourth category is further divided into two sub-groups: functional status and multidimensional instruments. This taxonomy is used in Table 3.1 to categorize the generic QL measures currently available for use with children and adolescents.

STANDARDS FOR EVALUATING THE PSYCHOMETRIC ADEQUACY OF GENERIC MEASURES

Increased interest in measuring QL over the past decade or so has resulted in a number of new measures, with varying degrees of attention paid to test construction. Consequently, it is important when selecting a QL measure to consider its psychometric adequacy as well as its ability to tap outcomes of primary interest to a particular investigation. The most important reliability and validity issues, as well as special concerns of psychometric properties pertinent to QL measures, are reviewed below.

RELIABILITY

Reliability is a necessary but not sufficient condition for determining whether an instrument is valid. The intended purpose of the measure dictates the reliability estimate of most importance. The reliability

TABLE 3.1 GENERIC QUALITY OF LIFE MEASURES AVAILABLE FOR USE WITH CHILDREN AND ADOLESCENTS

MEASURE	DOMAINS	RESPONDENT	AGE (YEARS)	NO. OF ITEMS (MINS. TO COMPLETE)	FORMAT
EPIDEMIOLOGIC SURVEY MEASURES					
NATIONAL HEALTH INTERVIEW SURVEY (NEWACHECK & TAYLOR, 1992)	SCHOOL DAYS MISSED TIME IN BED DOCTOR VISITS HOSPITALIZATIONS MEDICATION USE PAIN/DISCOMFORT	PARENT	< 18 YEARS	9	TELEPHONE INTERVIEW
ONTARIO CHILD HEALTH STUDY (BOYLE ET AL., 1987)	FUNCTIONAL LIMITATIONS	PARENT	4–16 YEARS	304	INTERVIEW
UTILITY MEASURES					
QUALITY OF WELL-BEING SCALE (KAPLAN, BUSH, & BERRY, 1978)	PHYSICAL SYMPTOMS MOBILITY PHYSICAL ACTIVITY FUNCTIONAL STATUS	PARENT	ALL AGES	23–38 (12–15)	INTERVIEW
HEALTH PROFILES					
CHILD HEALTH AND ILLNESS PROFILE ADOLESCENT EDITION (STARFIELD ET AL., 1995)	RISKS DISCOMFORT SATISFACTION DISORDERS ACHIEVEMENT RESILIENCE	ADOLESCENT	11–17	153 (30)	QUESTIONNAIRE
RAND HEALTH STATUS MEASURE FOR CHILDREN (EISEN ET AL., 1979)	PHYSICAL HEALTH MENTAL HEALTH SOCIAL HEALTH GENERAL HEALTH SOMATIC SYMPTOMS BEHAVIOR PROBLEMS	PARENT	0–4 5–13	38 59	QUESTIONNAIRE

TABLE 3.1 GENERIC QUALITY OF LIFE MEASURES AVAILABLE FOR USE WITH CHILDREN AND ADOLESCENTS (*CONTINUED*)

MEASURE	DOMAINS	RESPONDENT	AGE (YEARS)	NO. OF ITEMS (MINS. TO COMPLETE)	FORMAT
16D HEALTH MEASURE (APAJASALO ET AL., 1996A)	MOBILITY, VISION HEARING, BREATHING SLEEPING, EATING SPEECH, ELIMINATION USUAL ACTIVITIES FRIENDS PHYSICAL APPEARANCE MENTAL FUNCTION DISCOMFORT/SYMPTOMS DEPRESSION, DISTRESS VITALITY	ADOLESCENT	12–15	16 (5–10)	QUESTIONNAIRE
17D HEALTH MEASURE (APAJASALO ET AL., 1996B)	ALL 16D DOMAINS + LEARNING/MEMORY CHRONIC ILLNESS FUNCTIONAL HEALTH HEALTH-RELATED QOL	CHILDREN	8–11	17 (<30)	PICTORIAL INTERVIEW
WARWICK CHILD HEALTH AND MORBIDITY PROFILE (SPENCER & COE, 1996)	GENERAL HEALTH ACUTE MINOR ILLNESS BEHAVIORAL ACCIDENT ACUTE SIG. ILLNESS HOSPITAL ADMISSION IMMUNIZATION	PARENT	0–5	16 (10)	INTERVIEW
CLINICAL OUTCOMES MEASURES **FUNCTIONAL STATUS INSTRUMENTS** COOP CHARTS (WASSON ET AL., 1994)	PHYSICAL FITNESS EMOTIONAL FEELINGS	ADOLESCENT	12–21	6 (< 5)	PICTORIAL CHARTS

54

TABLE 3.1 GENERIC QUALITY OF LIFE MEASURES AVAILABLE FOR USE WITH CHILDREN AND ADOLESCENTS (CONTINUED)

MEASURE	DOMAINS	RESPONDENT	AGE (YEARS)	NO. OF ITEMS (MINS. TO COMPLETE)	FORMAT
	SCHOOLWORK SOCIAL SUPPORT FAMILY COMMUNICATIONS HEALTH HABITS				
FUNCTIONAL STATUS (II) R (STEIN & JESSOP, 1990)	COMMUNICATION MOBILITY, MOOD, ENERGY PLAY, SLEEP EATING, TOILETING	PARENT	0–16	43, 14 (< 30)	INTERVIEW
PLAY PERFORMANCE SCALE FOR CHILDREN (LANSKY ET AL., 1985)	PLAY	PARENT	1–16	1 (< 5)	QUESTIONNAIRE
STANFORD CHILDHOOD HEALTH ASSESSMENT QUESTIONNAIRE (SINGH ET AL., 1994)	DRESSING/GROOMING ARISING, EATING WALKING, HYGIENE REACH, GRIP, AND ACTIVITIES	PARENT CHILD	8–19 8–19	30	QUESTIONNAIRE
MULTIDIMENSIONAL INSTRUMENTS ADOLESCENT ILLNESS IMPACT MEASURE (SPIETH & HARRIS, 1998)	PHYSICAL, PSYCHOLOGICAL, AND SOCIAL FUNCTIONING IMPACT OF MEDICAL CARE PULMONARY AND DIABETES HEALTH ISSUES	PARENT ADOLESCENT	11–18 11–18	47 47 (< 17)	QUESTIONNAIRE

TABLE 3.1 GENERIC QUALITY OF LIFE MEASURES AVAILABLE FOR USE WITH CHILDREN AND ADOLESCENTS (CONTINUED)

MEASURE	DOMAINS	RESPONDENT	AGE (YEARS)	NO. OF ITEMS (MINS. TO COMPLETE)	FORMAT
CHILD HEALTH QUESTIONNAIRE (LANDGRAF, ABETZ, & WARE, 1996)	GLOBAL HEALTH PHYSICAL FUNCTION ROLE/SOCIAL LIMITATIONS (EMOTIONAL AND PHYSICAL) BODILY PAIN/DISCOMFORT BEHAVIOR, MENTAL HEALTH SELF-ESTEEM, GENERAL HEALTH PERCEPTIONS CHANGE IN HEALTH PARENTAL IMPACT (EMOTIONAL AND TIME) FAMILY ACTIVITIES FAMILY COHESION	PARENT CHILD	5–18 5–13	98, 50, 28 87	QUESTIONNAIRE
CHILD HEALTH RATING INVENTORIES (KAPLAN ET AL., 1995)	PHYSICAL FUNCTIONING ROLE FUNCTIONING GENERATED COGNITIVE FUNCTIONING EMOTIONAL WELL-BEING	CHILD	5–12	18 (20)	COMPUTER IMAGES
HOW ARE YOU? (MAES & BRUIL, 1995)	PHYSICAL, COGNITIVE, AND SOCIAL FUNCTIONING PHYSICAL COMPLAINTS HAPPINESS	PARENT	7–13		
QUALITY OF LIFE PROFILE—ADOLESCENT VERSION (RAPHAEL ET AL., 1996)	BEING BELONGING BECOMING	ADOLESCENT	14–20	54	QUESTIONNAIRE

estimates most pertinent to QL measures are internal consistency, interrater/intrarater reliability and sensitivity. Other reliability estimates, such as alternate forms reliability, are less important because different forms of QL measures are rarely available (Bergner & Rothman, 1987). Similarly, test-retest reliability estimates may not be as relevant because QL scores are expected to change over time especially with concomitant changes in health status. Consequently, acceptable test-retest reliability correlation coefficients for QL measures may be lower than those typically accepted due to the effect of health status changes on QL scores over time. A more relevant estimate of reliability is the sensitivity of the QL measure in detecting health-related changes in QL.

Internal consistency

Internal consistency is an estimate of how well an instrument measures a single construct or characteristic. The calculation is based on all correlations between two items in a test, or correlations between items within a conceptually distinct subscale of a measure. An internal consistency coefficient, most commonly Cronbach's alpha, of .70 or greater is an acceptable level for a measure used to describe a population (Nunnally, 1978). However, when assessing an individual's level of health, and changes in health over time, higher coefficients (.90 and above) are desirable (Bergner & Rothman, 1987). Because QL measures are often comprised of multiple scales of functioning across different domains, emphasis should be placed on the internal consistency of each subscale rather than on the internal consistency of the measure as a whole.

Inter-rater reliability

Interrater reliability is an estimate of how well two or more trained interviewers or observers agree with each other's ratings. An interrater reliability coefficient of .80 or above is the standard usually applied as acceptable. This reliability estimate is most relevant when evaluating QL measures that use an interview format. Due to the need to train interviewers so as to achieve acceptable levels of interrater reliability, instruments that use an interview format are sometimes considered less practical by researchers.

A different type of interrater reliability is that calculated between a child and a parent's report, or between a parent's and a physician's report. Reports provided by respondents other than the patient (i.e., the child) are commonly referred to as proxy reports. The low associations typically obtained between patient and proxy respondents have plagued QL researchers. However, such findings are consistent with other areas of research in that reports of overt behaviors (e.g., physical mobility) are often more highly correlated than reports of covert behaviors (e.g., feelings of sadness). See the section in this chapter on the use of proxy respondents for a more detailed discussion of this issue.

General considerations in reviewing reliability criteria

Other questions to consider when evaluating the reliability of a QL instrument are: (1) If a few subscales are to be selected from a longer measure, are reliability estimates available for the specific combination of subscales to be used? (2) Was the sample used in measure development comparable to the planned study population and are reliability estimates available for different chronic disease populations? and (3) Is the range of item scores, including floor and ceiling effects for the subscales, appropriate for the proposed study? (Scientific Advisory Committee, 1995). These considerations, particularly the latter, will affect the measure's sensitivity to change, a key consideration in many QL studies.

VALIDITY

For the purposes of QL assessment, validity usually addresses the question, "Does the measure accurately assess the theoretical construct of interest?" This is a difficult question to answer given the inconsistencies in QL definitions and theoretical models (Eiser, 1995; Spieth & Harris, 1996). Notwithstanding this fundamental problem, three types of validity most pertinent to QL measures are content, criterion, and construct validity.

Content validity

Content validity refers to whether the selected items appear to measure what the scale as a whole is purported to measure (face validity) and cover the important aspects of the construct under study (item sampling validity). The generation of scale items through interviews and/or focus groups with a sample of individuals from the target population enhances content validity. Similarly, a careful review of the selected items by a panel of judges (usually health professionals with relevant expertise) may be used to assess content validity. Nonetheless, it is important to review a scale's content, item-by-item, to determine if the category labels accurately tap the construct of interest in a proposed project.

Criterion-related validity

Criterion-related validity, either concurrent or predictive, refers to the correlation of the measure with another established measure designed to assess the same construct. Due to the lack of a gold standard and the multidimensional nature of most QL measures, a variety of unidimensional criterion measures (e.g., measures of anxiety, social functioning) are often used to establish the validity of particular QL subscales or domains. If two multidimensional instruments, both of which purportedly assess QL, do not correlate highly with one another, there are several possible explanations: (1) the new instrument is not as good as the established measure; (2) the new instrument is better than the criterion; or (3) the two instruments do not measure the same aspects of QL. These latter two concerns are particularly problematic in QL assessment due to the varying domains included in a comprehensive assessment of QL and the lack of a "gold standard" against which to establish criterion validity.

Construct validity: convergent

Construct validity addresses the question of what is actually being measured by the scale. More specifically, convergent validity is the extent to which a QL measure is related to other data in a manner that is consistent with a priori, theoretically derived hypotheses. The multitrait-multimethod matrix paradigm (Campbell & Fiske, 1959) is often invoked as a framework for establishing the convergent validity of QL measures. For example, evidence of convergent validity may be derived by correlating different measures of the same construct (monotrait-heteromethod). For example, scores on a physical functioning scale might be correlated with involvement in sports activities or school attendance records.

Construct validity: divergent

The discriminant, or divergent, validity (Campbell & Fiske, 1959) of QL instruments is examined by determining the extent to which there is little or no correlation with a test that measures a different construct. For example, the lack of a significant association between a measure of QL and a measure of social desirability would provide support for the discriminant validity of the QL measure. Unfortunately, discriminant validity is rarely reported in QL investigations.

Divergent validity is often confused with discriminative validity which is another important type of validity for QL instruments. Discriminative validity, or known group comparisons, refers to an instrument's ability to accurately discriminate between known groups of patients (Van Knippenberg & De Haes, 1988). The discriminative validity of a measure is investigated by determining whether or not scores on a measure accurately distinguish between children and adolescents known to differ in health status (e.g., oncology patients on and off chemotherapy).

Sensitivity

A crucial aspect of construct validity for a QL instrument is its ability to detect change within the same population over time (Hays & Hadorn, 1992). Sensitivity to changes in QL is an important aspect of validity in longitudinal projects examining QL. Effect sizes, a standard unit used to evaluate the magnitude of before/after changes in a scale, should be reviewed to determine whether the measure's responsiveness to change is sufficient for the project being planned.

EVALUATION OF GENERIC MEASURES CURRENTLY AVAILABLE FOR USE WITH CHILDREN AND ADOLESCENTS
EPIDEMIOLOGIC HEALTH STATUS SURVEYS

The impact of chronic childhood illness was first assessed by way of large scale epidemiologic surveys. These surveys were designed to quickly and broadly evaluate the degree of childhood dysfunction within the general population due to a variety of pediatric illness conditions.

National Health Interview Survey (NHIS)

The National Health Interview Survey (NHIS) (Newacheck & Taylor, 1992) consists of nine questions used to estimate the prevalence of childhood chronic illness in a nationally representative sample. An adult member (usually a parent), of each of the 17,110 households, surveyed completed the NHIS on a sample child up to 18 years old. Parents first reported whether the child had one of 19 childhood health conditions. If a condition was reported, nine questions were used to gauge the impact of the condition over the prior year. Questions cover days missed from school, time spent in bed, doctor visits, hospitalizations, medication use, and pain/discomfort. Three of the questions use a yes/no format, four ask about the number of days a problem existed, and the two questions on pain and discomfort use four and three point Likert scales as response formats.

Reliability and validity studies have not been conducted with the NHIS. The authors note, however, that studies with the adult version of the NHIS found that 35% to 45% of conditions found in medical records were not reported by survey participants, while 8 to 12% of conditions reported in interviews were not found in medical records (Newacheck & Taylor, 1992). Nonetheless, this scale provides a brief, overall assessment of the burden of an illness on children that may be suitable for broad surveys of functioning.

Ontario Child Health Study (OCHS) Survey

The Ontario Child Health Study (OCHS) (Boyle et al., 1987; Cadman et al., 1986) instrument was developed for use in an epidemiologic survey designed to determine the prevalence and distribution of mental health problems in Ontario children 4 to 16 years old. As part of this survey, information on health and medical conditions was obtained. The 10 questions regarding health were adapted from the RAND Corporation's Measure of Children's Health Status (Eisen, Ware, & Donald, 1979), checklists of chronic illness conditions (Haggerty, Roghmann, & Pless, 1975; Walker, Gortmaker, & Weitzman, 1981), and the Canada Health Survey (Statistics Canada, 1981). Parents were asked to indicate whether there was a limitation of function due to an illness, injury, or medical condition for at least six months, which affected physical activity (four questions), mobility (two questions), self-care (one question), roles (e.g., in play or schoolwork) or school attendance (three questions). The authors do not present any data on reliability. They also did not compare parent report to physical exams or clinic records. The OCHS items have been used in additional studies to examine psychiatric disorders and social adjustment among children with chronic disorders (Cadman et al., 1987). However, the OCHS items are similar to those found in other epidemiologic surveys which have established psychometric properties so these more well developed surveys may be more appropriate for use than the OCHS survey.

UTILITY MEASURES

The most salient feature of utility measures is that they are rooted in economic decision theory and involve weighting trade-offs between length and quality of life. As noted earlier, utility measures are most appropriately used to evaluate the impact of health care services at the level of the general population, although they have been adapted for use within clinical investigations.

Quality of Well-Being Scale (QWB)

The Quality of Well-being Scale (QWB) (Kaplan, Bush, & Berry, 1978; Bush, Kaplan, & Berry, 1982) is a utility measure developed to evaluate health policies for both children and adults by comparing health outcomes in different disease populations (Kaplan, 1989; Kaplan, Atkins, & Timms, 1984). The QWB interview, which is comprised of four scales that focus on the physical impact of an illness, takes an average of 12 minutes to complete (Harris et al., 1994). The measure utilizes a six-day follow-back format wherein a parent reports on the child's status on each of the preceding six days.

Extensive preparation is required to administer the QWB, as interviewers must be trained to criterion through practice with audiotaped interviews available from its developers. The scoring of interviews is also somewhat labor-intensive in that a single index score results from a complicated scoring procedure in which levels of mobility, physical activity, social activity and a symptom complex score are aggregated (see Richards & Hemstreet, 1994, for a conceptual description of the index score). A computerized scoring program is available which facilitates the scoring of QWB interviews.

QWB index scores have been shown to be reliable over a one-year period (Kaplan et al., 1978), and interday reliability has been demonstrated across the seven days assessed (Anderson et al., 1989). Low to moderate correlations (r's = .23 to .55, p < .05) between parent and adolescent reports have been found in a sample of cystic fibrosis patients (Czyzewski et al., 1994). The convergent validity of the QWB was supported by significant positive correlations between scores on the QWB and self-rated well-being (r's = .42 to .49), as well as negative correlations between QWB scores and age (r = −.75), number of chronic medical conditions (r = −.75), and number of physician contacts (r = −.55) (Kaplan et al., 1976). Children with a greater number of prior hospitalizations and surgeries were rated by their parents as more impaired on the QWB in another study (Bradlyn et al., 1993).

Although there is some evidence to support the convergent validity of the measure (Kaplan et al., 1976), questions have arisen regarding the measure's apparent insensitivity to disease status and variations in health status (Ware, 1984). The QWB seems most useful in assessing individuals with high levels of impairment and is relatively insensitive in assessing low levels of impairment (Czyzewski et al., 1994; Richards & Hemstreet, 1994). A more general concern about the QWB is that only the "least desirable" symptom on each day is scored, thus attenuating the scores of patients who report several symptoms (Richards & Hemstreet, 1994).

Although the QWB has proven to be useful in health policy decision-making for adults, there are several limitations with respect to its use with children. First, the QWB is inappropriate for direct administration with children younger than 14 years of age because young children may have difficulty remembering physical symptoms for each of the previous six days (Hinds, 1990; Richards & Hemstreet, 1994). Second, the measure was developed using adult samples thus calling into question its applicability with pediatric populations (Rosenbaum, Cadman, & Kirpalani, 1990). Finally, the low concordance between patient and parent scores and the absence of significant correlations between the QWB and well-validated measures of psychosocial functioning may preclude its use with pediatric populations (Czyzewski et al., 1994).

HEALTH PROFILES

Health profiles are designed to capture descriptive ratings across a wide range of areas of functioning likely to be affected by an illness and its treatment. Like utility measures, health profiles are designed for use with large population-based samples. Unlike utility measures, health profiles do not involve weighting respondent preferences between length and quality of life. Rather, ratings of dysfunction are typically descriptive in nature. Health profiles are also somewhat more useful with clinical populations than are utility measures in that they result in a score for each of the different domains surveyed in addition to an aggregate index score.

Children's Health Inventory Profile, Adolescent Edition (CHIP-AE)

The Children's Health Inventory Profile, Adolescent Edition (CHIP-AE) (Starfield et al., 1995) is the revised version of the original Child Health and Illness Profile (CHIP; Starfield et al., 1993). The original version, which took 45 minutes to 1 hour to complete, was judged to be too long to be practical. Both versions of these self-report measures, for use with 11 to 17 year olds, are designed to assess health status in epidemiologic surveys, identify high-risk populations, and assess the effects of health services and public policy on child health (Starfield et al., 1993). The revised CHIP-AE assesses six domains: Risks, Discomfort, Satisfaction,

Disorders, Achievement, and Resilience. Each domain also has subdomains, 20 in total. For example, Discomfort includes Physical Discomfort, Emotional Discomfort, and Limitations on Activity; Resilience includes Family Involvement, Problem-Solving, Physical Fitness, and Home Safety/Health. There are 107 items, plus 46 disease/injury specific questions. The revised scale can be completed in about 30 minutes.

The CHIP-AE was rationally derived through reviews of the existing literature, focus groups, and a convenience sample of 121 adolescents. Each item on the CHIP-AE is rated on a three point scale with higher scores indicating more satisfaction and lower scores indicating less satisfaction in the particular domain. The CHIP-AE was developed with four groups of adolescents, grades 6 through 12, in both urban and rural communities (N = 3451). Internal consistency was .80 or above for 8 of the 13 subdomains where internal consistency was expected, and in two or more of the four samples. One week test-retest reliability ranged from .53 to .87 for the different subdomains. The developers conclude that the stability of responses for a population-based measure are adequate with the exception of the Home Safety and Health domains. Thus, the developers predict that changes over time in a group's subdomain score are likely to reflect real changes in health status, although there is no evidence to support this to date.

The developers theorized that parents are the most informed source about many aspects of their adolescent's health. Therefore, criterion validity was assessed by comparing adolescent responses to parent and school responses. Correlation coefficients ranged from .11 to .45, kappa coefficients averaged .30. Although these correlations are lower than desirable for a test of criterion validity, they are comparable to other correlations of parent/child reports (Achenbach, McConaughy, & Howell, 1987). Concurrent validity was demonstrated by correlations ranging from .59 to .68 on selected subdomains with established measures (e.g. the Children's Depression Inventory) tapping similar constructs. Construct validity was assessed by comparing the CHIP-AE responses of 877 school children to 70 general medical clinic patients and 74 chronically ill patients (Starfield et al., 1996). Acutely ill adolescents reported more physical discomfort, minor illness, and decreased physical fitness than adolescents in the school sample. Chronically ill adolescents reported more limitations on activity, long-term medical disorders, dissatisfaction with their health and less physical fitness than adolescents in the school sample.

There are good psychometric data to support the use of the CHIP-AE as a health profile of adolescent QL. The developers note that it is most suitable for evaluations of populations or clinical groups, but not individuals, although a shorter version of the CHIP-AE that may be suitable for clinical management is being developed. Audio-taped and computerized versions of the CHIP-AE, to increase ease of administration, are also being considered.

RAND Health Status Measure for Children (HSMC)

The RAND Health Status Measure for Children (HSMC) was developed to assess the impact of different insurance plans on the health status of children in the general population (Eisen et al., 1979; 1980). The HSMC is a parent-report questionnaire based on a multidimensional model of child health that assesses the four core QL domains (disease state, physical, psychological, and social functioning) as well as general health perceptions and behavior problems (Eisen et al., 1979). There are two versions of the measure, one for children aged 0–4, and the other for children aged 5–13. There is some evidence to support the psychometric properties of the HSMC (Eisen et al., 1979; 1980). Specifically, the internal consistency for all scales, was found to be fair for both the 0–4 version (r's = .53–.77) and the 5–13 version (r's = .57–.87) (Eisen et al., 1980). Interrater reliability has not been demonstrated.

The HSMC has been determined to have content, face, and construct validity, and the separate scales contribute unique information to the assessment of child health status (Eisen et al., 1980). In terms of concurrent validity, a modified version of the HSMC correlated significantly and in the expected direction with three of four global QL ratings and with the Cystic Fibrosis Problem Checklist (Sanders et al., 1991) in a sample of cystic fibrosis patients (Harris et al., 1994). That is, more positive QL ratings were associated with reports of less dysfunction and fewer behavior problems.

The HSMC may not be sensitive to different levels of dysfunction in pediatric populations (Pantell & Lewis, 1987), due to the fact that the normative sample was primarily comprised of healthy children (Eisen et al., 1979). Norms for chronically ill children are not available. However, the HSMC was not designed for diagnostic purposes, nor to detect differences between specific treatments in specific disease populations, but rather to measure changes in children's health status due to health care financing arrangements (Eisen et al., 1980).

Overall, the RAND HSMC holds substantial promise as a generic QL instrument for children. Its strengths include its multidimensional and developmental framework and the fact that there is some empirical support for its validity. Furthermore, the profile scoring system of the HSMC is useful for identifying specific areas of dysfunction. The primary weakness of the HSMC is the lack of norms for pediatric populations.

Sixteen-Dimensional Health-Related Measure (16D)

The Sixteen-Dimensional Health-Related Measure (16D) (Apajasalo et al., 1996a) is a downward extension of a measure designed for adults (Sintonen & Pekurinen, 1993). The developers limited the scale to early adolescence, ages 12 to 15, in order to describe a more developmentally homogeneous sample than is typically used in QL measures. The content and items were selected by a group of physicians and health economists in Helsinki, Finland. The items and dimensions were then further refined after pilot testing the preliminary instrument with 60 adolescents. The measure consists of 16 multiple choice questions about functioning in the following health-related domains: Mobility, Vision, Hearing, Breathing, Sleeping, Eating, Speech, Elimination, Usual Activities (i.e., school and hobbies), Friends, Physical Appearance, Mental Function, Discomfort/Symptoms, Depression, Distress, and Vitality. All items are ranked on a 1 to 5 scale which takes about 5 to 10 minutes to complete.

The developers administered the scale to 263 healthy controls and devised an item weighting system by having these subjects rank order the 16 dimensions on a 0 to 100 importance scale. The sum of the 16 weights then total to one score. Breathing, Friends, Mobility, and Mental Functioning were the highest rated dimensions on this importance scale. Parent ratings on the same dimensions were very similar. Overall scores were slightly higher for the male control subjects than for the female control subjects. One week test-retest reliability with 35 of these subjects revealed a statistically significant difference between administrations. However, 91% of the subjects scored within two standard deviations of the mean difference which Apajasalo et al. (1996a) describe as an acceptable repeatability coefficient.

The 16D is noteworthy because it was developed for adolescents within a specific developmental phase and because of its weighted index score. Its self-report format ensures that the adolescent's perception of his or her QL is evaluated rather than by proxy (i.e., parent-reported) which, by definition, cannot adequately capture such subjective rankings. However, each domain is represented by only one item which likely limits its reliability and validity as a measure of QL. Thus, the 16D is still in the early phases of development and more research on its psychometric properties are necessary before widespread use can be recommended.

Seventeen Dimensional Health-Related Measure (17D)

The Seventeen Dimensional Health-Related Measure (17D) was adapted from the 16D (described above) for use with children 8 to 11 years old (Apajasalo et al., 1996b). The items were first adapted from the 16D by a group of professionals and then four items were further modified after pilot testing with 79 children. This pilot testing also resulted in raising the lower age limit from 7 to 8 years of age, because 7 year-olds had difficulty completing the measure. The 17 multiple-choice items represent the same dimensions as those included in the 16D with the addition of a Learning Ability and Memory dimension. However, unlike the 16D, the 17D is illustrated with pictures and is completed using a structured interview format rather than self-report. The interview takes about 20 to 30 minutes to complete. A weighting system (similar to that used for the 16D) was developed based on the responses of 115 parents. Parents were used instead of children because the child respondents had difficulty ranking the dimensions in relation to one another.

The final version of the 17D was administered to 244 school-aged children. Total scores on the 17D were slightly higher for female control subjects than for male control subjects, although the profiles themselves were very similar. Two week test-retest reliability was calculated using 42 control subjects and revealed a slight, but statistically significant improvement in 17D scores. The repeatability coefficient revealed that 95% of the subjects fell within two standard deviations of the mean difference.

The 17D was also administered to 23 survivors of organ transplants and 20 patients with skeletal dysplasias. Discriminative validity was supported by the fact that patients had significantly lower scores than did controls on the 17D total score and on most of the predicted dimensions. Like the 16D, further work on the psychometrics of the 17D is needed before conclusions regarding its reliability and validity can be reached.

Warwick Child Health and Morbidity Profile

The Warwick Child Health and Morbidity Profile (WCHMP) (Spencer & Coe, 1996) is a parent-completed measure for infants and preschool children. The WCHMP was developed in the United Kingdom as a quick, easy to administer measure of health and morbidity for use in both research and service projects, either cross-sectionally or long-itudinally. The WCHMP uses an interview format to examine 10 domains, labeled as: General Health, Acute Minor Illness, Behavioral, Accident, Acute Significant Illness, Hospital Admission, Immunization, Chronic Illness, Functional Health status, and Health-Related QL. A single global question is used to tap each domain, with secondary questions used to obtain more in-depth information in 6 of the domains. Four categories of responses are scored for each domain in this 10 minute interview. The WCHMP is not a health index but rather a "single summary of a child's health and illness experience" (p. 369, Spencer & Coe, 1996).

The WCHMP was developed in three phases with 228 preschool children. Two week to three month test-retest kappa coefficients were very good (greater than .80) for 2 domains, good (between .61 and .80) for 4 domains, and moderate (between .41 and .60) for 4 domains. In the original study, interrater reliability was perfect on 6 of the domains, with only one kappa below .80 (.76) for the remaining four domains. Construct validity was tested by validating parental responses on the WCHMP against pediatric clinic records. Parental reports, in general, correlated well with clinic records. Kappa coefficients ranged from .696 for chronic illness status to .854 for acute minor illness.

The WCHMP field testing included a significant sample of parents from low SES backgrounds suggesting it can be used across SES categories. The developers of the scale note that the validation of the WCHMP must be considered preliminary at present. In particular, a principal components or factor analytic procedure is needed to provide support for the independence of the hypothesized domains. Further studies are planned by the developers, but investigations of the WCHMP by independent investigators have yet to be reported.

CLINICAL OUTCOMES MEASURES: FUNCTIONAL STATUS INSTRUMENTS

In general, functional status measures are designed to assess, in relatively objective terms, a patient's ability to complete activities of daily living (ADLs). Thus, the primary intent of such measures is to assess levels of mobility, pain, and general physical functioning.

Functional status measures also tend to be comprised of fewer items so as to better serve as brief and easy to score screening tools. Given the practicality of functional status measures, they often serve as proxy measures for true QL measures despite the absence of one or more of the core QL domains (e.g., psychological functioning). Moreover, functional status measures are useful in primary care settings because responses can be linked directly to patient management at the time of the clinic visit (Wasson et al., 1992).

COOP charts — adolescent version

The adolescent version of the COOP was modeled after an adult measure which uses nine pictorial charts to assess overall patient functioning in areas including physical condition, emotional condition, pain, QL, and social activities. The measure is named after the Dartmouth COOP project, the primary care research network that developed and tested the measure (Nelson et al., 1990). The adult measure has been shown to be reliable and valid, easy to use in office settings, and relatively sensitive to changes in health status (Nelson et al., 1990). The adolescent version of the COOP was developed on a sample of 658 youths ranging in age from 12 to 21 years of age.

This self-administered scale was initially pilot tested using a measure covering 17 functional areas. Focus groups of primary care physicians and adolescents resulted in the elimination of three areas. Field testing reduced the number of areas even further to six picture-and-word charts. The six areas (Physical Fitness, Emotional Feelings, Schoolwork, Social Support, Family Communications, and Health Habits) are each rated on a five point Likert scale with corresponding pictorial representations for each point on the scale. This brief measure takes less than five minutes to complete. Test-retest reliability assessed on consecutive days in a sample of 199 adolescents, revealed an average correlation of .77 (range, .71 to .80). Concurrent validity was assessed by examining the association between each of the six areas and items selected from existing questionnaires tapping the same content domain. The average correlation for the corresponding area was .62 which was comparable to the correlation (.64) found in the adult COOP validation study (Nelson et al., 1990), and .32 for the noncorresponding areas. Discriminant validity was demonstrated by the ability of the Health Habits chart of the adolescent COOP to discriminate between adolescents with a history of drug use and adolescents who did not report drug use after controlling for age, gender, and race.

The adolescent version of the COOP is praiseworthy for its ease of administration and its potential for use in a busy clinical practice setting. The pictorial nature of the scale is appealing, although it has not been demonstrated that the pictures improve responding or increase the validity of the measure. In addition, the developers note that the six functional areas are important but not inclusive and may miss some important areas of functioning, especially at the individual level (Wasson et al., 1994). This measure is clearly best utilized as a screen for health problems and is not likely to be sensitive to changes over time except to detect significant changes in health status (Wasson et al., 1994). The developers of the scale suggest that a score of three or above on a functional area indicates the need for further inquiry by the physician.

Functional Status-II-R

The Functional Status-II-R, or FS II(R) (Stein & Jessop, 1990), is a revised version of the Functional Status Measure (FS I) (Stein & Jessop, 1985). The FS II (R) is a parent interview suitable for children from birth to 16 years of age with chronic physical disorders. The FS I and FS II (R) were modeled on the Sickness Impact Profile (SIP; Bergner et al., 1981). Like the SIP, the FS II (R) is designed to cut across diseases, focus on observable behavior, and cover a broad range of functioning. Four age categories are included on the measure: infants (0–9 months), toddlers (10–23 months), preschoolers (2 to 5 years) and school age (greater than 5 years of age). The FS II (R) contains items related to Communication, Mobility, Mood, Energy, Play, Sleep, Eating, and Toileting. Each item has two parts. First, it is determined whether the child demonstrates the particular behavior "never or rarely", "some of the time", or "almost always". Second, if there is dysfunction, probes are used to determine if it is due "fully", "partly", or "not at all" to a health problem. The FS II (R) takes less than 30 minutes to complete. The FS II (R) score is the percentage of all possible points on the scale for a particular age group. The scale is available in English, Spanish, and Dutch.

The FS II (R) was developed with a sample of 462 children with a chronic condition and 276 healthy children. The original scale consisted of 53 items but 10 items which were consistently misunderstood were eliminated resulting in a 43 item final version with a 14 item short form also available. Factor analyses with the chronically ill sample revealed a two factor solution, with factor one labeled General Health at all age levels. Factor two was labeled Responsiveness in the two youngest age groups, Activity for the 2 to 3 year olds, and Interpersonal Functioning in the oldest group. Internal consistency was 0.80 or greater for all factors, at all age levels, in both the chronically ill and combined samples, including the short form. The mean scores for the healthy sample were significantly higher than the mean scores for the chronically ill group, demonstrating discriminant validity. Concurrent validity was demonstrated by high correlations between the FS II (R) and morbidity (days in hospital, days absent from school) for all age groups on both the short and long version of the scale. In addition, there is evidence to support the measure's discriminative validity in that when children with various types of impairments were compared against each other, those with more severe impairments scored worse on the FS II (R) than those with less severe impairments. Finally, physician ratings on day-to-day limitations correlated moderately with the FS II (R) (Stein & Jessop, 1990).

Although the FS II (R) is an improvement over the FS I, the scale developers do not present any data on test-retest reliability. In addition, the interview format, especially the need for probes, makes the FS II (R) somewhat more time consuming and expensive to administer than similar measures which use a self-report format.

Play Performance Scale for Children (PPSC)

The Play Performance Scale for Children (PPSC) (Lansky et al., 1985; Lansky et al., 1987), although developed specifically for pediatric oncology patients, is a global rating of QL. The PPSC consists of a one-item rating of a child's functional status, based on changes in the child's play. The PPSC is an 11-point scale from 0 to 100, with anchors provided for each decile, ranging from 0 = unresponsive to 100 = fully active, normal.

Validation studies of the PPSC have shown good interrater reliability between mothers and fathers (r = .71; Lansky et al., 1987), and between parents and physicians (r = .74; Mulhern et al., 1990). However, Mulhern et al. (1990) found low absolute agreement (kappa = .30, p < .01) between health care professionals and parents. Significant correlations between PPSC ratings for cancer inpatients and outpatients with age-corrected total adaptive behavior composite scores on the Vineland Adaptive Behavior Scale (Sparrow, Balla, & Cicchetti, 1984), and three global QL scales (Mulhern et al., 1990) support concurrent validity.

Strengths of the PPSC include its developmental framework (an integral issue in the assessment of QL in children) and minimal response bias because it is designed to be a relatively objective rating of behavior (Lansky et al., 1987). However, because the PPSC is a one-item rating scale, rather than a multidimensional measure of QL, it yields only a gross estimate of functioning (Mulhern et al., 1990).

Stanford Childhood Health Assessment Questionnaire

The Stanford Childhood Health Assessment Questionnaire (CHAQ) (Singh et al., 1994) is an adaptation of the Stanford Health Assessment Questionnaire (HAQ; Ramey, Raynauld & Fries, 1992), a well-validated, frequently used measure for adults with arthritis. The CHAQ is both a parent-administered and self-administered instrument (for children from 8 to 19 years of age) designed to measure functional status, specifically in children with juvenile rheumatoid arthritis (JRA). The authors adapted the items of the CHAQ from the HAQ in order to compare functional status across age groups and conduct longitudinal studies. The disability section of the CHAQ consists of 30 items which represent 8 subscales: Dressing and Grooming (4 items), Arising (2 items), Eating (3 items), Walking (2 items), Hygiene (5 items), Reach (4 items), Grip (5 items) and Activities (5 items). In each of the 8 areas, ratings are obtained on: a) difficulty performing the function (0 = no difficulty, 1 = some difficulty, 2 = much difficulty, or 3 = unable to perform); b) use of special aids or devices; and c) activities requiring the assistance of others. The highest (worst) score on any question in an area determines the score for that area. If help or aids/devices are needed in an area, a minimum score of 2 is assigned. The scores from the 8 areas are averaged to calculate a Disability Index. A Discomfort score is calculated using a visual analog scale (VAS), ranging from "no pain" (0) to "very severe pain" (100). Additionally, a Global Arthritis Score is calculated on a VAS ranging from "very well" (0) to "very poor" (100).

Scale development was conducted with a sample of 72 JRA patients. Excellent internal consistency was obtained for the scale as a whole (alpha = .94) and each of the functional areas (range .92 to .93). The mean correlation coefficient across functional areas was .60 (range = .38 to .79). Parent-child reliability was determined by having 29 parent/child pairs, for children 8 to 19 years of age, complete the CHAQ. The Spearman correlation coefficient was .84 between parents and children. Test-retest reliability was calculated after a two week interval for 13 patients resulting in a correlation coefficient of .79. Because there is not a gold standard for measuring arthritis severity, the authors demonstrated convergent validity of the Disability Index with a rating scale used with JRA patients, the Steinbrocker functional class. The correlation between the two measures was .77. The Disability Index also correlated highly with a number of involved joints (.67) and morning stiffness (.54).

Although specifically devised for arthritis, the areas covered on the CHAQ may make it applicable to other chronic illnesses, especially other chronic physical disorders. The CHAQ is notable because of the authors attention to developmental differences. There is at least one question in each functional area relevant to children of all ages. By devising a rating scale in which scores are derived from the highest rated item, questions not relevant to certain ages (e.g., opening car doors for a 3 year old) do not invalidate the score in an area. Thus, the CHAQ is a measure that can be used longitudinally. Future studies are needed to determine whether the CHAQ will be sensitive to change secondary to clinical improvement or deterioration.

CLINICAL OUTCOME MEASURES: MULTIDIMENSIONAL INSTRUMENTS

There is consensus that true QL instruments are multidimensional and assess the four core domains of disease state, physical, psychological, and social functioning. Such measures allow clinicians and researchers to comprehensively evaluate the impact of a chronic illness and its treatment on children and adolescents without requiring the administration of a lengthy battery of measures.

Adolescent Illness Impact Measure (AIM)

The Adolescent Illness Impact Measure (AIM) assesses quality of life in chronically ill adolescents, ages 11 through 18 (Spieth & Harris, 1998). Parallel self-report and parent-report versions of the AIM are available. The measure is comprised of 47 items that represent 7 factor analytically-derived QL domains (Physical, Psychological, and Social Functioning, Functional Status, Impact of Medical Care, and Pulmonary and Diabetes-Related Health Issues). Preliminary evidence supports the psychometric adequacy of the AIM. Both the self-report and parent-report versions were found to be internally consistent (alphas = .84 and .89, respectively). The measure also has good inter-rater reliability ($r = .62$, $p < 0.001$). Concurrent validity for the AIM has been demonstrated in that total scores from both versions of the AIM and a measure of children's health status (i.e., the RAND HSMC) correlated significantly (r = .33, p < 0.005; r = .55, p < 0.001). Finally, a significant difference in AIM scores for 42 healthy and 42 chronically ill adolescents (matched on sex and age) was obtained, providing evidence for the AIM's discriminative validity.

Child Health Questionnaire (CHQ)

The Child Health Questionnaire (CHQ) is a family of measures that have resulted from over 30 independent, but complementary, studies conducted in 10 countries over a period of approximately 5 years (Landgraf, Abetz, & Ware, 1996). The CHQ is designed to evaluate physical and psychosocial functioning along the three parameters of: (1) health status, (2) disability, and (3) personal evaluation of well-being. Factor analyses consistently identified two orthogonal factors which accounted for 59.2% of the total measured variance: Physical Health and Psychosocial Health. This two-dimensional model of health is further represented by 10 subscales: Physical Functioning, Role/Social Functioning (Physical), General Health Perceptions, Bodily Pain/Discomfort, General Behavior, Mental Health, Self-Esteem, Role/Social Functioning (Emotional), Parental Impact (Emotional), and Parental Impact (Time). Family functioning, as related to the child's physical health, is assessed by the inclusion of two additional items: Family Activities and Family Cohesion. Finally, a global item, Change in Health, designed to assess changes in the child's health during the previous year may be included. There is a child-report form and three parallel parent forms available. The self-administered child form is available for children ages 10 to 18 years and includes 87 items. Short forms and summary scores for the child completed form are not yet available (Landgraf, Abetz, & Ware, 1996). The full-length parent form assesses 12 concepts and includes 98 items. There is also a 50-item (CHQ-PF50) and a 28-item (CHQ-PF28) parent form available. The age range for the child targeted by the parent forms is 5 to 18 years.

There are data from several studies supporting the psychometric properties of the 50- and 28-item parent forms and the 87-item child form of the CHQ. For the CHQ-PF50, internal consistency estimates (i.e., alpha coefficients) from a normative sample of 379 parents ranged from .66–.94, with a median reliability estimate of .84. In six of ten clinical samples (i.e., asthma, epilepsy, cystic fibrosis, and psychiatric), alpha coefficients ranged from .69 to .89. For the eight multi-item scales that comprise the CHQ-PF28, the median alpha coefficient was .75. Estimates of internal consistency for the CHQ-CF87 ranged from .73 to

.97, across three clinical samples (i.e., ADHD, cystic fibrosis, end-stage renal disease) and a school-based sample. Finally, the CHQ has good demonstrated discriminative validity in that the scales can discriminate children with clinically defined conditions from a representative sample of healthy children (Landgraf, Abetz, & Ware, 1996).

The utility of the CHQ is enhanced by several practical features included in the manual. First, the CHQ manual presents norms obtained across several studies and diseases. Second, confidence intervals for scores obtained from the CHQ-PF50 and CHQ-PF28 are presented. Finally, a SAS-based computer scoring algorithm is available. However, further work on this scoring program is required as one user reported spending several hours devising scoring templates, after which data from each CHQ form could be entered into a database and scored in approximately 20 minutes (B.J. Masek, personal communication, May 14, 1998). Overall, the CHQ promises to be a useful and versatile measure of QL.

Child Health Rating Inventories (CHRI)

The Child Health Rating Inventories (CHRI) is an 18-item computer illustrated self-report questionnaire for school-aged children ages 5–12 (Kaplan et al., 1995). A principal components and factor analytic procedure resulted in 4 domains: Physical Functioning, Role Functioning (e.g., school attendance), Cognitive Functioning, and Emotional Well-Being (i.e., fun and overall QL). Each item is comprised of an animated cartoon image of a child engaging in 5 levels of functioning representing the range from not limited at all to very limited by health problems. It takes young children, who need not be literate, approximately 20 minutes to complete the assessment.

Only preliminary evidence on the psychometric adequacy of the CHRI is currently available. The initial validation study was conducted with a sample of 196 healthy elementary school children and 241 children with a chronic illness (i.e., 73 with diabetes, 50 with asthma, 70 with cardiac disease, and 48 who had undergone bone marrow transplantation). Internal consistency estimates for the 4 domains were acceptable (Cronbach's alphas > .70). Evidence to support the concurrent validity of the CHRI was suggested by significant correlations between physician ratings of the chronically ill children's disease severity and child CHRI ratings (p's < .01). However, in terms of interrater reliability, there was little agreement between child and parent reports. Although further evidence to support the psychometric properties of the CHRI is needed, it promises to fulfill a unique niche in QL assessment due to its appealing format, its brevity, and its utility with pre-literate children.

How Are You? (HAY)

The How Are You? (HAY) (Bruil et al., 1997; Maes & Bruil, 1995) is a self-report and parent-report instrument developed in the Netherlands for 7 to 13 year old children. The items were generated by reviewing the literature and interviewing children with a chronic illness and their families as well as health professionals. There are also items specific to JRA, asthma, diabetes, and epilepsy. The generic portion of the HAY covers functioning in daily life including: Physical Functioning, Cognitive Functioning, Social Functioning, Physical Complaints, and Happiness. The response format varies by item but is typically on a four point scale with different verbal descriptors (e.g., never, sometimes, often, very often; good, not so good, not good, not good at all) and sometimes pictorial representations (happy to very sad faces). Items typically examine prevalence, as well as other characteristics of an activity such as quality of the child's performance of an activity and feelings about the activity. Most questions refer to the child's behavior and feelings over the prior seven days. The disease-specific section of the HAY consists of four components of disease states: Physical Symptoms, Self-Management, Emotion Related to the Disease, and Effects of Disease on Self-Concept. Separate child and parent versions of the HAY are available. The forms are identical except parents do not rate their child's feelings. The HAY takes about 20 minutes to complete.

The authors report scale development data from a pilot project of 89 children with a chronic illness and 134 healthy children (Maes & Bruil, 1995) and a larger study with a slightly revised version of the HAY which included 569 children with a chronic illness and 344 healthy children (Bruil et al., 1997). Bruil et al. (1997) report that 92% of the children were able to complete the HAY without difficulty. A confirmatory factor analysis and inspection of alpha coefficients eliminated three domains from the generic scale (Social Problems, General Treatment, and Negative Emotions), but the four domains of the disease-specific scale were retained (Bruil et al., 1997). Alpha coefficients for the nine final domains ranged from .76 to .86. The correlations between child and parents ratings ranged from .49 to .72 for observable behavior. Children with chronic illness also scored significantly lower than healthy children on the prevalence and quality of performance items of the physical and social activities domain. The correlation between the cognitive competence scale of the Child Behavior Checklist and cognitive functioning domain of the HAY was .59, but the correlations between the physical and social competence scale of the CBCL and the corresponding HAY domains were lower.

The authors note that further analyses need to be conducted but the preliminary data suggest that the HAY has potential for use in assessing QL in clinical populations. The generic and disease-specific components will also be valuable when comparing children with different chronic diseases. A final caveat in considering this measure is that there may be cultural differences between the validation sample and a proposed sample that would affect response patterns. For example, a majority of children in the Netherlands rely on their ability to bicycle as a means for getting to school. Thus, they would likely weight the importance of the item relating to this area of functioning differently than would children in other countries who bicycle strictly for recreation.

Quality of Life Profile — Adolescent Version (QOLPAV)

The Quality of Life Profile — Adolescent Version (QOLPAV) is a self-report measure for adolescents developed on a sample ranging in age from 14 to 20 years (Raphael et al., 1996). The QOLPAV is based on a unique model of QL defined as "the degree to which the person enjoys the important possibilities of his/her life" (Raphael et al., 1996; p. 367). Three domains of functioning are encompassed by this model: Being (physical, psychological and spiritual), Belonging (physical, social and community), and Becoming (practical, leisure and growth). The initial item pool was developed using focus groups and pilot tested with 20 adolescents. The final sample item pool consisted of 54 items, six in each of 9 domains described above. All items are rated on "Importance" and "Satisfaction" scales ranging from not at all important or satisfied (1) to extremely important or satisfied (5). A weighted scoring procedure is used such that items rated as high in importance, but low in satisfaction receive the worst QL scores while items high on importance and high in satisfaction scores receive high QL scores. Single items, not included in the computation of the total score, address degree of control and opportunities perceived as available in each of the domains.

Internal consistency was calculated with a sample of 150 adolescents. Correlation coefficients for the overall score and the three domains all exceeded .80. The QOLPAV correlated moderately with several brief measures of self-esteem, life satisfaction, social support, and life chances. The correlations between these measures and the subdomains of the QOLPAV were comparable across domains with little differentiation. The QOLPAV was consistently correlated with adolescent report of their health status, especially physical being. Tobacco use was significantly negatively correlated ($r = -.27$) with physical being, but no other subdomains, and alcohol use was negatively correlated with the majority of the subdomains and total score of the QOLPAV (range $-.15$ to $-.28$).

The QOLPAV is distinct from the other QL measures reviewed here because of its focus on subjective versus objective aspects of QL. The authors developed the measure to tap their theoretical model of subjective QL (Woodill et al., 1994), but the validation conducted to date has been limited. It has not been tested on a sample of chronically ill adolescents, and initial analyses did not support the specificity of the subdomains. This latter difficulty may indicate that the subdomains do not have differential predictive validity or the measures against which the QOLPAV was validated were too brief or nonspecific to detect differences. The relationship between the QOLPAV and objective measures of QL will also be important to investigate in future studies.

PRACTICAL AND METHODOLOGIC CONSIDERATIONS WHEN SELECTING A GENERIC MEASURE

When selecting a generic QL measure, it should be considered against the ideal standards proposed in a recent consensus conference (Bradlyn et al., 1996). A comprehensive QL instrument should assess physical, social, and emotional functioning, have a patient report version whenever applicable, be sensitive to change over time, and across the lifespan, be peer reviewed, and be easily administered (i.e., the burden to staff and patients should be minimal) (Bradlyn et al., 1996). Generic QL measures should be applicable to a wide range of healthy and ill populations, questions should be broad-based, and the items should be comparable across disease populations. The hypotheses of a given study should drive instrument selection, both in terms of content (i.e., do the items on the measure reflect the questions of interest?), and psychometric properties (e.g., in a repeated measures design, is the instrument sufficiently sensitive to changes over time?). In longitudinal designs, a developmentally sensitive instrument with consistency of domains across age levels will be an important selection criteria. General considerations and special concerns when assessing child and adolescent QL are discussed below.

GENERAL CONCERNS WHEN ASSESSING QUALITY OF LIFE

Staff burden

Simple QL measures, that utilize only one item and/or a pictorial format, can usually be self-administered (even by persons with limited English), or administered by office staff, are easy to score and are directly interpretable. These qualities make such measures attractive for use in office and clinic settings (Nelson et al., 1990). However, although the demands of a busy clinical setting make brevity a necessity in many instances, precision of measurement is lost. One solution to this problem is to use brief screening measures initially to identify problem areas, and to then administer longer, more detailed measures to assess a specific functional area more accurately if indicated (Nelson et al., 1990).

Interpretation of Quality of Life scores

Most papers reporting the development of a QL measure do not present norms.[2] Consequently, the interpretation of QL scores poses difficulties for clinicians and researchers alike (Wasson et al., 1992). In most cases, if a measure is used consistently, health care professionals will develop their own thresholds for indicating the need for further assessment/ referral.

However, clinicians may initially have difficulty determining whether a QL score, or change in a QL score, indicates a need for further assessment or treatment. Similarly, researchers may encounter problems in establishing the clinical significance of QL scores. A related concern for researchers is the precision of a measurement obtained in a study examining a population parameter. One way to address this problem is for instrument developers to present confidence intervals in descriptive papers so readers can estimate the degree of variability expected when administering the instrument to a similar population. That is, the greater the variability reflected by the confidence interval of a particular instrument's scores, the less likely the same result will be obtained in a comparable study. Such information would be useful to investigators conducting validation studies or research projects using a QL measure.

SPECIAL CONCERNS WHEN ASSESSING QUALITY OF LIFE IN CHILDREN AND ADOLESCENTS

Use of proxy respondents: implications for validity of measurement

Assessment of QL in children may be problematic when proxy respondents (e.g., parents) are used due to the low concordance often obtained between parent and child reports (Achenbach, McConaughy, & Howell, 1987). Parents ratings of their child's QL may be confounded by their own emotional state regarding their child's disease. For example, the degree to which a parent feels responsible for his or her child's condition may affect the ratings. Similarly, maternal depression or perception of burden due to the child's illness and treatment likely affect parental proxy ratings (Ennett et al., 1991; Richters, 1992). Investigators may address this issue to some extent by explicitly assessing for these factors. For example, a measure of family burden, such as the Impact on Family Scale (Stein & Reissman, 1980), may be included in investigations of pediatric QL.

Furthermore, the assessment of QL is, by definition, a subjective process. There is general consensus in the QL literature that the patient should be the primary source of such information (Aaronson et al., 1991; Bradlyn et al., 1996; Cella & Tulsky, 1990; Moinpour, et al., 1989; Ware, 1984). A national panel of experts agreed that the patient's report provides the most relevant clinical and scientific QL data, specifically with regard to the impact of oncology treatments (Nayfield & Hailey, 1990). Although this position is based on the assumption that the patient is an adult, Pantell and Lewis (1987) hold that children should also be asked to provide QL information as they may be more aware of certain aspects of their present functional status than are their caretakers and physicians. In the psychological literature there is substantial evidence that children's self-reports are an important source of information that can add significantly to the understanding of a variety of behavioral and psychological events (Achenbach, McConaughy, & Howell, 1987; Moretti et al., 1985; Peterson, Harbeck, & Moreno, 1993). However, despite agreement that QL assessment (in adults) necessarily presumes a subjective evaluation (Kaplan & Anderson, 1990), self-reports from children are often viewed with skepticism by the medical community (Hollandsworth, 1988), and children and adolescents, in particular, have historically been seen as unreliable sources of information (Stone & Lemanek, 1990).

In an attempt to address these concerns, the concordance between patient self-reported QL and proxy-reported QL has been investigated. Unfortunately, reports across informants (i.e., patients, caregivers, physicians) are often divergent (e.g., Czyzewski et al., 1994; Mulhern et al., 1990). This raises the obvious concern as to which report is more accurate. There is general agreement that such discrepancies are due to the fact that each informant draws upon different information when assessing QL. Correspondence between raters tends to be high with respect to overt behaviors (Eisen et al., 1980; Rosenbaum, Cadman, & Kirpalani, 1990), but drops dramatically with respect to covert, or subjective states. For example, the information used by physicians may be primarily physiologic, whereas a patient's ratings may be primarily subjective (i.e., based on affective states) (Mulhern et al., 1990). Thus, variations in ratings may be a function of different perspectives and different concerns and each report may be partially accurate (Ware et al., 1981). Further, because patients and health care professionals rely on different information in their assessments of QL, high agreement between their ratings should not be expected. Finally, each report may be partially inaccurate because informants may be subject to different response biases. It is possible that parents are motivated to present themselves and the QL of their child in a favorable manner, whereas children may be less subject to socially desirable responding (Eisen et al., 1980). On the other hand, children may be less experienced than parents in describing their subjective states.

When conducting QL assessment, information from multiple sources helps ensure that a comprehensive and accurate assessment has been obtained, particularly in the absence of a definitive criterion measure or gold- standard. Children's self-reports of their physical and mental status are an integral component of such an assessment. Ware et al. (1981) suggest that until a better understanding of the associations between objective and subjective measures of QL are achieved, both self-report and proxy measures are necessary.

Importance of a developmental framework

There are at least three reasons to use a developmental framework when assessing pediatric QL: (1) because children's cognitive abilities change across development; (2) because children's subjective experience of their own well-being changes; and (3) due to difficulties in interpreting deviations from normal developmental functioning. Each of these considerations will be discussed in turn.

First, the use of a developmental framework when assessing pediatric and adolescent QL is necessitated by changes in cognitive and language abilities (i.e., reading and comprehension) that affect the accuracy and reliability of self-reports. Such skills are prerequisites for responding to questions about QL (Pantell & Lewis, 1987; Rosenbaum et al., 1990). Two primary developmental considerations include the age and abstract reasoning of the respondent and the temporal proximity of the event (Hinds, 1990).

After about the age of nine, children are believed to be capable of accurately reporting their emotions. Most adolescents have the ability to incorporate abstract concepts when describing themselves and can evaluate their own thoughts and behaviors critically (Stone & Lemanek, 1990). However, adolescent reports of cognitions, behaviors, and emotions, should be cued through the use of age-appropriate language. Thus, particular attention to the reading level of self-administered instruments is recommended and the reading level of new instruments should be assessed by using "readability formulas" (Stone & Lemanek, 1990). When assessing the QL of children and adolescents, it is also important to consider their understanding of time. Children and adolescents are more oriented to the present as compared with adults, and may have difficulty providing information about the distant past or future projections (Hinds, 1990; Kamphuis, 1987). For this reason, the time frame utilized in QL assessment may be shortened to facilitate accurate reporting. Additionally, strategies that aid in the recall of specific events are recommended, for example, keying questions to holidays or personal or national events (cf. Sobell et al., 1980).

Second, in addition to the need to consider the cognitive abilities of the child respondent, it is equally important to consider how the meaning of QL changes for children throughout childhood (Eiser, 1995). For example, there are qualitative changes that occur in the nature of social interactions across childhood. A 7-year-old child may perceive an extended hospitalization as distressing due to separation from her parents, whereas a 17-year-old youth may be more distressed by being separated from peers. Similarly, changes in appearance (e.g., alopecia) may differentially affect children at different stages of development (Bradlyn et al., 1996). Thus, the most appropriate measures for evaluating childhood and adolescent QL are those that take into account normative changes in abilities and roles across developmental phases (Apajasalo et al., 1996; Bradlyn et al., 1996; Eiser, 1995). At a theoretical level, this latter point is well taken, but at a practical level it presents several challenges.

It seems obvious that QL scores obtained from chronically ill children at several points in time will reflect developmental changes. Moreover, childhood health, functional status, and QL are often defined as the child's capacity to perform *age-appropriate* roles and tasks. However, the typical sequence of age-appropriate psychological, social, and intellectual development in healthy children is as yet ill-defined. Hence, comparisons of development (and QL scores) between chronically ill and healthy children are problematic due to the fact that there are not well-defined developmental norms for healthy children (Stein & Jessop, 1982). Furthermore, decelerations or deviations in developmental sequences secondary to a debilitating chronic illness may be normative within the context of that illness (Pal, 1996). One way to address this difficulty in score interpretation, is for instrument developers to begin developing norms for scores on pediatric QL measures across illnesses.

Because consideration of developmental issues is important to the assessment of childhood QL, for a variety of reasons, the availability of different versions of a measure at the various developmental phases (e.g., infants, toddlers, school-age children, and adolescents) is useful, particularly when tracking QL longitudinally. A measure that purportedly assesses QL from childhood through adulthood is likely to be less sensitive to the issues outlined here than are measures validated for use with children at particular developmental phases (Eiser, 1995).

CONCLUSION
THE ADVANTAGES OF USING A GENERIC QUALITY OF LIFE MEASURE

Generic measures have two primary advantages. First, they allow for the comparison of QL outcomes across different diseases and disorders (Patrick & Deyo, 1989). This is particularly important when working with pediatric populations given the difficulty any one investigator typically encounters when attempting to obtain sufficiently large samples within specific disease populations. Moreover, particular areas of investigation may be best studied across illness groups, in which case, the use of generic measures is advantageous in that it allows for the application of a noncategorical approach (Stein et al., 1993) to the study of health outcomes in chronic childhood illness. Second, generic measures are designed to assess all areas of childhood functioning most likely to be affected by an illness and its treatment and are thus more comprehensive. Because such comprehensive QL assessments have been conducted infrequently within the context of clinical trials or medical research (Bradlyn, Harris, & Spieth, 1995), the outcomes obtained are often unexpected (McSweeny & Creer, 1995). That is, either subjective QL ratings have contradicted a priori hypotheses, or the medical intervention resulted in decreased ratings in another QL domain than was unanticipated. At least two QL investigations with adults resulted in unexpected findings (Rockey & Griep, 1980; Sugarbaker et al., 1982) which will likely facilitate improved treatment, better health outcomes and more informed clinical decision-making. Similarly, for children and adolescents diagnosed with bone tumors of the extremities, treatment may involve amputation of the affected limb or a limb-salvaging procedure. It might be hypothesized that better QL outcomes would be obtained from children whose limb was saved versus amputated. In fact, the opposite may be true as was found by Sugarbaker et al. (1982) in a study with adult patients. Thus, the importance of such comprehensive assessments should not be underestimated.

DISADVANTAGES OF USING A GENERIC QUALITY OF LIFE MEASURE

The disadvantages of a particular QL measure will likely vary considerably depending on its intended purpose (e.g., to obtain individual health outcomes versus to collect epidemiologic data). In general, the primary disadvantages to using generic QL measures are that they may be less sensitive in tapping condition-specific symptoms and in detecting health status changes in particular disease conditions. That is, it cannot be assumed that a generic instrument will be sensitive to QL changes across all disease conditions. However, supplementing a generic measure with a condition-specific measure is a widely recommended approach. Similarly, instruments that use a modular approach in which different subscales may be combined according a particular investigation's needs may address this issue.

In conclusion, there is substantial support in the literature for the systematic assessment of QL as an important outcome measure with pediatric populations. Medical efforts to extend the length of children's lives should be augmented by efforts to improve the qualitative aspects of their lives as well. There is a very real need for the inclusion of QL measures in pediatric and adolescent clinical and research trials, particularly given the fact that normal childhood development can be profoundly affected by the toxicities and untoward effects of aggressive medical treatments. It is hoped that the categorization and evaluation of the generic measures included here will facilitate future efforts to systematically assess the QL of children and adolescents.

NOTES

[1] It should be noted that although every attempt was made to provide a comprehensive review of pediatric QL measures, there has been a recent increase in the number of newly developed measures some of which may not have been available for evaluation at the time of writing.

[2] A notable example is the CHQ manual which includes QL score norms for several illness populations.

AUTHOR NOTE

The author extends her gratitude to Dr. Anthony Spirito for his careful readings and helpful comments at several points during the preparation of this chapter.

References

Aaronson, N.K., Meyerowitz, B.E., Bard, M., Bloom. J.R., Fawzy, F.I., Feldstein, M., Fink, D., Holland, J.C., Johnson, J.E., Lowman, J.T., Patterson, W.B., & Ware, J.E. (1991). Quality of life research in oncology: Past achievements and future priorities. *Cancer, 67,* 839–843.

Achenbach, T.M., McConaughy, S.H., & Howell, C.T. (1987). Child/adolescent behavioral and emotional problems: Implications of cross-informant correlations for situational specificity. *Psychological Bulletin, 101,* 213–232.

Anderson, J.P., Kaplan, R.M., Berry, C.C., Bush, J.W., & Rumbaut, R.G. (1989). Interday reliability of function assessment for a health status measure: The Quality of Well-Being Scale. *Medical Care, 27,* 1076–1084.

Apajasalo, M., Sintonen, H., Holmberg, C., Sinkkonen, J., Aalberg, V., Pihko, H., Siimes, M.A., Kaitila, I., Mäkelä, A., Rantakari, K., Anttila, R., & Rautonen, J. (1996a). Quality of life in early adolescence: A sixteen-dimensional health-related measure (16D). *Quality of Life Research, 5,* 205–211.

Apajasalo, M., Rautonen, J., Holmberg, C., Sinkkonen, J., Aalberg, V., Pihko, H., Siimes, M., Kaitila, I., Mäkelä, A., Erkkilä, K., & Sintonen, H. (1996b). Quality of life in pre-adolescence: A 17-dimensional health-related measure (17D). *Quality of Life Research, 5,* 532–538.

Bergner, M., Bobbitt, R.A., Carter, W., & Gilson, B. (1981). The Sickness Impact Profile: Development and final revision of a health status measure. *Medical Care, 19,* 787–805.

Bergner, M., & Rothman, M. (1987). Health status measures: An overview and guide for selection. *Annual Review of Public Health, 8,* 191–210.

Boyle, M.H., Offord, D.R., Hofmann, H.G., Catlin, G.P., Byles, J.A., Cadman, D.T., Crawford, J.W., Links, P.S., Rae-Grant, N.I., & Szatmari, P. (1987). Ontario Child Health Study: Methodology. *Archives of General Psychiatry, 44,* 826–831.

Bradlyn, A.S, Harris, C.V., & Spieth, L.E. (1995). Quality of life assessment in pediatric cancer trials: A retrospective review of Phase III cooperative group reports. *Social Science and Medicine, 4,* 1463–1465.

Bradlyn, A.S., Harris, C.V., Warner, J.E., Ritchey, A.K., & Zaboy, K. (1993). An investigation of the validity of the Quality of Well-Being Scale with pediatric oncology patients. *Health Psychology, 12,* 246–250.

Bradlyn, A.S., Ritchey, A.K., Harris, C., Moore, I., O'Brien, R., Parsons, S., Patterson, K., & Pollock, B. (1996). Quality of life research in pediatric oncology. Research methods and barriers. *Cancer, 78,* 1333–1339.

Bruil, J., Maes, S., le Coq, E., & Boeke, A. (April, 1997). *Assessing quality of life among children with a chronic illness: the development of a questionnaire.* Paper presented at the Sixth Florida Conference on Child Health Psychology, Gainesville, FL.

Bush, J., Kaplan, R., & Berry, C. (1982). A standardized quality of well-being scale for cost-utility and policy analysis in health: Reliability and generalizability, *Medical Care, 20.*

Cadman, D., Boyle, M., Offord, D., Szatmari, P., Rae-Grant, N., Crawford, J., & Byles, J. (1986). Chronic illness and functional limitations in Ontario children: Findings of the Ontario Child Health Study. *Canadian Medical Association Journal, 135,* 761–767.

Cadman, D., Boyle, M., Szatmari, P., & Offord, D. (1987). Chronic illness, disability, and mental and social well-being: Findings of the Ontario Child Health Study. *Pediatrics, 79,* 805–813.

Campbell, D.T., & Fiske, D.W. (1959). Convergent and discriminant validation by the multitrait-multimethod matrix. *Psychological Bulletin, 56,* 81–105.

Cella, D., & Tulsky, S. (1990). Measuring quality of life today: Methodological aspects. *Oncology, 4,* 29–38.

Czyzewski, D.I., Mariotto, M.J., Bartholomew, K., LeCompte, S.H., & Sockrider, M.M. (1994). Measurement of quality of well-being in a child and adolescent cystic fibrosis population. *Medical Care, 32,* 965–972.

Eisen, M., Ware, J., & Donald, C. (1979). Measuring components of children's health status. *Medical Care, 17*, 902–921.

Eisen, M., Donald, C.A., Ware, J.E., & Brook, R.H. (1980). *Conceptualization and measurement of health for children in the Health Insurance Study.* RAND Corporation: #R–2313-HEW.

Eiser, C. (1995). Choices in measuring quality of life in children with cancer: A comment. *Psycho-oncology, 4*, 121–131.

Ennett, S., DeVellis, B., Earp, J., Kredich, D., Warren, R., & Wilhelm, C. (1991). Disease experience and psychosocial adjustment in children with juvenile rheumatoid arthritis: children's views versus mothers' reports. *Journal of Pediatric Psychology, 16*, 557–568.

Haggerty, R.J., Roghman, K.J., & Pless, I.B. (1975). *Child health and the community*, pp. 345–350. Wiley: Toronto.

Harris, C.V., Bradlyn, A.S., Aronoff, S., Spieth, L.E., Warner, J.E., & Pinzone, H. (October, 1994). *Quality of life in cystic fibrosis.* Poster presented at the Annual North American Cystic Fibrosis Conference, Orlando, FL.

Hays, R., & Hadorn, D. (1992). Responsiveness to change: An aspect of validity, not a separate dimension. *Quality of Life Research, 1*, 73–75.

Hinds, P. (1990). Quality of life in children and adolescents with cancer. *Seminars in Oncology Nursing, 6*, 285–291.

Hollandsworth, J.G. (1988). Evaluating the impact of medical treatment on the quality of life: A 5-year update. *Social Sciences and Medicine, 26*, 425–434.

Kamphuis, R.P. (1987). The concept of quality of life in pediatric oncology. In N.K. Aaronson and J. Beckmann (Eds.), *The quality of life of cancer patients* (pp. 141–151). New York: Raven Press.

Kaplan, R.M. (1989). Health outcome models for policy analysis. *Health Psychology, 8*, 723–735.

Kaplan, R.M., & Anderson, J.P. (1990). The general health policy model: an integrative approach. In B. Spilker (Ed.), *Quality of life in clinical trials* (pp. 131–149). New York: Raven Press, Ltd.

Kaplan, R.M., Atkins, C.J., & Timms, R. (1984). Validity of the Quality of Well-Being Scales as an outcome measure in chronic obstructive pulmonary disease. *Journal of Chronic Diseases, 37*, 85–95.

Kaplan, R.M., Bush, J.W., & Berry, C.C. (1976). Health status: Types of validity and the Index of Well-Being. *Health Services Research, 11*, 478–507.

Kaplan, R.M., Bush, J.W., & Berry, C.C. (1978). The reliability, stability, and generalizability of a Health Status Index. *American Statistical Association, Proceedings of the Social Statistics Section*, 704–709.

Kaplan, S.H., Barlow, S., Spetter, D., Sullivan, L., Khan, A., & Grand, R. (1995). Assessing functional status and health-related quality of life among school-aged children: Reliability and validity of a new self-reported measure [Abstract]. *Quality of Life Research, 4*, 444.

Landgraf, J.M., Abetz, L., & Ware, J.E. (1996). *The CHQ user's manual.* First Edition. Boston, MA: The Health Institute, New England Medical Center.

Lansky, S.B., List, M.A., Lansky, S.B., Cohen, M.E., & Sinks, L.B. (1985). Toward the development of a Play Performance Scale for Children (PPSC). *Cancer, 56*, 1837–1840.

Lansky, S.B., List, M.A., Lansky, L.L., Ritter-Sterr, C., & Miller, D.R. (1987). The measurement of performance in childhood cancer patients. *Cancer, 60*, 1651–1656.

MacKeigan, L.D., & Pathak, D.S. (1992). Overview of health-related quality of life measures. *American Journal of Hospital Pharmacology, 49*, 2236–2245.

Maes, S., & Bruil, J. (1995). Assessing the quality of life in children with a chronic illness. In J. Rodriguez-Marin (Ed.), *Health psychology and quality of life research* (pp. 637–652). Alicante, Spain: Health Psychology Department, University of Alicante.

McSweeny, A.J., & Creer, T.L. (1995). Health-related quality of life assessment in medical care. *Disease-a-Month, XLI(1)*, 6–71.

Moinpour, C., Feigl, P., Metch, B., Hayden, K., Meyskens, F., & Crowley, J. (1989). Quality of life endpoints in cancer clinical trials: review and recommendations. *Journal of the National Cancer Institute, 81*, 485–495.

Moretti, M.M., Fine, S., Haley, G., & Marriage, K. (1985). Childhood and adolescent depression: Child-report versus parent-report information. *Journal of the American Academy of Child Clinical Psychiatry, 24*, 298–302.

Mulhern, R.K., Fairclough, D.L., Friedman, A.G., & Leigh, L.D. (1990). Play performance scales as an index of quality of life of children with cancer. *Psychological Assessment, 2,* 149–155.

Nayfield, S., & Hailey, B. (1990, July). *Quality of life assessment in cancer clinical trials: Report of the workshop on quality of life research in cancer clinical trials.* Bethesda, MD: National Cancer Institute and Office of Medical Applications of Research, National Institutes of Health.

Nelson, E.C., Landgraf, J.M., Hays, R.D., Wasson, J.H., & Kirk, J.W. (1990). The functional status of patients. How can it be measured in physicians' offices? *Medical Care, 28,* 1111–1126.

Newacheck, P.W., & Taylor, W.R. (1992). Childhood chronic illness: Prevalence, severity and impact. *American Journal of Public Health, 82,* 364–371.

Nunnally, J. (1978). *Psychometric theory.* New York: McGraw-Hill.

Pal, D.K. (1996). Quality of life assessment in children: a review of conceptual and methodological issues in multidimensional health status measures. *Journal of Epidemiology and Community Health, 50,* 391–396.

Pantell, R.H., & Lewis, C.C. (1987). Measuring the impact of medical care on children. *Journal of Chronic Diseases, 40(S),* 99S–108S.

Patrick, D.L., & Deyo, R.A. (1989). Generic and disease-specific measures in assessing health status and quality of life. *Medical Care, 27,* S217–S232.

Peterson, L., Harbeck, C., & Moreno, A. (1993). Measures of children's injuries: Self-reported versus maternal-reported events with temporally proximal versus delayed reporting. *Journal of Pediatric Psychology, 18,* 133–147.

Ramey, D.R., Raynauld, J.-P., & Fries, J.F. (1992). The Health Assessment Questionnaire 1992: status and review. *Arthritis Care and Research, 5,* 119–129.

Raphael, D., Rukholm, E., Brown, I., Hill-Bailey, P., & Donato, E. (1996). The Quality of Life Profile-Adolescent version: Background, description and initial validation. *Journal of Adolescent Health, 19,* 366–375.

Richards, J., & Hemstreet, M.P. (1994). Measures of life quality, role performance, and functional status in asthma research. *American Journal of Respiratory and Critical Care Medicine, 149,* S31–S39.

Richters, J. (1992). Depressed mothers as informants about their children: A critical review of the evidence for distortion. *Psychological Bulletin, 112,* 485–499.

Rockey, P.H., & Griep, R.J. (1980). Behavioral dysfunction in hyperthyroidism: Improvement with treatment. *Archives of Internal Medicine, 140,* 1194–1197.

Rosenbaum, P., Cadman, D., & Kirpalani, H. (1990). Pediatrics: Assessing quality of life. In B. Spilker (Ed.), *Quality of life assessments in clinical trials* (pp. 205–215). New York: Raven Press, Ltd.

Sanders, M.R., Gravestock, F.M., Wanstall, K., & Dunne, M. (1991). The relationship between children's treatment-related behaviour problems, age, and clinical status in cystic fibrosis. *Journal of Paediatric Child Health, 27,* 290–294.

Scientific Advisory Committee (September, 1995). Instrument review criteria. *Medical Outcomes Trust Bulletin,* 1–4.

Singh, G., Athreya, B., Fries, J., & Goldsmith, D. (1994). Measurement of health status in children with juvenile rheumatoid arthritis. *Arthritis & Rheumatism, 37,* 1761–1769.

Sintonen, H., & Pekurinen, M. (1993). A fifteen-dimensional measure of health-related quality of life (15D) and its applications. In S.R. Walker and R.M. Rosser (Eds.), *Quality of life assessment: Key issues in the 1990s* (pp. 185–195). Dordrecht: Kluwer Academic Publishers.

Sobell, M.B., Maisto, S.A., Sobell, L.C., Cooper, A.M., Cooper, T., & Sanders, B. (1980). Developing a prototype for evaluating alcohol treatment effectiveness. In L.C. Sobell, M.B. Sobell, and E. Ward (Eds.), *Evaluating alcohol and drug abuse treatment effectiveness: Recent advances* (pp. 129–150). New York: Pergamon Press.

Sparrow, S.S., Balla, D.A., & Cicchetti, D.V. (1984). *Vineland Adaptive Behavior Scales.* Circle Pines, MN: American Guidance Service.

Spencer, N.J., & Coe, C. (1996). The development and validation of a measure of parent-reported child health and morbidity: The Warwick Child Health and Morbidity Profile. *Child: Care, Health & Development, 22,* 367–379.

Spieth, L.E., & Harris, C.V. (1996). Assessment of health-related quality of life in children and adolescents: an integrative review. *Journal of Pediatric Psychology, 21,* 175–193.

Spieth, L.E., & Harris, C.V. (1998). *Assessment of adolescent quality of life: Development and preliminary validation of a self-report measure.* Manuscript in preparation.

Starfield, B., Bergner, M., Ensminger, M., Riley, A., Ryan, S., Green, B., McGauhey, P., Skinner, A., & Kim-Harris, S. (1993). Adolescent health status measurement: Development of the Child Health and Illness Profile. *Pediatrics, 91,* 430–435.

Starfield, B., Forrest, C., Ryan, S., Riley, A., Ensminger, M., & Green, B. (1996). Health status of well versus ill adolescents. *Archives of Pediatric and Adolescent Medicine, 150,* 1249–1256.

Starfield, B., Riley, A., Green, B., Ensminger, M., Ryan, S., Kelleher, K., Kim-Harris, S., Johnston, D., & Vogel, K. (1995). The Adolescent Child Health and Illness Profile. A population-based measure of health. *Medical Care, 33,* 553–566.

Statistics Canada & Department of National Health and Welfare (1981). *Canada Health Survey. The Health of Canadians. (Cat.# 82–538).* Minister of Supply and Services: Ottowa, Canada.

Stein, E.L., Bauman, L., Westbrook, L., Coupey, S., & Ireys, H. (1993). Framework for identifying children who have chronic conditions: The case for a new definition. *The Journal of Pediatrics, 122,* 342–347.

Stein, R.E.K., & Jessop, D.J. (1982). A noncategorical approach to chronic childhood illness. *Public Health Reports, 97,* 354–362.

Stein, R.E.K., & Jessop, D.J. (1985). Assessing the functional status of children. In D.K. Walker & J.B. Richmond (Eds.), *Monitoring child health in the United States: Selected issues and policies.* Cambridge, MA: Harvard University Press.

Stein, R.E.K. & Jessop, D.J. (1990). Functional status II(R): A measure of child health status. *Medical Care, 28,* 1041–1055.

Stein, R.E.K., & Reissman, C.K. (1980). The development of an impact-on-family scale: Preliminary findings. *Medical Care, 18,* 465–472.

Stone, W.L., & Lemanek, K.L. (1990). Developmental issues in children's self-reports. In A.M. La Greca (Ed.), *Through the eyes of the child: Obtaining self-reports from children and adolescents* (pp. 18–56). Boston: Allyn & Bacon.

Sugarbaker, P.H., Barofsky, I., Rosenberg, S.A., & Gianola, F.J. (1982). Quality of life assessment of patients in extremity sarcoma clinical trials. *Surgery, 91,* 17–23.

Temkin, N., Dikmen, S., Machamer, J., & McLean, A. (1989). General versus disease-specific measures: Further work on the Sickness Impact Profile for head injury. *Medical Care, 27,* S44–S53.

Van Knippenberg, F.C.E., & De Haes, J.C.J.M. (1988). Measuring the quality of life of cancer patients: Psychometric properties of instruments. *Journal of Clinical Epidemiology, 41,* 1043–1053.

Walker, D., Gortmaker, S., & Weitzman, M. (1981). *Chronic illness and psychosocial problems among children in Genesee county.* School of Public Health, Harvard University, Boston, MA.

Ware, J. (1984). Conceptualizing disease impact and treatment outcomes. *Cancer, 15(S),* 2316–2323.

Ware, J.E., Brook, R.H., Davies, A.R., & Lohr, K.N. (1981). Choosing measures of health status for individuals in general populations. *American Journal of Public Health, 71,* 620–625.

Wasson, J.H., Kairys, S.E., Nelson, E.C., Kalishman, M., & Baribeau, P. (1994). A short survey for assessing health and social problems of adolescents. *The Journal of Family Practice, 38,* 489–494.

Wasson, J., Keller, A., Rubenstein, L., Hays, R., Nelson, E., & Johnson, D. (1992). Benefits and obstacles of health status assessment in ambulatory settings. *Medical Care, 30,* MS42–49.

Woodill, G., Renwick, R., Brown, I., & Raphael, D. (1994). Being, belonging, and becoming: An approach to the quality of life of persons with developmental disabilities. In D. Goode (Ed.), *Quality of life for persons with disabilities: International issues and perspectives.* Boston: Brookline Press.

World Health Organization. (1948). *Constitution of the World Health Organization basic document.* Geneva, Switzerland: World Health Organization.

Chapter 4

QUALITY OF LIFE IN CHILDREN: A HEALTH CARE POLICY PERSPECTIVE

Robert M. Kaplan

Evaluating health outcomes in children and adolescents has been particularly challenging. Most assessments of health outcome are derived from a model of health care that focuses on disease and curative medicine, however, an emerging view of health care goes beyond identifying and curing diseases. An adequate conceptualization of health for children and adolescents requires new models of health and health care. The purpose of this chapter is to review a General Health Policy Model (GHPM) and to discuss its applicability to the assessment of outcomes for children and adolescents. The first portion of the chapter will review some of the conceptual issues that challenge the use of traditional measures. The next section will describe why traditional psychometric approaches may not always be applicable for studies of health outcome in children and youth. Then, the General Health Policy Model will be presented and its potential uses for studies of children and youth will be discussed. In presenting these issues, it will be argued that most contemporary approaches to the conceptualization and treatment of child health outcomes are based on a disease model. As a result these approaches neglect a large portion of health care for children and adolescents.

CONCEPTUAL ISSUES

The measurement of health outcomes for children and adolescents has typically been conceptualized using a curative biomedical model. This model assumes that most health problems have identifiable pathology. Measurement is usually related to physician appraisal of disease activity using physiological measures. These might include blood chemistry, physical examination, or radiographic evidence of disease pathology. Behavioral factors, such as cigarette smoking, high risk behaviors, or consumption of high fat diets might be recognized as predictors of later disease pathology. However, they are rarely recognized as important on their own (Kaplan, 1990). The two cornerstones of the traditional curative model of medical care are diagnosis and treatment. Diagnosis is linked to pathophysiology and treatment is based on experimental clinical trials.

There are a variety of reasons why this traditional model has limitations for evaluating policies for children and adolescents. First, despite the predominance of the curative model of medical care, the goals of health care are typically much broader. In addition to curing disease, the goals of health care include promoting health, preventing illness and injury, restoring functional capacity, avoiding premature death, and taking care of people for whom a cure is not available (Fox, 1997). The traditional biomedical or curative model values some types of information more than others. Patient reports, for example, may have little value in the traditional model because biological tests are trusted to detect underlying disease pathology. If disease can be detected with a laboratory measure, how a patient experiences or reports symptoms is of little value. Thus, patient self-reports are regarded as unscientific and untrustworthy. Symptoms that cannot be verified or linked to their pathophysiology might be disparagingly regarded as "all in the patient's head" (Fox, 1997).

In the model, diagnosis defines the problem and provides direction for cure. Despite the importance of diagnosis, there are at least three reasons why diagnosis might not necessarily lead to the resolution of health care problems. First, diagnosis does not always lead to better health outcomes. There are many cases in which diagnostic tests identify a problem for which there is no effective treatment (Kaplan, 1997a). In other cases, health outcomes may be the same or even better if treatment is withheld. Most acute illnesses in childhood are self-limiting and will get better without treatment. When treatment is applied, children are exposed to side effects without any clear assurance of benefit. Second, diagnoses are not always correct. Some problems are overlooked while, in other cases, the wrong diagnosis is given and an incorrect treatment might be applied. The third problem with diagnosis dependent health care is that there are many cases in which health care might be enhanced even though a disease cannot be diagnosed. For example, the goal of preventive medicine is to keep people from having a diagnosable condition. Children who smoke cigarettes or who engage in dietary behaviors that increase their risk for adult diseases do not have a diagnosis. However, investing in the prevention of these behaviors will enhance health outcomes over the life cycle.

THE OUTCOMES MODEL

As an alternative model for health care, we have proposed an outcomes model (Kaplan, 1990, 1994, 1996, 1997a). The outcomes model is similar to the curative model in several ways. However, the ultimate outcome is not a measure of disease process. The goal of health care is to extend the duration of life or to improve the QL. Disease processes are of interest because pathology may either shorten life expectancy or make life less desirable. The same variables that predict disease process may also predict life expectancy or QL. However, in contrast to the traditional biomedical model, behaviors or biological events may affect life expectancy independently of disease process. Further, the measures of success in the outcomes model are different than those in the traditional biomedical model. The outcomes model emphasizes QL and life duration instead of clinical measures of disease process. As similar as these two models appear, they lead to substantially different approaches to health care (Kaplan, 1990). These distinctions are addressed in the following sections.

Valuing health service

The traditional biomedical model uses procedures to fix biological problems. The greater use of procedures in the US than in other countries resulted in the disproportionate cost in the American system. By 1990, it was clear that cost control would dominate the health policy agenda throughout the decade. Often, cost reduction is considered the major objective of health care reform. Pauly (1995) for example, argues that cost should be the central consideration in policy analysis. However, too much attention on cost may neglect the basic mission of health care. For example, if cost is the only criterion, the development of guidelines for appropriate care may exclude expensive services. In order to choose between alternative health programs, it is best to evaluate not only the costs but also the benefits (Strum & Wells, 1995). Such an evaluation recognizes all financial and health outcomes as either a cost or a benefit. Financial outcomes are easily understood, but patient reported clinical outcome measures are rarely taken and are often misunderstood. For example a change in an arterial blood gas value is not an ideal health outcome measure because it may not mean much to a patient or to a public policy maker. On the other hand, restoration or preservation of the ability to perform activities of daily living is the goal of many therapies. Patient-centered outcomes are measurable and the emerging outcomes research paradigm is beginning to develop momentum.

Despite the improvements in measuring patient outcomes, determining the value of health services has been particularly difficult. In contrast to cost–benefit analysis, which focuses on the dollar returns for investing in particular programs, cost-utility analysis focuses on patient reported health outcomes in relation to the financial costs of the program. In economics the value of a product is related to the willingness of consumers to pay for it. For example, the value of a house is set by the price consumers are willing to pay for the home. If the price is too high, few houses are sold. Health services are difficult to value in this manner because consumers rarely pay for them directly. Instead, the charges are paid by third parties. Third party payment cuts the connection between the desire for services and the need to pay for them. This leads to a "taboo" against acknowledging that costs are a factor in health care (Eddy, 1997). In contrast to the traditional biomedical model that values outcomes from the provider's perspective, the outcomes model emphasizes patient or consumer reports.

Diagnosis and prevention

The traditional model is designed to treat sick patients. Contacts with the system are patient initiated and there are few incentives to care for people who are not feeling sick or do not have a diagnosis. Focusing on diagnosis often directs attention away from activities that have the greatest potential to benefit public health.

Major non genetic contributors to mortality were examined in an important analysis by McGinnis and Foege (1993). When these external factors are considered independent of the disease model, clear priorities for prevention emerge. A summary of the estimates for actual causes of death in the United States is presented in Table 4.1. Tobacco use is associated with more than 400,000 deaths each year, while diet and activity patterns account for an additional 300,000. These dwarf the

TABLE 4.1   ACTUAL CAUSES OF DEATH — U.S. 1990

FACTOR	DEATHS	PERCENT
TOBACCO	400,000	19
DIET-ACTIVITY PATTERNS	300,000	14
ALCOHOL	100,000	5
MICROBIAL AGENTS	90,000	4
TOXIC AGENTS	60,000	3
FIREARMS	35,000	<2
SEXUAL BEHAVIOR	30,000	1
MOTOR VEHICLES	25,000	1
ILLICIT USE OF DRUGS	20,000	<1
TOTAL	1,060,000	50

SOURCE: MCGINNIS & FOEGE, *JAMA*, 270: 2207–2212, 1993.

number of deaths associated with problems that the public is generally concerned about, such as illicit drug use. The McGinnis and Foege analysis challenged us to think differently about how we evaluate public health programs. Only a small fraction of the trillion dollars the US spend annually on health care is devoted to the control of the major factors which cause premature mortality in the United States. Estimates suggest that less than 5% of the total annual health care budget is devoted to prevention efforts (Rothenberg et al., 1987). Shifting attention from diagnosis and treatment to helping people live longer and better makes it clear that preventive efforts to reduce tobacco, drug and alcohol and to promote physical activity deserve greater attention.

One of the major challenges in developing outcome indicators for young people is in quantifying the benefits of preventive programs. There are several reasons why the potential for disease prevention has often been overlooked by public policy makers. Preventive services rarely make headlines or gain the same attention as high technology medical interventions. For example, transplantation of a diseased heart attracts the media and brings public adulation for the providers. A patient who survives such transplantation is thought to have benefited from the miracles of modern medical science and the surgeons are handsomely rewarded. When an illness is prevented, no one is aware that a problem has been avoided. There are no headlines because there is no news, and there are no fees for the experts who helped avoid a catastrophe. Yet preventive services have the potential for a huge impact. An estimated 400,000 Americans die prematurely each year as a result of tobacco use. Substantial numbers of cancer and heart disease deaths may be prevented or at least delayed through modification of tobacco use. Many of the health habits that cause poor health outcomes later in life are established in the adolescent years. Programs that alter these detrimental behaviors are often completely overlooked by traditional evaluation strategies because the interventions do not require the diagnosis of a disease.

How the outcomes model leads to different decisions than the traditional biomedical model

The outcomes model redefines the goal of health care to concentrate on life expectancy and QL. In contrast to the traditional medical model that emphasizes biological measures, the outcomes model embraces patient-reported measures of functioning and QL. Although the traditional biomedical model and the outcomes model are similar in many ways, they lead to different decisions about the use of resources for prevention.

The use of tonsillectomy helps illustrate differences between a traditional biomedical approach and outcome approach to health care. Tonsillectomy was once the most common surgical procedure for children and adolescents. According to the traditional biomedical model, chronic inflammation of the tonsils could be found through examination and fixed with a simple surgical procedure. However, there was no evidence that children who underwent tonsillectomy suffered fewer respiratory infections. Further, there was some evidence that the procedure did harm. To some observers tonsillectomy was regarded as "ritualistic surgery" (Bolando, 1969). Once questions about the value of the procedure were raised, the rate of the procedure began to vary. Some studies showed that the chances of having the procedure were 200 times greater in some communities than in others (Wennberg, 1990). Yet, adolescents or children living in areas with a high volume of tonsillectomies appeared to have about the same rate of respiratory infections as those living in areas where few tonsillectomies were performed. Some traditional approaches using measures of inflammation might have concluded that tonsillectomy is valuable because it gets rid of chronically diseased tissue. An outcomes perspective suggests that the procedure uses resources without necessarily providing health benefits. Today, the procedure is used rarely, except in cases where children or adolescents have severe sleep apnea (Kaplan, 1998).

CURRENT OUTCOME MEASURES FOR CHILDREN AND ADOLESCENTS

This book concentrates on QL assessment for children and adolescents. In the past, most attempts to develop outcome measures for children and adolescents embraced the traditional curative biomedical model (Drotar, 1997). Disease specific measures have been developed specifically for particular medical diagnoses. There are now measures for children with cystic fibrosis, diabetes, asthma, growth abnormalities, or other chronic illnesses (Drotar, 1997).

Bullinger and Ravens-Sieberer (1995) reviewed the literature and found only a few measures that assess QL outcomes for children. More recently, they reported that among 20,000 publications on health-related QL, only about 13% related to children (N = 3050) (Ravens-Sieberer & Bullinger, 1997). One of the few attempts to measure population based QL in children has been described by Starfield and colleagues (1996). These investigators developed a child specific health and illness profile-adolescent edition (CHIP-AE), a measure that includes six domains: discomfort, satisfaction with health, disorders, achievement of social expectations, risks and resilience. Teenagers who are acutely ill reported more physical discomfort and minor illnesses. They also reported lower physical fitness. Chronically ill teenagers reported more activity limitation and long-time medical disorders. They were also less satisfied with their health and were less physically fit than adolescents without chronic medical problems. The CHIP-AE is an important development because it is one of the few attempts to offer a child centered rather than disease centered measure. The CHIP-AE has been evaluated in several studies (Starfield et al, 1993, 1995). Another child specific measure is the "How are you?" (HAY) that was created in the Netherlands. The HAY was designed for children with chronic illnesses such as asthma, arthritis, diabetes mellitus or epilepsy (Bruil, Maes, le Coq & Boeke, 1997).

Evaluation of current measures

The literature on outcomes assessment for children considers a variety of methodological issues. Landgraf and Abetz (1996) questioned who the appropriate respondent should be. Although some investigators believe that five year olds can provide reliable reports, more conservative estimates suggest that children must be nine or ten years of age before they can report for themselves. Similarly, sick children may not be able to complete self-administered questionnaires and reading level must also be taken into consideration. Landgraf and Abetz evaluated 11 instruments on the basis of content that they felt was appropriate. The categories of content included conditions/symptoms, functioning, mental health, current health, and behavioral issues. When Varni and colleagues (1998) created a new 32 item Pediatric Cancer QL Inventory (PCQL-32), they began with the assumption that separate dimensions were required to represent symptoms, physical functioning, psychological functioning, social functioning, and cognitive functioning.

As is often the case in literature reviews, Landgraf and Abetz simply tabulated whether or not they thought the various instruments included the content represented by their categories. Presumably, measures associated with the most check marks are most desirable. However, the conclusion of these reviews are completely determined by the review criteria. Unfortunately, measures can appear to have missed areas of content even though that content is clearly included. For example, one of the categories in the Landgraf and Abetz review is mental health.

Measures are regarded as including mental health if they have a subcategory identified as "mental health". However, other measures that include mental health items under a general category of symptoms are reported not to include mental health. Unfortunately, the matrix approach to evaluating health outcomes measures is often of little value. For example, general measures, such as the Health Utility Index (HUI) often provide sensitive, valid, and reliable estimates of child health status (Saigal et al., 1996).

Perhaps of greater concern is that most current measures of child health status are derived from conceptual models that ignore child wellness. Despite the appeal of developing specific measures for children, most health care offered for children and adolescents is for acute illnesses or for self-limiting medical conditions. The three most common reasons for adolescents to use health care services are for physical examinations, acne, and sore throats (US Department of Health and Human Services, 1988). The great majority of adolescents have no chronic medical illnesses and must be regarded as very healthy. In a population such as the US, there are about 870 deaths per 100,000 people in the population each year. Among adolescents, there are approximately 27 deaths per 100,000 persons. In other words, the mortality rate for adolescents is about 3% of that for the general population. Further, deaths among adolescents are often not associated with diseases, but rather the result of untimely accidents.

In addition to the problem that the content of many measures may be irrelevant to most health issues in children and adolescents, many of the measurement theories and methods may also be problematic.

Psychometric tradition

In addition to being dependent on the dominant medical model, the creation of new measures has also been driven by psychometric methods. Measures are often evaluated for psychometric properties, such as reliability and validity. Despite the appeal of traditional psychometric evidence, reviewers rarely recognize that some psychometric criteria may not be relevant to the evaluation of health status measures.

Item sampling. One of the basic tenants of psychometric theory is that each item in a test or measure is an unbiased and representative sample from the domain under study. In the construction of an intelligence test, for example, there are an infinite number of items that might represent intellectual ability. The Domain Sampling Model (Nunnally, 1967) assumes that items are sampled from this domain and performance and that each item is assumed to be an unbiased estimate of the underlying trait. Reliability is estimated from the inter-item correlations and the extent to which the items are intercorrelated characterizes the reliability of the measure. Reliable measures are those for which the component items measure the same construct.

Measures of health status may be derived from a very different theoretical model. Items may not be considered random samples from a large domain because each may have a very specific meaning. For example, report of a severe headache offers very specific information. The item is not randomly sampled from all possible symptoms and the meaning of reporting a headache is very different from the meaning of reporting difficulty urinating. Thus, item sampling, as known in psychometric theory, is not necessarily relevant to many health status measures.

A second type of reliability in psychometric theory concerns time sampling. Psychological traits are considered to be stable over the course of time. If Sally is intelligent today, we expect her to be equally intelligent in two weeks. Variation in her performance across the two weeks might be attributable to sampling error. Thus, test-retest estimates are an important source of information.

This same logic may not apply to health status measures. If Sally is very sick today, we may not expect her to be equally sick in two weeks. Differences between health scores taken at two points in time may mean that she recovered from her illness or that she got sicker. When the underlying construct is expected to change over time, test-retest evaluations have very little meaning.

Validity studies. It is common in the evaluation of health status and QL measures to estimate concurrent validity. Most often a QL measure is correlated with a physiological variable, and the QL measure is assumed validated if it corresponds with some aspect of physiology. As attractive as this approach is, the poor validity of many physiological measures is a major justification for measuring QL in the first place.

Given the conceptual and measurement problems described above, alternative approaches to health outcomes assessment should be considered. In the next section, a general health policy model, based on an alternative measurement strategy, will be reviewed.

A general health policy model

Comprehensive models of health status are needed to understand health outcomes. The major aspects of the model include mortality (death) and morbidity (health-related QL). In several papers, we have suggested that diseases and disabilities are important for two reasons. First, illness may cause the life expectancy to be shortened. Second, illness may make life less desirable at times prior to death (diminished health-related QL) (Kaplan, 1993; Kaplan & Anderson, 1996).

Over the last two decades, a group of investigators at the University of California, San Diego, has developed the General Health Policy Model (GHPM). Central to the Model is a general conceptualization of QL. The model separates aspects of health status and life quality into distinct components. These are life expectancy (mortality), functioning and symptoms (morbidity), preference for observed health states (utility), and duration of stay in health states (prognosis).

Mortality. A model of health outcomes necessarily includes a component for mortality. Indeed, many public health statistics focus exclusively on mortality through estimations of crude mortality rates, age-adjusted mortality rates, and infant mortality rates.

Morbidity. Health-related QL is also an important outcome. Most public health indicators are relatively insensitive to variations toward the well end of the continuum. Measures of mortality, to give an extreme example, ignore all variations of morbidity: a person in a coma is considered equivalent to an asymptomatic person at full function. In addition, disability measures often ignore those who are relatively healthy. For example, the RAND Health Insurance Study reported that about 80% of the general populations have no dysfunction. Thus, they would estimate that 80% of the population is well. In studies where symptoms and function are assessed only about 12% of the general population report no symptoms on a particular day (Kaplan et al., 1976). In other words, health symptoms or problems are a very common aspect of the human experience. Some might argue that symptoms are unimportant because they are subjective and unobservable. However, symptoms are highly correlated with the demand for medical services, expenditures on health care, and motivations to alter lifestyles. Thus, we feel that the quantification of symptoms is very important when assessing morbidity. The General Health Policy Model, using the Quality of Well-Being (QWB) scale mentioned later, considers functioning in three areas (mobility, physical activity, and social activity) and symptoms.

Utility (relative importance). Not all outcomes are equally important. For example, a treatment in which 20 of 100 patients die is not equivalent to one in which 20 of 100 patients develop nausea. Given that mortality and the various components of morbidity can be tabulated, it is important to consider their relative importance. A key component of the General Health Policy Model attempts to scale the various health outcomes according to their relative importance. This exercise adds the "quality" dimensions to health status. In the preceding example, the relative importance of dying would be weighted more than developing nausea. The weighting is accomplished by rating all states on a quality continuum ranging from 0 (for dead) to 1.0 (for optimum, asymptomatic functioning). These ratings are typically provided by independent judges who are representative of the general population. Using this system it is possible to express the relative importance of states in relation to the life–death continuum. A point halfway on the scale (0.5) is regarded as halfway between optimum function and death.

Prognosis. Another dimension of health status is the duration of a condition. A headache that lasts one hour is not equivalent to a headache that lasts one month. A cough that lasts three days is not equivalent to a cough that lasts three years. In considering the severity of illness, duration of the problem is central. As basic as this concept is, most contemporary models of health outcome measurement completely disregard the duration component. In the General Health Policy Model, the term prognosis refers to the probability of transition among health states over the course of time. In addition to consideration of duration of problems, the model considers the point at which the problem begins. A person may have no symptoms or dysfunctions currently but may have a high probability of health problems in the future. The prognosis component of the model takes these transitions into consideration. A discount rate is used for future outcomes if the utility of a future outcome is not the same as that of a present outcome. For example, a headache that will begin a year from now may be less of a concern than a headache that will start immediately.

Discount rates for health outcomes are very important in under-standing investments in child health services. Many of these services require current investments in order to obtain a future benefit. For example, preventive programs for children and youth require that we invest money in programs such as sex education, tobacco use prevention, or physical activity. The purpose of these programs is to establish habits that will reduce the chances of future health problems. Thus, current assets are being used to achieve a benefit that might not be obtained for many years. However, expenditure of resources to avoid future problems may divert use of funds from current health problems. Future benefits may be valued lower than current benefits and these differences can be explicitly included in the analysis.

The components of the model can be integrated to express outcomes in terms of quality-adjusted life years (QALYs). A QALY is defined as the equivalent of a completely well year of life, or a year of life free of any symptoms, problems, or health-related disabilities. A principal advantage of the QALY is that it provides a common metric that allows different programs to be directly compared. The quality-adjusted life expectancy is the current life expectancy adjusted for diminished QL associated with dysfunctional states and the duration of stay in each state.

Quality of Well-being Scale (QWB)

The Quality of Well-being scale (QWB) is one of several different approaches for computing the quality-adjusted life years that are required for the GHPM (Kaplan & Anderson, 1996). Using this method children (and adults) are classified according to objective levels of functioning. These levels are represented by scales of mobility, physical activity, and social activity (see Table 4.2). In addition to classification into these observable levels of function, individuals are also classified by their least desirable symptom or problem (see Table 4.3). On any particular day, nearly 80% of the general population is optimally functional. However, fewer than half of the population experience no symptoms. Symptoms or problems may be severe, such as wheezing from asthma, or minor such as having to take medication or adhering to a prescribed diet for health reasons.

The observable states of health and functioning and symptoms describe current status, but may offer little information on quality. In order to map these states onto a preference continuum for the desirability of various conditions, "quality" rating between 0 for death and 1.0 for completely well are obtained from judges. These weights are shown in Tables 4.2 and 4.3. A quality adjusted life year is defined as the equivalent of a completely well year of life, or a year of life free of any symptoms, problems, or health-related disabilities. The well-life expectancy (sometimes called the quality adjusted life expectancy) is the current life expectancy adjusted for diminished QL associated with dysfunctional states and the durations of stay in each state. It is possible

TABLE 4.2 QUALITY OF WELL-BEING/GENERAL HEALTH POLICY MODEL: ELEMENTS AND CALCULATING FORMULAS (FUNCTION SCALES, WITH STEP DEFINITIONS AND CALCULATING WEIGHTS)

STEP NO.	STEP DEFINITION	WEIGHT
	MOBILITY SCALE (MOB)	
5	NO LIMITATIONS FOR HEALTH REASONS	–.000
4	DID NOT DRIVE A CAR, HEALTH RELATED; DID NOT RIDE IN A CAR AS USUAL FOR AGE (YOUNGER THAN 15 YR), HEALTH RELATED, *AND/OR* DID NOT USE PUBLIC TRANSPORTATION, HEALTH RELATED; *OR* HAD OR WOULD HAVE USED MORE HELP THAN USUAL FOR AGE TO USE PUBLIC TRANSPORTATION, HEALTH RELATED	–.062
2	IN HOSPITAL, HEALTH RELATED	–.090
	PHYSICAL ACTIVITY SCALE (PAC)	
4	NO LIMITATIONS FOR HEALTH REASONS	–.000
3	IN WHEELCHAIR, MOVED OR CONTROLLED MOVEMENT OF WHEELCHAIR WITHOUT HELP FROM SOMEONE ELSE; *OR* HAD TROUBLE OR DID NOT TRY TO LIFT, STOOP, BEND OVER, OR USE STAIRS OR INCLINES, HEALTH RELATED; *AND/OR* LIMPED, USED A CANE, CRUTCHES, OR WALKER, HEALTH RELATED; *AND/OR* HAD ANY OTHER PHYSICAL LIMITATION IN WALKING, OR DID NOT TRY TO WALK AS FAR AS OR AS FAST AS OTHERS THE SAME AGE ARE ABLE, HEALTH RELATED	–.060
1	IN WHEELCHAIR, DID NOT MOVE OR CONTROL THE MOVEMENT OF WHEEL-CHAIR WITHOUT HELP FROM SOMEONE ELSE, *OR* IN BED, CHAIR, OR COUCH FOR MOST OR ALL OF THE DAY, HEALTH RELATED	–.077
	SOCIAL ACTIVITY SCALE (SAC)	
5	NO LIMITATIONS FOR HEALTH REASONS	–.000
4	LIMITED IN OTHER (E.G., RECREATIONAL) ROLE ACTIVITY, HEALTH RELATED	–.061
3	LIMITED IN MAJOR (PRIMARY) ROLE ACTIVITY, HEALTH RELATED	–.061
2	PERFORMED NO MAJOR ROLE ACTIVITY, HEALTH RELATED, BUT DID PERFORM SELF-CARE ACTIVITIES	–.061
1	PERFORMED NO MAJOR ROLE ACTIVITY, HEALTH RELATED, *AND* DID NOT PERFORM OR HAD MORE HELP THAN USUAL IN PERFORMANCE OF ONE OR MORE SELF-CARE ACTIVITIES, HEALTH RELATED	–.106

to consider mortality, morbidity, and the preference weights for the various observable states of function.

A mathematical model integrates components of the model to express outcomes in a common measurement unit. Using information on current functioning and duration, it is possible to express the health outcomes in terms of equivalents of well-years of life, or as some have described them, Quality-Adjusted Life Years (QALYs). The model for point in time Quality of Well-being is:

QWB = 1 – (observed mobility × mobility weight)
  – (observed physical activity × physical activity weight)
  – (observed social activity and social activity weight)
  – (observed symptom/problem × symptom/problem weight).

TABLE 4.3 QUALITY OF WELL-BEING/GENERAL HEALTH POLICY MODEL: SYMPTOM/PROBLEM COMPLEXES (CPX) WITH CALCULATING WEIGHTS

CPX NO.CPX DESCRIPTION	WEIGHTS
1 DEATH (NOT ON RESPONDENT'S CARD)	−.727
2 LOSS OF CONSCIOUSNESS SUCH AS SEIZURE (FITS), FAINTING, OR COMA (OUT COLD OR KNOCKED OUT)	−.407
3 BURN OVER LARGE AREAS OF FACE, BODY, ARMS, OR LEGS	−.387
4 PAIN, BLEEDING, ITCHING, OR DISCHARGE (DRAINAGE) FROM SEXUAL ORGANS — DOES NOT INCLUDE NORMAL MENSTRUAL (MONTHLY) BLEEDING	−.349
5 TROUBLE LEARNING, REMEMBERING, OR THINKING CLEARLY	−.340
6 ANY COMBINATION OF ONE OR MORE HANDS, FEET, ARMS, OR LEGS EITHER MISSING, DEFORMED (CROOKED), PARALYZED (UNABLE TO MOVE), OR BROKEN — INCLUDES WEARING ARTIFICIAL LIMBS OR BRACES	−.333
7 PAIN, STIFFNESS, WEAKNESS, NUMBNESS, OR OTHER DISCOMFORT IN CHEST, STOMACH (INCLUDING HERNIA OR RUPTURE), SIDE, NECK, BACK, HIPS, OR ANY JOINTS OR HANDS, FEET, ARMS, OR LEGS	−.299
8 PAIN, BURNING, BLEEDING, ITCHING, OR OTHER DIFFICULTY WITH RECTUM, BOWEL MOVEMENTS, OR URINATION (PASSING WATER)	−.292
9 SICK OR UPSET STOMACH, VOMITING OR LOOSE BOWEL MOVEMENT, WITH OR WITHOUT CHILLS, OR ACHING ALL OVER	−.290
10 GENERAL TIREDNESS, WEAKNESS, OR WEIGHT LOSS	−.259
11 COUGH, WHEEZING, OR SHORTNESS OF BREATH, *WITH* OR *WITHOUT* FEVER, CHILLS, OR ACHING ALL OVER	−.257
12 SPELLS OF FEELING, UPSET, BEING DEPRESSED, OR OF CRYING	−.257
13 HEADACHE, OR DIZZINESS, OR RINGING IN EARS, OR SPELLS OF FEELING HOT, NERVOUS OR SHAKY	−.244
14 BURNING OR ITCHING RASH ON LARGE AREAS OF FACE, BODY, ARMS, OR LEGS	−.240
15 TROUBLE TALKING, SUCH AS LISP, STUTTERING, HOARSENESS, OR BEING UNABLE TO SPEAK	−.237
16 PAIN OR DISCOMFORT IN ONE OR BOTH EYES (SUCH AS BURNING OR ITCH-ING) OR ANY TROUBLE SEEING AFTER CORRECTION	−.230
17 OVERWEIGHT FOR AGE AND HEIGHT OR SKIN DEFECT OF FACE, BODY, ARMS, OR LEGS, SUCH AS SCARS, PIMPLES, WARTS, BRUISES OR CHANGES IN COLOR	−.188
18 PAIN IN EAR, TOOTH, JAW, THROAT, LIPS, TONGUE; SEVERAL MISSING OR CROOKED PERMANENT TEETH — INCLUDES WEARING BRIDGES OR FALSE TEETH; STUFFY, RUNNY NOSE; OR ANY TROUBLE HEARING — INCLUDES WEAR-ING A HEARING AID	−.170
19 TAKING MEDICATION OR STAYING ON A PRESCRIBED DIET FOR HEALTH REASONS	−.144
20 WORE EYEGLASSES OR CONTACT LENSES	−.101
21 BREATHING SMOG OR UNPLEASANT AIR	−.101
22 NO SYMPTOMS OR PROBLEM (NOT ON RESPONDENT'S CARD)	−.000
23 STANDARD SYMPTOM/PROBLEM	−.257
X24 TROUBLE SLEEPING	−.257
X25 INTOXICATION	−.257
X26 PROBLEMS WITH SEXUAL INTEREST OR PERFORMANCE	−.257
X27 EXCESSIVE WORRY OR ANXIETY	−.257

The net cost/utility ratio is defined as

$$\frac{\text{net cost}}{\text{net QWB} \times \text{duration in years}} = \frac{\text{cost of treatment} - \text{cost of alternative}}{[\text{QWB}_2 - \text{QWB}_1] \times \text{duration in years}},$$

where QWB_2 and QWB_1 are measures of quality of well-being taken after and before treatment. The model quantifies the health activity or treatment program in terms of the quality adjusted life years that it produces or saves.

Consider, for example, a child who has rare metabolic disease who is in a state of wellness that is rated by community peers as 0.5 on the 0 to 1.0 utility scale. If the child remains in that state for one year, he or she would have lost the equivalent of 1/2 of one year of life. However, a child who has a respiratory infection might also be rated as 0.50. In this case, the illness might only last three days and the total loss in QALYs might be $3/365 \times 0.50$ which is equal to 0.004 QALYs. By itself it is clear that the respiratory infection does not produce as significant a health outcome as the rare metabolic disease. But suppose that 5,000 children in a community get bad respiratory infections. The QALYs lost would then be $5,000 \times 0.004$ which is equal to 20 years. The loss to the community is greater than the one person with the severe rare metabolic disease. This indicates that the common respiratory infection may be a greater health policy problem than the rare disease.

Now suppose that a vaccination becomes available and that the threat of the respiratory infection can be eliminated by vaccinating the 35,000 people in the community. The cost of the vaccine is $5.00 per person or $175,000. The average cost/utility of the program would be $8,750/QALY.

Further, suppose that treatment of the metabolic condition costs $10,000 and produces .20 QALYs for one person. Thus, the cost/utility for treatment of the metabolic condition would be $10,000/.20 = $50,000/QALY. In other words, the cost to produce a QALY would be higher for treatment of the metabolic condition than it would be for the community vaccination program. On the other hand, given the cost utility of other programs, it is likely that both programs would be deemed worthy of support. Typically, programs are regarded as a good investment if they produce a QALY for less than $100,000.

The QWB has been used in a wide variety of population studies (Anderson, et al., 1989; Erickson, et al., 1989). In addition, the methods have been used in clinical trials and studies to evaluate therapeutic interventions in a wide range of medical and surgical conditions. These include chronic obstructive pulmonary disease (Kaplan et al., 1984), AIDS (Kaplan, et al., 1995), cystic fibrosis (Ornstein, et al., 1989), diabetes mellitus (Kaplan, et al., 1987), atrial fibrillation (Ganiats, et al., 1993), lung transplantation (Squier, et al., 1994), arthritis

(Bombardier et al., 1986: Kaplan, et al., 1992), cancer (Kaplan, 1993c), Alzheimer's disease (Kerner et al., 1998), sinus disease (Hodgkin, 1994) and a wide variety of other conditions (Kaplan, 1993b). Further, the method has been used for health resource allocation modeling and has served as the basis for an innovative experiment on rationing of health care by the state of Oregon.

The General Health Policy Model and the QWB have been used in several studies of children. One example of validity evidence of the QWB in a child population concerns cystic fibrosis (CF), a serious genetic disease with a prevalence of 1 in 2,000 live births. Clinical studies of CF typically use pulmonary function tests, chest roentgenograms, and clinical judgment to assess treatment effectiveness. Although pulmonary function testing and exercise evaluations provide objective physiologic measures of disease severity, they may not be sensitive to important aspects of disease progression and treatment effects. During acute exacerbations of pulmonary infection, CF patients are commonly treated with potent intravenous antibiotics. Although these improve pulmonary function, they may have undesirable side effects, in some cases causing irreversible deafness or renal dysfunction.

Thus, although measures of outcome in terms of pulmonary function may show improvement in that clinical domain, an overall measure of well-being should consider both the benefits and consequences of the powerful treatments. Furthermore, many of the important consequences of CF may be overlooked with traditional measures and pulmonary function tests. These include upset stomachs, headaches, chest pain, bone and joint pain, coughing, and shortness of breath. Considering the goals of extending life and improving quality of life, a general health status measure seems quite appropriate for studies of CF patients.

In preparation for a clinical trial evaluating exercise treatments for CF patients, Orenstein and his colleagues (1989) completed a QWB validity study for a group of CF patients. They administered the QWB to 44 child and adolescent CF patients (19 female, 25 male). Pulmonary function was measured using standard spirometric methods.

There were highly significant correlations between QWB scores and representative tests of pulmonary function: forced expired volume in one second (FEV_1) ($r = .55$, $p < .0001$) and maximal midexpiratory flow rate (MMEFR) ($r = .48$, $p < .001$). The QWB also was administered to 15 patients who performed progressive exercise tests; their scores were plotted against one representative test of exercise tolerance (peak oxygen consumption, VO_2 max). Again, there was a significant association between QWB and VO_2max ($r = .57$, $p < .01$). The associations appeared to be equally strong for CF patients across different age groups. However, the correlation was not perfect ($r < 1.0$), indicating that QWB captures aspects of life quality in addition to pulmonary function. Pulmonary function and exercise testing do provide objective measures of disease severity and progression. However, they may not be sensitive to many other important aspects of the disease and within the same level of pulmonary function, patients may show considerable variability in their daily activities (Orenstein et al., 1989, Kaplan & Anderson, 1996).

In the next section some of the conceptual issues will be reviewed. In particular, we review how the model stimulates different thinking about health policies for children and adolescents. Particular attention is devoted to programs in disease prevention.

NON DISEASE OUTCOMES

There are many reasons why measurement strategies that are useful for characterizing adult health status, may not be valuable for studies of children and adolescents. Many threats to adolescent health status are not diseases. Instead, they are high risk behaviors and bad behavioral choices. More than 75% of all deaths for individuals between 10 and 20 years of age are caused by unintentional injuries, homicides, and suicides. In contrast to threats from bacteria, viruses, or genetic diseases, the real threats to teenagers are guns, cigarettes, and other illegal substances.

Resnick and colleagues (1997) reported results from the U.S. National Longitudinal Study of Adolescent Health. The results were a cross-sectional analysis of 12,118 adolescents in grades 7–12 from a representative sample of students in the United States. The results confirmed the remarkably high rate of high risk behaviors among children and adolescents. More than 10% of the female and 7.5% of the males have considered suicide in the last year. Approximately 5% of the females and 2% of the males had attempted suicide. Pregnancy history was common with 11.8% of the seventh and eighth graders and 19.4% of the ninth through twelfth graders having experienced at least one pregnancy. About half of the ninth through twelfth grade students were sexually active. About a quarter of the students reported having been a victim of violence and 12.4% had admitted carrying a weapon within the last 30 days.

In the following sections several examples will be used to illustrate why the outcomes model may lead to different policy decisions than the traditional biomedical model. The first example considers a medical decison about screening for a disease — cystic fibrosis. The second example is about using community interventions to reduce diseases associated with cigarette smoking. The third example goes outside the traditional medical model to prevent loss of QALYs by reducing injuries. The examples are connected through the use of QALYs and outcomes thinking for the analysis. In all of these cases, it would be difficult to conceptualize the benefits of these public health programs using traditional QL outcome measures.

SCREENING FOR CYSTIC FIBROSIS

Cystic fibrosis (CF) is the most common genetic childhood disease in Caucasians for which a clear genetic linkage has been established (Welsh et al., 1995). Although life expectancies for CF children have been improving, there is no cure for CF and treatment remains burdensome and expensive. Because there is no cure, prevention through genetic screening must be explored as a policy option.

Most studies on QL in CF focus on the current impact of the disease. However, this disease might be preventable and current measures can not quantify the potential benefit of preventing the disease. The gene associated with CF has been identified (CFTR). The cloning of the CFTR gene created the possibility of preventing CF by averting the birth of affected children. It remains to be determined whether population screening for CF carriers will be valuable. Screening has been limited because of provider resistance, patient anxiety, and the resistance to invest resources to test a large number of women in order prevent a small number of affected children. Screening for genetic diseases may yield a substantial number of false positive results that may create unnecessary anxiety. Screening also raises the difficult issue of pregnancy termination when affected fetuses are identified.

The cloning of the CFTR gene has made population carrier screening possible. Three features of CF screening have raised serious concerns: 1) the very large number of potential testees, 2) the imperfect sensitivity of the test, and 3) the significant cost of the test.

Systematic policy analysis can be used to weigh the benefits of these programs against their costs. One study in Rochester, New York (Loader et al., 1996), attempted to offer screening to all pregnant women and assessed what proportion physicians actually offer screening to pregnant women. If the providers agreed to screen their patients, they were offered free testing to all their female patients of reproductive age, 18 years or over, and free counseling of all carriers. If a patient was found to be a carrier, she was invited to participate in an evaluation of CF carrier screening. At the time of counseling, the manifestations, inheritance, and treatment of CF and the patient's options were presented, the patient's questions answered, and the patient offered carrier testing for the father of the fetus.

If the partner was tested and found negative, the patient was informed that the residual probability of having a child with CF in any given pregnancy was about one in 666. If the partner tested positive, the couple was invited for a more detailed description of the clinical manifestations and management of CF and offered prenatal diagnosis. Of the 4879 women tested, 124 were found to be CF carriers. Of the 124, 106 partners (85%) were tested. In five of the 106 couples the partner was also shown to be a carrier, and prenatal diagnosis was chosen by four of these five. At least three of the four couples having prenatal diagnosis said they would terminate if the fetus were affected, but none of the fetuses proved to be affected. Ninety percent of the 4879 women tested were pregnant. Providers typically did not find offering testing to nonpregnant women to be important. Among pregnant women, only 57% of those offered the test actually completed it.

When analyzed to estimate the cost to produce a QALY, screening produced a QALY for about $12,175. This compared very favorably with widely used medical procedures. For example, total hip replacement costs about $293,029 per QALY (Liang, 1987), while screening mammography costs about 10 times as much as screening for CF (Eddy, 1990). On the other hand, some services, such as pneumococcal vaccine for the elderly produce a QALY at about one-eighth the cost of CF screening. Among the total mix of programs, screening seems to be a reasonable option (Rowley et al., 1998).

The analysis is based on several assumptions. Although the cost/utility model incorporates parental anxiety and a variety of other QL factors, the estimates of cost to produce a QALY depended on assumptions about replacement pregnancy. If we assume that a family loses life years by terminating a pregnancy, then the program causes a loss of life years and would not be advised because the use of resources would result in a net loss of family QALYs. However, if the pregnancy was replaced, the program would produce QALYs and appear to be very cost effective. The curative medical model would simply advocate screening and treatment of all women because that is the best way to eradicate disease. The outcomes model requires difficult philosophical assumptions. These philosophical assumptions can have very important implications for the interpretation of the analysis.

Perhaps the most complex issue is in accounting for the aborted fetus. The results of our analysis are very sensitive to assumptions about the replacement of a pregnancy. Typically, cost/utility analysis begins at birth. Thus, therapeutic abortion is not associated with either gains or losses in life years. Once a child is born, years of life accrue. A child with cystic fibrosis would have fewer Quality-Adjusted Life Years than a well child. In the analysis above, it was assumed that an aborted child would be replaced and the appropriate comparison would be an unaffected child.

An alternative scheme begins accounting at conception, or at the time a fetus is physiologically viable. Thus, an aborted fetus could accrue the number of Quality-Adjusted Life Years equal to the total life expectancy (Ganiats, 1996). Similarly, the estimate of the family life years would be those of the parents, less those that would have accrued to the aborted fetus. Another way to do the analysis is "without replacement". Considering the small number of terminated pregnancies, the replacement variable had only a small effect on average live years per family, but did swing the conclusion away from screening if there would be no replacement and toward screening if replacement was assumed. The outcomes model requires that these difficult issues be made explicit and that they become a component of the analysis.

There is some inconsistency in the literature with regard to accounting for costs of a terminated pregnancy. Ganiats (1996) reviewed the 41 English-language papers that appeared in Medline between 1986 and 1993 under the terms amniocentesis, cost, and QL. The dominant methodology was to value impact on patients without attempting to consider life lost for the aborted fetus. The difficulty is that the analyses often account for medical savings that are prevented through pregnancy termination without considering any potential benefits that would accrue if the pregnancy were completed.

These issues are challenging and relate to valuation of life and its quality. However, these issues are ignored by most approaches to measurement because most measures consider only current health and do not incorporate a full life perspective. The outcomes model and the traditional biomedical model might lead to different conclusions about the value of screening for CF. While the traditional model favors screening, the recommendations based on the outcomes model depend on some difficult assumptions about QL and about the appropriateness of assuming that pregnancies can be replaced.

SMOKING

Cigarette smoking remains the greatest single cause of preventable deaths in contemporary society. The health consequences of tobacco use have been documented in thousands of studies. Although cigarette smoking has declined in the United States and the United Kingdom within recent years, the worldwide trend is towards increased use of tobacco products. Peto and colleagues (Peto et al., 1992) project that world wide there will be 10 million tobacco related deaths per year by the Year 2010. Current estimates suggest that tobacco use in the US is responsible for 434,000 deaths each year (McGinnis & Foege, 1993). Smoking is a major factor in poor pregnancy outcomes. Estimates suggest that 17 to 26% of low birthweight deliveries are associated with maternal tobacco use and that 5 to 6% of prenatal deaths can be attributed to maternal tobacco use (USDHHS, 1988, 1989, 1990). Deaths associated with tobacco use account for over 20 times the number associated with drug use, 16 times the number associated with auto crashes, and 15 times the number of homicides (McGinnis & Foege, 1993).

Virtually, all smokers initiate the habit during youth. Estimates suggest that approximately 3,000 young people in the US start smoking each day (Pierce, 1991). The number of adults who are age 20 years or older who begin smoking has declined in recent years (Lee et al., 1993). Initiation of tobacco use during adulthood is rare: more than 90% of all smokers started when they were children or teenagers (Gilpin, Lee, Evans, & Pierce, 1994).

The tobacco industry has agreed not to market tobacco to youth. Thus, most countries have a legal age for cigarette purchase and these policies have been in effect throughout the twentieth century. Nevertheless, studies repeatedly demonstrate that children and teenagers can easily obtain cigarettes (Centers for Disease Control, 1990).

The importance of the cigarette smoking problem is summarized in recent data reported by McGinnis and Foege (1993). There are approximately 2,150,000 deaths in the United States each year. Deaths are accounted for according to major and underlying cause. The traditional biomedical model emphasizes disease-specific causes of death, and pathways to prevention typically consider risk factors for particular diseases. For example, cigarette smoking is associated with deaths from cancer of the lung. Thus, efforts to reduce lung cancer concentrate on smoking cessation. However, most of the major causes of death are associated with a variety of different risk factors. Further, many risk factors are associated with death from a variety of different causes. For example, tobacco use causes not only lung cancer, but a wide variety of other malignancies, heart disease, stroke, and birth complications (Kaplan et al., 1995).

There are several approaches to the reduction of cigarette smoking available to policymakers, and in current use in varying degrees and combinations by the federal government, several states and local governments. Among these policy tools are mass media education campaigns, bans on cigarette advertising, school programs, quitting assistance, localized grass-roots interventions, and the imposition of excise taxes on cigarettes. Economists argue that, by increasing the price of cigarettes, the imposition of excise taxes is one of the most effective ways to control cigarette use (Lewit, Coate, & Grossman, 1981; Hu, Sung, & Keeler, 1995; Chaloupka & Grossman, 1996).

Employing a series of different assumptions to estimate the impact of increasing the tobacco tax, it is possible to estimate the effects of tobacco tax policies. We assumed an elasticity (a change in the percentage demand divided by the change in the percentage price) of –.26, a very conservative estimate. The assumption used here suggests, for example, that if there is a 20% increase in price, there will be approximately a 5% decrease in demand. The –.26 value was taken from the low estimates among published studies. The estimates of price elasticity for smokers of all ages as reported in the US Surgeon General's report in 1989 was –.47 (p. 537). Other estimates for the sensitivity analysis are based on three studies by Lewit and Coate (1983) and are consistent with other estimates (Hu et al., 1991).

In one analysis that used Monte Carlo simulation, we assumed that there are about 56 million smokers in the US and that one in four of these smokers will eventually die of a tobacco related disease, and a tax increase of 20% (considerably less than that proposed). Using a computer to generate data under various assumptions, this analysis considers the expected change in life expectancy for smokers and builds in a model of reduced health-related QL for smokers beginning at age 50. These methods combine death and reduced life quality into a single Quality-Adjusted Life Year (QALY) index. A death premature by one year is represented by the loss of one QALY. A year of life in which quality is reduced by one-half because of a disease, is represented by the loss of 0.50 QALYs. The QL has not been included in most previous studies. QL is included because the tobacco users experience loss of everyday functioning and devastating symptoms before their premature

deaths. The prevalences rate for reduced life expectancy and dysfunction are based on estimates from the US National Health Interview
Survey. According to the analysis, there is a 50% chance that we could
save 6.4 million Quality-Adjusted Life Years in the US by increasing
tobacco taxes by 20%. The model shows that there is a 90% chance of
saving about three million Quality-Adjusted Life Years. To put these
figures into perspective, the total annual health effect of arthritis is
estimated to cost society 5 million Quality-Adjusted Life Years, while
the impact of homicide is about 1.5 million years. In other words, the
public health benefits of an increased tobacco tax may well exceed the
benefit of having a whole year without arthritis or of eliminating our
epidemic of homicide for one year. We know of no other health services
that can improve the public health to the extent estimated to be
attributable to an increased tobacco tax (Kaplan, 1993b).

Overall, the analysis suggests that there is a public health advantage
to raising tobacco taxes and that, even under the most conservative
assumptions, the model appears to support the advantages of tobacco
taxes in relation to the traditional medical programs. Similar conclusions have been reached by several authors and have been summarized
by Warner (1986). However, these analyses are very preliminary. There
is considerable uncertainty about many different pieces in the model.
For example, the elasticity estimates may not be accurate. Further, there
is uncertainty about some of the relationships between consumption
and disease. Finally, previous experience with the model comes
primarily from the white or general population.

INJURY PREVENTION

Experts make the distinction between accidents and unintentional
injuries. The word accident implies that there is a random event over
which we have no control. The alternative term, unintentional injury,
distinguishes carelessness from intentional injuries such as assault and
murder. Although injuries may be unintentional, they might be
preventable.

Young children are rarely prepared to protect themselves from
hazardous environments. As a result, there are substantial numbers of
unintentional poisonings, falls, and assaults resulting in significant loss
of Quality-Adjusted Life Years. Older children may place themselves at
risk for injury through risky behaviors such as climbing, in-line skating,
or skateboarding. They might also expose themselves to excessive
injuries by failing to take precautions like wearing a helmet while

participating in these activities. Teenagers often expose themselves to greater risk by using drugs or alcohol.

The disease model emphasizes the use of resources to combat diagnosed pathologies. When figures for deaths from cancer, heart disease, and unintentional injuries are depicted as a function of age, unintentional injuries appear to be the leading cause of death for individuals prior to age 45. For adolescents and young adults, deaths from injury are significantly more common than deaths from cancer and heart disease (Committee on Trauma Research, 1985).

A variety of policy changes may be effective in reducing morbidity and mortality from unintentional injuries. For example, countries differ in standards used to regulate child labor. In the United States, for example, there is strict federal regulation that protects child laborers who are under 14 years of age and work in non-agricultural industries. On the other hand, children can work in agricultural production without protection of these same laws. Children can be employed in agricultural production when they are as young as 10 years of age. Work on family farms is often completely unregulated. The US Department of Labor Statistics reported 114 agricultural work-related deaths for youths 16–19 years of age during the interval 1992–1996 (Rivara & Grossman, 1997). Other evidence suggests that each year nearly 100,000 children in the United States suffer non-fatal injuries associated with agricultural production (Rivara, 1997). With the development of age-appropriate guidelines for work protection, it may be possible to substantially reduce deaths and injury among young children. These prevention strategies might include combinations of education and policy change. For example, extension of child labor protection laws from non-agricultural to agricultural sectors may result in significant reductions in childhood injuries. However, since many injuries occur on family farms, achieving these changes may be difficult.

Other legislative changes have been shown to be successful. For example, when motorcycle riders are required by law to wear helmets and the law is strictly enforced, more than 90% of riders wear the helmets and there are decreases in morbidity and mortality. However, these laws are not universally enforced in different communities. Areas with poor enforcement also have higher rates of head trauma (Waller, 1986). There is some evidence that community-wide intervention may prevent injuries in children. For example, in the late 1980s, the community of Seattle, Washington experienced approximately 400,000 emergency room visits due to bicycle crashes in children and adolescents. Many of these involved serious head injuries. While it is well known that helmets reduce brain injuries by 85%, only about 2–3% of children were wearing helmets. Community-wide media campaigns significantly increased the use of helmets (Bergman et al., 1990). Later analyses in the same community showed that nearly half of all riders wore a helmet at the time of the crash (Rivara, Thompson, & Thompson, 1997). The pay-off in terms of reduced mortality and morbidity seems likely, but has yet to be firmly established (Rivara et al., 1997), in part because helmets are not used properly (Ching, Thompson, Thompson, Thomas, Chilcott, & Rivara, 1997).

In the United States, the most challenging problem involves injury from firearms. Handgun violence is associated with 40,000 deaths and 240,000 injuries each year in the United States. The annual costs exceed $14 billion and 80% of these charges are paid for by tax payers (Wintemute, 1994).

Firearm homicides in the US among adolescent males tripled between 1985 and 1993 (Wintemute, 1994). There were 99,025 non-fatal firearm related injuries during the period from June 1, 1992 through May 31, 1993. The age category 15–24 has disproportionate injuries and deaths associated with firearm use. Further, there are strong differences by racial and ethnic groups. African-Americans, for example, are about three times as likely as non-Hispanic Caucasians to be killed using a firearm. However, African-Americans are more than nine times as likely to be injured by a firearm (Annest et al., 1995). If current trends continue, we could expect 350,000 firearms deaths in the United States by the year 2000. Depending on the assumptions, it would be anticipated that, in addition to those who are killed, between 1 and 2 million individuals would sustain non-fatal injuries.

It has been popular to argue that increases in violence can be attributed to violence portrayed on television. However, experimental studies on TV violence do not provide a firm foundation for these attributions (Kaplan & Singer, 1976). It is informative to compare US homicide rates to countries that have similar television consumption patterns. In Australia, for example, where children are exposed to a steady diet of violent American television, there were only 13 homicides caused by handguns in 1992. In the United Kingdom, there were 33 handgun associated fatalities despite relative common exposure to television violence. In the United States, however, there were 13,220 handgun related fatalities. In Canada there are significantly fewer guns, but television and culture are similar to the US. Yet the Canadian homicide rate is only a fraction of what it is in the US (Centerwall, 1991). The difference may be attributable to the availability of handguns, not the availability of television sets.

Firearm related injuries are expensive. In one study, the mean hospital charge per firearm related hospital admission was $52,271. Using the figure of 240,000 injuries per year, the estimated costs are about $12.5 billion. Since the majority of victims are uninsured, hospitals need to recover the costs for caring for injury patients from other sources. In particular, costs are shifted from patients admitted to the hospital for other reasons (Kizer et al., 1995).

In summary, firearm related violence is clearly a public health problem affecting adolescents. Thus, a comprehensive health policy for adolescents should include some approach to violence control.

Several years ago, violence was declared a public health emergency in the United States (Koop & Lumberg, 1992). To a large extent, violence is everyone's problem. The billions of dollars of uncompensated care for firearm related injury victims are shifted to insured patients. Thus, at a certain level, the costs are shared by the entire population. Several public policy proposals have been offered. The simplest proposals are recommendations to limit the availability of guns (Adler et al., 1994; Mock et al., 1994). The difficulty with these proposals is that the number of hand guns available is overwhelming. For example, some evidence suggests that nearly half of all American households maintain one or more firearms (US Bureau of Justice Statistics, 1994). Although, many gun owners report that they keep guns for this purpose, systematic studies show that firearms are rarely used to protect from invading criminals. Other steps, such as measures to make it more difficult to invade a home may offer better protection (Kellermann et al., 1995).

Although a total ban on handguns is unlikely, aggressive programs to restrict sales and to remove other weapons are worthy of consideration as public health options. Several experiences have demonstrated that people are willing to turn in guns if they are paid. One proposal involves offering a substantial cash fee of $1,000 for the return of any handgun — no questions asked. Such a program might serve as an incentive for criminals to steal guns from one another in order to retrieve the award. The cost of the program to retrieve 100 million guns would be 100 million × $1,000 equals $100 billion (plus administrative costs). In other words, costs would be equivalent to about one-tenth of what the US spends annually on health care. Of course, not all 100 million guns could be purchased, and it would be optimistic to say that half would be returned. Under that assumption, the cost of the program would be $50 billion.

Dividing the costs of the program by the number of years it produces gives a cost/utility ratio. The health benefits from the program would be substantial. Totally eliminating homicide is approximately 2 million life years and reducing mortality by 50% would produce about one million life years. A rough estimate of the quality-adjusted life years produced by reducing non-fatal injuries would produce 3 to 6 million life years. Assuming a total health benefit of about 5 million life years suggests that the program would be relatively expensive in comparison to other health programs. It would cost about $25 million to produce each life year. However, the costs occur in the first year and the benefits would be repeated every year. In other words, over time the total health benefits would multiply and the costs would not (Kaplan, 1984).

Other benefits of the program are not considered in this analysis. For example, most adults experience some reduction in QL because they are afraid of being victimized (Department of Justice, 1994). If reduced fear and anxiety improved QL by 1% for 250 million American citizens, there would be a public health benefit of about 2.5 million Quality-Adjusted Life Years at a cost of about $100 billion. The cost/utility ratio would be about $40,000 to produce a Quality-Adjusted Life Year. This is clearly within the range of other public health programs that are commonly supported. It is likely that the program would be less expensive because not all gun owners would participate. On the other hand the program would also produce benefits in terms of savings on medical care costs. If it saved half of the current amount spent, that would reduce the total costs by about $6 to 7 billion the first year. Over time, the cost/effectiveness of the program would improve because the benefits would accrue each year while the costs would be only in the initial year.

We recognize that these analyses are highly speculative. Since implementation would require a total ban on all new gun sales and strict penalties for gun possession, it may not be politically feasible. However, these rough analyses do help place the problem in perspective.

SUMMARY AND CONCLUSIONS

This book is about QL measures for children and adolescents. The predominant trend has been to apply psychometric methods to the development of disease and age specific measures. This work represents the dominant psychometric and medical models. Despite remarkable achievements in child health status measurement, contemporary approaches fail to capture the issues in maintaining population health status. Considerable effort in child health care is devoted to preventive efforts. In order to quantify the impact of these programs, it is necessary to apply different conceptual models. These models are usually not disease specific and may recognize expected changes in health over the course of time.

Disease specific measures arise from a traditional biomedical model that is centered on disease pathology. With disease specific and multiple dimension measures, we may neglect the most important threats to population health status. Improvements in population health status might result from preventing poor health outcomes among people who are currently well. The greatest threats to population health status include unintentional injuries, suicides, and the acquisition of the risky habits of substance abuse or unprotected sex. Quantifying these issues requires a model that combines morbidity and mortality, includes the expected trajectory of wellness over the life span, and offers a summary index. These approaches are controversial, and the methodologies are not well worked out. However, the conceptual models may be valuable for identifying ways to maximize population health status.

References

Adler, K.P., Barondess, J.A., Cohen, J.J., Farber, S.J., Foreman, S., Gambuti, G., Hamburg, M., Kase, N.G., Messite, J., & Michels, R. (1994). Firearm violence and public health. Limiting the availability of guns. *JAMA, 71,* 1281–1283.

Anderson, J.P., Kaplan, R.M., & DeBon, M. (1989). Comparison of responses to similar questions in health surveys. In F. Fowler (Ed.), *Health survey research methods* (pp. 13–21). Washington, DC: National Center For Health Statistics.

Annest J.L., Mercy, J.A., Gibson, D.R., & Ryan, G.W. (1995). National estimates of nonfatal firearm-related injuries — beyond the tip of the iceberg. *JAMA, 273,* 1749–1754.

Bergman, A.B., Rivara, F.P., Richards, D.D., & Rogers, L.W. (1990). The Seattle children's bicycle helmet campaign. *American Journal of Diseases in Children, 144,* 727–731.

Bolande, R.P. (1969). Ritualistic surgery: Circumcision and tonsillectomy. *New England Journal of Medicine, 280,* 591.

Bombardier, C., Ware, J., Russell, I.J., et al. (1986). Auranofin therapy and Quality of Life for patients with rheumatoid arthritis: Results of a multicenter trial. *American Journal of Medicine, 81,* 565–578.

Bruil, J., Maes, S., Coq, J., & Boeke, J. (1997). The development of the How Are You? (HAY), A Quality of Life questionnaire for children with a chronic illness. *MAPI Quality of Life Newsletter Sept–Dec 1997,* 9.

Bullinger, M., & Ravens-Sieberer, U. (1995). Grundlagen, Methoden und Anwendungsgebiete der Lebensqualitätsforschung bei Kindern [General principles, methods and areas of application of Quality of Life research in children]. *Praxis der Kinderpsychologie und Kinderpsychiatrie, 44,* 391–399.

Bureau of Justice Statistics (1994). *National Crime Victimization Survey Redesign.* Washington, DC: US Department of Justice, BJS Clearinghouse.

Centers for Disease Control and Prevention. (1994). Deaths resulting from firearm and motor-vehicle-related injuries: United States, 1968–1991. *Morbidity, Mortality Weekly Report, 43,* 37–41.

Centerwall, B.S. (1991). Homicide and the prevalence of handguns — Canada and the United States, 1976 to 1980. *American Journal of Epidemiology, 134,* 1245–1260.

Centerwall, B.S. (1995). Race, socioeconomic status, and domestic homicide. *JAMA, 127,* 1755–1758.

Chaloupka, F.J., & Grossman, M. (1996). *Price, tobacco control policies, and youth smoking.* Working Paper 5740, National Bureau of Economic Research.

Ching, R.P., Thompson, D.C., Thompson, R.S., Thomas, D.J., Chilcott, W.C., & Rivara, F.P. (1997). Damage to bicycle helmets involved with crashes. *Accident Analysis and Prevention, 29,* 555–562.

Committee on Trauma Research. (1985). *Injury in America: A continuing public health problem.* Washington, DC: National Academy Press.

Drotar, D. (1997). Relating parent and family functioning to the psychological adjustment of children with chronic health conditions: What have we learned? What do we need to know? *Journal of Pediatric Psychology, 22,* 149–165.

Eddy D.M. (1989). Screening for breast cancer. *Annals of Internal Medicine, 111,* 389–99.

Eddy, D.M. (1997). Balancing cost and quality in fee-for-service versus managed care. *Health Affairs, 16,* 162–173.

Erickson, P., Kendall, E.A., Anderson, J.P., & Kaplan, R.M. (1989). Using composite health status measures to assess the nation's health. *Medical Care, 27* (Suppl 3), S66–S76.

Fox, E. (1997). Predominance of the curative model of medical care: A residual problem. *JAMA, 278,* 761–763.

Ganiats, T.G. (1996). Justifying prenatal screening and genetic amniocentesis programs by cost-effectiveness analyses: A re-evaluation. *Medical Decision Making, 16,* 45–50.

Ganiats, T.G., Palinkas, L.A., & Kaplan, R.M. (1992). Comparison of Quality of Well-being scale and functional status index in patients with atrial fibrillation. *Medical Care, 30,* 958–964.

Gilpin, E.A., Lee, L., Evans, N., & Pierce, J.P. (1994). Smoking initiation rates in adults and minors: United States, 1944–1988. *American Journal of Epidemiology, 140,* 535–543.

Hodgkin, P.S. (1994). Health impact of endoscopic sinus surgery assessed by the Quality of Well-being (QWB) Scale. Unpublished paper, University of California, San Diego.

Hu, T.W., Sung, H.Y., & Keeler, T.E. (1995). Reducing cigarette consumption in California: Tobacco taxes vs an anti-smoking media campaign. *American Journal Public Health, 85,* 1218–1222.

Kaplan, R.M. (1984). The measurement of human aggression. In R.M. Kaplan, V.J. Konecni, & R.W. Novaco (Eds.), *Aggression in children and youth* (pp. 44–72). The Hague, Netherlands: Martinus Nijhoff International.

Kaplan, R.M. (1990). Behavior as the central outcome in health care. *American Psychologist, 45,* 1211–1220.

Kaplan, R.M. (1993a). Quality of Life assessment for cost/utility studies in cancer. *Cancer Treatment Reviews, 19* (Suppl A), 85–96.

Kaplan, R.M. (1993b). Application of a general health policy model in the American health care crisis. *Journal of the Royal Society of Medicine, 86,* 277–281.

Kaplan, R.M. (1993c). *Hippocratic predicament: Affordability, access, and accountability in health care.* San Diego, CA: Academic Press.

Kaplan, R.M. (1994). An outcomes-based model for directing decisions in women's health care. *Clinical Obstetrics and Gynecology, 37,* 192–206.

Kaplan, R.M. (1996). Measuring health outcome for resource allocation. In R.L. Glueckauf, R. Frank, G.R. Bond, & J.H. McGrew (Eds.), *Psychological practice in a changing health care system: Issues and new directions* (pp. 101–133). New York, NY: Springer.

Kaplan, R.M. (1997a). Decisions about prostate cancer screening in managed care. *Current Opinion in Oncology, 9,* 480–486.

Kaplan, R.M. (1997b). Implications of Quality of Life assessment in public policy for child and adolescent health. In D. Drotar (Ed.), *Assessing pediatric health-related quality of life and functional status: Implications for research, practice, and policy.* Mahwah, NJ: Lawrence Erlbaum.

Kaplan, R.M., & Anderson, J.P. (1996). The general health policy model: An integrated approach. In B. Spilker (Ed.), *Quality of life and pharmacoeconomics in clinical trials* (pp. 309–322). New York, NY: Raven.

Kaplan, R.M., Anderson, J.P., Patterson, T.L., McCutchan, J.A., Weinrich, J.D., Heaton, R.H., Atkinson, J.H., Thal, L., Chandler, J., & Grant, I. (1995). Validity of the Quality of Well-being Scale for persons with HIV infection. *Psychosomatic Medicine, 57,* 138–157.

Kaplan, R.M., Atkins, C.J., & Timms, R. (1984). Validity of a quality of well-being scale as an outcome measure in chronic obstructive pulmonary disease. *Journal of Chronic Diseases, 37,* 85–95.

Kaplan, R.M., Bush, J.W., & Berry, C.C. (1976). Health status: Types of validity and the index of well-being. *Health Services Research, 11,* 478–507.

Kaplan, R.M., Coons, S.J., & Anderson, J.P. (1992). Quality of Life and policy analysis in arthritis. *Arthritis Care and Research, 5,* 173–183.

Kaplan, R.M., Hartwell, S.L., Wilson, D.K., & Wallace, J.P. (1987). Effects of diet and exercise interventions on control and Quality of Life in non-insulin-dependent diabetes mellitus. *Journal of General Internal Medicine, 2,* 220–228 (republished in *Diabetes Spectrum,* 1989, *2(1),* 20–25).

Kaplan, R.M., Orleans, C.T, Perkins, K.A., & Pierce, J.P. (1995). Marshaling the evidence for greater regulation and control of tobacco products: A call for action. *Annals of Behavioral Medicine, 17,* 3–14.

Kaplan, R.M., & Singer, R.D. (1976). Television violence and viewer aggression: A reexamination of the evidence. *Journal of Social Issues, 34,* 35–70.

Keeler, T.E., Hu, T.W., Barnett, P.G., Manning, W.G., & Sung, H.Y. (1996). Do cigarette producers price-discriminate by state? An empirical analysis of local cigarette pricing and taxation. *Journal of Health Economics, 15,* 499–512.

Kellermann, A.L., Westphal, L., Fischer, L., & Harvard, B. (1995). Weapon involvement in home invasion crimes. *JAMA, 273,* 1759–1762.

Kerner, D.N., Patterson, T.L., Grant, I., & Kaplan, R.M. (1998). Validity of the Quality of Well-being scale for patients with Alzheimer's Disease. *Journal of Aging and Health, 10,* 44–61.

Kizer, K.W., Vassar, M.J., Harry, R.L., & Layton, K.D. (1995). Hospitalization charges, costs and income for firearm-related injuries at a university trauma center. *JAMA, 273,* 1768–1773.

Koop, C.E. & Lundberg, G.B. (1992). Violence in America: A public health emergency. Time to bite the bullet. *JAMA, 267,* 3075–3076.

Lee, L.L., Gilpin, E.A., & Pierce, J.P. (1993). Changes in the patterns of initiation of cigarette smoking in the United States: 1950, 1965, and 1980. *Cancer Epidemiology Biomarkers and Prevention, 2,* 593–597.

Lewit, E.M., & Coate, D. (1982). The potential of using excise taxes to reduce smoking. *Journal of Health Economics, 1,* 121–145.

Loader, S., Caldwell, P., Kozyra, A., Levenkron, J.C., Boehm, C.D., Kazazian, H.H.J., & Rowley, P.T. (1996). Cystic fibrosis carrier population screening in the primary care setting. *American Journal of Human Genetics, 59,* 234–247.

McGinnis, J.M., & Foege, W.H. (1993). Actual causes of death in the United States. *JAMA, 270,* 2207–2212.

Mock, C., Pilcher, S., & Maier, R. (1994). Comparison of the costs of acute treatment for gunshot and stab wounds: Further evidence of the need for firearms control. *Journal of Trauma, 36,* 516–521.

Nunnally, J. (1978). *Psychometric theory.* New York: McGraw-Hill.

Orenstein, D.M., Nixon, P.A., Ross, E.A., & Kaplan, R.M. (1989). The quality of well-being in cystic fibrosis. *Chest, 95,* 344–347.

Pauly, M.V. (1995). Valuing health care benefits in money terms. In F. Sloan (Ed.), *Valuing health care: Costs benefits and effectiveness of pharmaceuticals and other medical technologies* (pp. 99–124). New York: Cambridge University Press.

Peto, R., Lopez, A.D., Boreham, J., Thun, M., & Heath, C., Jr. (1992). Mortality from tobacco in developed countries: Indirect estimation from national vital statistics. *Lancet, 339,* 1268–1278.

Pierce, J.P. (1991). Progress and problems in internation public health efforts to reduce tobacco useage. *Annual Review of Public Health, 12,* 383–400.

Rescind, M.D., Bearman, P.S., Blum, R.W., Bauman, K.E., Harris, K.M., Jones, J., Tabor, J., Beuhring, T., Sieving, R.E., Shew, M. et al. (1997). Protecting adolescents from harm. Findings from the National Longitudinal Study on Adolescent Health. *JAMA, 278,* 823–832.

Rivara, F.P. (1997). Fatal and non-fatal farm injuries to children and adolescents in the United States, 1990–3. *Injury Prevention, 3,* 190–194.

Rivara, F.P., Grossman, D.C., & Cummings, P. (1997). Injury prevention: Second of two parts. *New England Journal of Medicine, 337,* 613–618.

Rivara, F.P., Thompson, D.C., & Thompson, R.S. (1997). Epidemiology of bicycle injuries and risk factors for serious injury. *Injury Prevention, 3,* 110–114.

Rothenberg, R., Masca, P., Mikl, J., et al. (1987). Cancer. *American Journal of Preventive Medicine, 3,* 30–42.

Rowley, P.T., Loader, S., & Kaplan, R.M. (1998). Prenatal screening for cystic fibrosis carriers: An economic evaluation. *American Journal of Human Genetics, 63,* 1160–1164.

Saigal, S., Feeny, D., Rosenbaum, P., Furlong, W., Burrows, E., & Stoskopf, B. (1996). Self-perceived health status and health-related quality of life of extremely low-birth-weight infants at adolescence. *JAMA, 276,* 453–459.

Squier, H., Ries, A.L., Kaplan, R.M., Prewitt, L.M., Smith, C.M., Kriett, J.M., & Jamieson, S.W. (1995). Quality of Well-being predicts survival in lung transplantation candidates. *American Journal of Respiratory and Critical Care Medicine, 152,* 2032–2036.

Starfield, B., Bergner, M., Ensminger, M., Riley, A., Ryan, S., Green, B., McGauhey, P., Skinner, A., & Kim, S. (1993). Adolescent health status measurement: development of the Child Health and Illness Profile. *Pediatrics, 91,* 430–435.

Starfield, B., Forrest, C.B., Ryan, S.A., Riley, A.W., Ensminger, M.E., & Green, B.F. (1996). Health status of well vs ill adolescents. *Archives of Pediatric and Adolescent Medicine, 150,* 1249–1256.

Starfield, B., Riley, A.W., Green, B.F., Ensminger, M.E., Ryan, S.A., Kelleher, K., Kim-Harris, S., Johnston, D., & Vogel, K. (1995). The adolescent child health and illness profile: A population-based measure of health. *Medical Care, 33,* 553–566.

Sturm, R., & Wells, K.B. (1995). How can care for depression become more cost-effective? *JAMA, 273,* 51–58.

U.S. Department of Health and Human Services (USDHHS). (1988). *The health consequences of smoking: Nicotine addiction.* Washington, DC: U.S. Government Printing Office.

U.S. Department of Health and Human Services (USDHHS). (1990). *The health benefits of smoking cessation.* Washington, DC: U.S. Government Printing Office.

U.S. Department of Justice, Bureau of Justice Statistics. (1993). *Crime victimization in the United States.* Washington, DC: U.S. Department of Justice.

U.S. Office on Smoking and Health. (1990). *Smoking and health, a national status report: A report to Congress (2nd Edition),* Department of Health and Human Services. Rockville, MD: U.S. Department of Health and Human Services, Public Health Service, Centers for Disease Control, Center for Chronic Disease Prevention and Health Promotion.

U.S. Surgeon General. (1989). *Reducing the health consequences of smoking: Twenty-five years of progress.* Rockville, MD: U.S. Department of Health and Human Services, Centers for Disease Control.

Varni, J.W., Katz, E.R., Seid, M., Quiggins, D.J.L., & Friedman-Bender, A. (1998). The pediatric cancer Quality of Life inventory (PedsQL-32): I Reliability and Validity. *Journal of Cancer, 82,* 1184–1196.

Vivier, P.M., Bernier, J.A., & Starfield, B. (1994). Current approaches to measuring health outcomes in pediatric research. *Current Opinion in Pediatrics, 6,* 530–537.

Waller, J.A. (1986). Prevention of premature death and disability due to injury. In J.M. Last (Ed.), *Public health and preventive medicine* (12th Edition) (pp. 1543–1576). Norwalk, CT: Appleton-Century-Crofts.

Warner, K.E. (1986). Smoking and health implications of a change in federal cigarette excise tax. *JAMA, 255,* 1028–1032.

Welsh, M.J., & Smith, A.E. (1995). Cystic fibrosis. *Scientific American, 273,* 52–59.

Wennberg, J.E. (1990). Small area analysis and the medical care outcome problem. In L. Secrest, E. Perrin, & J. Bunker (Eds), *Research methodology: Strengthening causal interpretations of nonexperimental data* (pp. 177–206). AHCPR, DHHS Publication No. (PHS) 90-3454. U.S. Department of Health and Human Services

Wintemute, G.J. (1994). Homicide, handguns, and the crime gun hypothesis: Firearms used in fatal shootings of law enforcement officers, 1980 to 1989. *American Journal of Public Health, 84,* 561–564.

CHRONIC CONDITIONS AS A GENERAL CLASS

Chapter 5

EPIDEMIOLOGY OF CHILDHOOD CHRONIC ILLNESS:
ISSUES IN DEFINITIONS, SERVICE USE, AND COSTS

Henry T. Ireys

Any effort to understand quality of life (QL) for children and adolescents in general must address issues specifically related to the prevalence, severity, and impact of chronic health conditions. A child's health status and the surrounding social environment may shape most directly the quality of that child's life, but broad population parameters and trends will play critical roles as well. Changes in the composition or demographic distribution of the population of young persons with chronic health conditions can affect dramatically the availability of resources for health and mental health care. Opportunities for a decent QL may be seriously eroded if needed services are unavailable to children and their families or are so costly that society is unwilling to pay for them.

This chapter reflects a public health perspective on the population of children with chronic illnesses and disabilities. It considers issues related to defining this population, its prevalence and demographic distribution, and associated patterns of service use and cost. The final section explores some of the implications of findings from epidemiologic and health services research for the study of QL in children and adolescents.

DEFINITIONS OF THE POPULATION: CONCEPTUAL AND METHODOLOGIC ISSUES

The prevalence of children with chronic health conditions is impossible to estimate without a clear definition of the conceptual boundaries of the population. Who should be included in this group of children? Children with certain disorders, such as spina bifida or sickle cell anemia, would be included in virtually every definition. Controversy arises when the more marginal conditions are considered: children with seasonal asthma who wheeze for a month, adolescents with long-standing acne, or infants with recurrent otitis media. Are these children part of the population?

One way to answer this question is to compare a child's condition with a list of conditions that have been determined *a priori* to define the set of chronic illnesses or disabilities. If the child's condition is on the list, then the child would be included. This approach is typically termed the condition-specific or list-based approach, and is often used for determining eligibility for services from public programs or for coverage in a health insurance plan.

This approach is limited by the large number of chronic conditions in childhood (well over 200) and lack of consensus concerning what should be on the list. Should "mild asthma" or chronic acne be included? Reasonable people, using different decision criteria, could easily disagree. Furthermore, some children have serious ongoing health problems long before an accurate diagnosis is made. Should these children be excluded from services simply because they have an obscure or unknown condition?

Another way to address the issue is to focus on the meaningful consequences of a health condition. If a child is limited in some way or has to use health or special education services more than usual, or is dependent on medical intervention to sustain health, then the child could be considered as having a special health care need. The functional and service use implications of a condition, rather than the diagnostic label, serves to define the population boundaries. This approach is typically termed the non-categorical or functional approach.

Over the past two decades, these different definitional approaches have been used in a wide variety of studies. As a result, prevalence estimates have varied widely. Based on studies in many countries, these estimates range from 2% of the population to 32% (see, for example, Boyle, Decoufle, & Yeargin-Alsopp, 1994; Cadman, Boyle, Szatmari, & Offord, 1987; Newacheck, 1994, and studies described below). Some studies rest on a condition-specific approach; others adopt a non-categorical perspective. These two approaches are complementary; each can be useful, depending on the research question or programmatic need. Understanding both approaches can help in selecting a method appropriate to the specific goals of a particular research effort.

Since the early 1990s, epidemiologic studies of this population of children have reflected greater consistency in national prevalence estimates because of (1) a greater consensus on how to define key concepts, (2) improved survey instruments, and (3) better population-based survey methods. These estimates indicate that 15% to 20% of the childhood population have some kind of ongoing health condition that has meaningful consequences for the child, and that 6% to 7% of all children have some kind of activity limitation or disability (Newacheck & Halfon, 1998; Stein, Westbrook, & Bauman, 1997; Westbrook, Silver, & Stein, 1998).

Availability of data from the disability supplement of the 1994–1995 National Health Interview Survey (NHIS) will provide the basis for numerous studies that will be available in the late 1990s and into the early part of the next century. These reports are unlikely to alter the basic estimate of 15% to 20% for children with chronic conditions (or 6% to 7% for children with limitations in activity), but they will provide more fine-grain analysis of the effects of specific demographic or health care system variables on prevalence rates in the United States. For readers interested in its methodologic details, the NHIS is described in Appendix A.

An increasingly important issue, at least in the United States, involves estimating the prevalence of children with chronic conditions in populations enrolled in managed care organizations (MCOs). Some managed care organizations, for example, may adopt coverage policies that discourage families from enrolling; as a result, MCOs will vary in the percent of enrolled children with chronic conditions. Those with higher percentages will be at a competitive disadvantage unless appropriate adjustments are made to capitation rates (Muldoon, Neff, & Gay, 1997; Neff & Anderson, 1995). An important challenge in the immediate future will involve identifying administratively feasible survey instruments and methods for this population of children who are enrolled in managed care systems.

NON-CATEGORICAL APPROACHES

Overview

The non-categorical approach emerges out of the common clinical observation that a particular diagnosis conveys little about the psychological and social functioning of a child or family. Most children with cystic fibrosis and their families, for example, function quite well by any measure of mental health status; others have numerous psychological problems that result from or are aggravated by the presence of the condition. Simply knowing that a child has cystic fibrosis is of little use in distinguishing between which children and families need mental health intervention and which do not. The same point can be made about health status. Some children with cystic fibrosis, for example, will require a great deal of medical intervention at every stage of life; other children with this disease will have periods of stability between periods of deterioration. Although children with chronic illnesses in general have poorer health status compared to children without these conditions, virtually every diagnostic group has wide variability in health status at any one point in time. These observations can be framed as a general hypothesis: variation in health status, mental health status, and social functioning is as great *within* a diagnostic group as it is *between* diagnostic groups (Stein & Jessop, 1982).

Another implication of a noncategorical approach is that children with diverse chronic health conditions share common experiences in responding to the challenges of living with the condition (Perrin et al., 1993; Pless & Perrin, 1985; Stein & Jessop, 1982; Stein, Coupey, Bauman, Westbrook, & Ireys, 1993). Parents of these children also share similar experiences, such as responding to the developmental and social challenges of raising a child who is "different", coping with the reactions that the condition creates in siblings, and dealing with multiple health, education, and financing systems. More than 20 years ago, Pless and Pinkerton (1975, p. 2) summarized this view succinctly:

> The chronicity of the illness and the impact that is has on the child, his parents, and his siblings, is more significant than the specific character of the disorder, be it diabetes, cerebral palsy, hemophilia, etc. In other words there are certain problems common to all chronic illness over and above particular challenges posed by individual needs.

If the diagnosis itself is not especially useful for predicting psychological functioning, might there be other variables that are predictive? Numerous conceptual models have been proposed and investigated to answer this question (e.g., Moos & Schaefer, 1989; Wallander, Varni, Babani, Banis, & Wilcox, 1989); these models typically identify several classes of variables, such as family character-istics, illness parameters, stressors, and availability of social support or other resources. A comprehensive review of these models is beyond the scope of this chapter.

It is useful, however, to examine the *consequences* for the child and family that can ensue from the presence of any chronic health condition. What does it mean to a child and family to have a chronic condition? For some families, it may mean the child has limitations in her or his ability to play with other children; for other families, it may mean going to doctors more often than other children; for still other families, it may have both of these consequences. For some families, the presence of a chronic condition may have no meaningful consequences; for example, a child with seasonal asthma may have few limitations and require minimal treatment. This child may be diagnosed as having asthma, but the consequences are so minimal that he or she has no "special" health care needs.

Epidemiologic use of a non-categorical approach

Stein and colleagues (Stein et al., 1993; Stein, Westbrook, & Bauman, 1997) proposed a non-categorical definition that has been used in several studies to estimate prevalence of children with ongoing health conditions. They define this group in the following manner (Stein et al., 1993):

"Children with an ongoing health condition have disorders that (1) have a biological, psychologic, or cognitive basis, and (2) have lasted or are virtually certain to last for at least 12 months, and (3) produce one or more of the following sequelae:

a) need for medial care or related services, psychologic services or educational services over and above the usual for the child's age, or for special ongoing treatments, interventions, or accommodations at home or in school,
b) limitation in function, activities or social role in comparison with healthy age peers in the general areas of physical, cognitive, emotional, and social growth and development, or
c) dependency on one of the following to compensate for or minimize limitation of function, activities, or social role: medications, special diet, medical technology, assistive device, or personal assistance."

This definition is useful because it distinguishes (based on the presence of relevant consequences) three groups of children: (1) those who require more services than usual, (2) those who have limitation in function, and (3) those who are dependent on interventions to compensate for functional limitations. A 39-item survey is now available that operationalizes this definition and can be used to assess prevalence rates of this population (Stein et al., 1997). This survey, termed the Questionnaire for Identifying Children with Chronic Conditions (QuICCC), determines whether children have none, one, two, or three of these consequences. An actual diagnosis is not necessary for a child to be classified as having a chronic health condition because the scale items focus on behavioral and health consequences, rather than the diagnosis.

Each of the 39 items in the QuICCC is a sequence of three parts. The first part asks about the specific consequences of having a chronic condition. There are 15 items related to the functional limitation domain (e.g., Is the child restricted in playing with other children?); 12 related to the compensatory domain (e.g., Does the child require a special diet?); and 12 in the service use or need domain (e.g., Does the child need or use physical therapy?). If a consequence is reported, the respondent is then asked in a second part whether the consequence is the result of a medical, behavioral, or other health condition. If this part is answered affirmatively, the final part of the item is asked: "Has this condition been going on or is it expected to go on for at least 1 year?" To meet the definition and be classifed as having a chronic condition, a child must qualify in each component (i.e., having a consequence that is related to a condition that will last at least 12 months) of at least one question sequence (Stein et al., 1997).

Several population-based studies using this survey have led to estimates of prevalence rates that range from 15% and 19% of the childhood population (Stein et al., 1997; Westbrook, Silver, & Stein, 1998). In one study (Westbrook et al., 1998), analyses were conducted on a national dataset representing a random sample of households with children; in total, 712 households with 1388 children were surveyed. Overall, 18% were identified as having a chronic health condition as operationally defined by the QuICCC. Of those children who were identified as having a chronic condition, about slightly less than half were included on the basis of one type of consequence; about a third reported two types of consequences; and about a fifth reported three types of consequences (Westbrook et al., 1998). Above-normal use of services was the consequence that contributed most to the inclusion of children into the target population, identifying 72% of all children classified by the QuICCC; compensatory items and functional limitation items identified 55% and 49% of the children, respectively. These results are generally consistent with other studies (Stein et al., 1997).

Other non-categorical definitions have been used for purposes of estimating prevalence. In a series of studies using National Health Interview Survey (NHIS) data from the 1980s, for example, Newacheck and colleagues used the construct, "limitation of activity" to define the population of children with disability (e.g., Newacheck & Taylor, 1992; Newacheck, Stoddard, & McManus, 1993). More recently, the United States Maternal and Child Health Bureau (MCHB, 1997) promulgated a non-categorical definition that emphasized the concepts of service use and risk status. This definition was developed to reflect and promote efforts for determining eligibility for state programs for children with special needs. It states:

> Children with special health care needs are those who have or are at an increased risk for chronic physical, developmental, behavioral, or emotional

conditions and who require health and related services of a type or amount beyond that required by children generally.

The concept of "at-risk" is important because it lays a foundation for identifying populations of children and families who may benefit from preventive interventions. For example, new developments in genetic testing have led to identification of conditions (e.g., ALS) that become symptomatic only in late adolescence or young adulthood. Children with HIV-infection represent another example of a group of young persons who are asymptomatic but incipient patients, and for whom interventions to preserve QL may be especially important.

CONDITION-SPECIFIC APPROACHES

Condition-specific approaches to estimating prevalence rates of particular chronic illnesses in childhood can serve a critical role in program planning. In many instances, studies using this approach bring much-needed attention to the issues of children with specific conditions or provide fine-grain analyses that serve particular clinical or programmatic purposes. In other instances, a condition-specific approach may be the only reasonable course of action given limitations in a particular data set.

The most common approach is to focus on a single diagnostic category and use multiple methods to detect true cases. Manners and Diepeveen (1996), for example, examined the prevalence of juvenile chronic arthritis (JCA) in 12 year old children in urban Australia. They combined a population-based survey with JCA-sensitive clinical examinations of 2,241 children and found a prevalence rate of 4.0 per 1,000. This rate is considerably higher than previous estimates, which range from 0.6 to 1.1 per 1,000. The authors suggest that lack of knowledge in the lay and professional communities contribute to undiagnosed JCA, which is accompanied by considerable morbidity in the form of substantial limitation of activity and higher use of general pediatric services.

This study is instructive for several reasons. First, it illustrates a sophisticated and epidemiologically sound multi-method strategy (population-based survey followed by clinical exam) for detection of children with JCA. Second, it underscores a serious lack of knowledge in the clinical and lay communities. Parents sought medical help for their children because of medical complaints, but physicians failed to correctly diagnose the complaints as related to JRA (Manners & Diepeveen, 1996). Third, the study illustrates a potential limitation of condition-specific approaches in that a child must have received a JCA-diagnosis before classification was possible. Thus, children with true cases of JCA may have been undercounted because they did not receive the correct label, even though they were experiencing symptoms and an ongoing need for services.

Numerous investigators in many different countries have pursued diagnostic-specific approaches (e.g., Haussler, Schafer, & Neugebaur, 1996; Landgren, Pettersson, Kjellman, & Gillberg, 1996). At first glance, a diagnostic approach would appear to be quite straightforward. The condition of interest is selected and strategies developed to survey a community or area to determine how many children have that condition. Implementing condition-specific prevalence studies, however, has numerous pitfalls. For example, a review of world-wide prevalence rates of severe mental retardation found 32 studies with prevalence rates ranging from 2.6 to 7.3 (Roeleveld, Zielhuis, & Gabreels, 1997). The authors note that despite over 25 years of research on the prevalence of mental retardation, there remains an urgent need for standardization of definitions and research methods.

One of the common methodologic strategies in calculating prevalence rates for specific conditions is to draw on programs that serve children with the condition of interest. Program-focused approaches to defining populations of children with chronic health problems involve counting and describing characteristics of individuals who use a particular service program or are known to service providers. From an epidemiologic perspective, this method is likely to underestimate the true prevalence of a population, possibly by a substantial margin, because not all potentially eligible individuals will actually enroll in a service program. Nonetheless, this approach may be the only feasible one in instances when resources are unavailable for prevalence studies using representative community-based or national samples. Furthermore, accurate counts and descriptions of program participants can have important implications for public policies.

Many condition-specific epidemiologic studies rely on program-based samples of children. An example of this strategy can be found in a study conducted in Atlanta, Georgia, in conjunction with the Centers for Disease Control and Prevention (Murphy, Yeargin-Allsopp, Decoufle, & Drews, 1995). The goal of this study was to determine the administrative prevalence (i.e., the number of children identified by the service system) of mental retardation among children who were 10 years old at any time in the period of 1985 through 1987. Ninety-five percent of the children were identified through review of school records, but numerous other sources were used, including hospitals, county health departments, state and county mental health service agencies, and private social service agencies. An administrative prevalence rate of 12.0 children per 1,000 children was found. The rate was higher in the African-American population (19.7 per 1,000 children) than in the white population (7.4) and was higher for boys (13.8 per 1,000) than for girls (10.1). The authors note (p. 321) that these figures are consistent with previous studies, but that their data set is "one of the few current population-based sources of information on children with developmental disabilities in the United States". In separate studies, this data set was used also to study the influence of sociodemographic and racial risk factors on prevalence rates of mental retardation (Drews, Yeargin-Allsopp, Decoufle, & Murphy, 1995; Yeargin-Allsopp, Drews, Decoufle, & Murphy, 1995).

Although this set of studies pertain to one urban area, and therefore may be limited in its generalizability, it does illustrate how service systems themselves can be used for epidemiologic purposes. With careful planning, data collected by service agencies can be a valuable source of information on broad social and demographic factors that can influence access to and use of services.

Another example of this approach may be found in a report on the changing prevalence of autism in one health district in Wales (Webb, Lobo, Hervas, Scourfield, & Fraser, 1997). This investigative team asked all school and child health professionals in a designated area to identify children who met specified criteria. Children who were nominated in this manner were further screened using a standardized checklist; children who were screened in were referred to a mental health clinic for comprehensive diagnosis and assessment. For younger children (those born between 1987 and 1989) the age specific prevalence figure was 9.2 per 10,000; for older children (those born between 1977 and 1979) the figure was 3.3 per 10,000. The authors note, "Our survey shows an apparent local increase in prevalence of AD [autistic disorder] in the decade 1978 to 1988, but in the context of the world literature our figures are in the mid-range of reported prevalence". The authors comment further that changes in how a condition is defined or in the assessment tools used in the diagnostic process can affect prevalence rates.

During the past several years, administrative data bases (i.e., data bases whose primary purpose is to pay bills or track patient-provider encounters) also have been used to calculate prevalence rates of children with specific conditions. The National Association of Children's Hospitals and Related Institutions (NACHRI), for example, has developed a list of ICD-9 codes that captures chronic health conditions of childhood that are associated with high rates of hospitalization and hospital-based service use. This approach has the advantage of using information (i.e., the ICD-9 code) that is already in the administrative data bases of health insurance companies, public health care programs, and managed care organizations. A preliminary report using data from the Washington State Medicaid program, found that 18.3% of enrolled children had one or more of the health conditions included on the list (Muldoon, Neff, & Gay, 1997). The conditions were classified further as either "physical health conditions" or "mental health conditions"; about 70% of the children were found to have physical health conditions, 20% to have mental health conditions, and about 10% were found to have both. In addition, conditions were classified into severity levels, based on expected need for services by a typical child with that condition.

From a health services research perspective, the strength of the list-based approach illustrated by the NACHRI effort to classify ICD-9 diagnostic codes is its feasibility. Because ICD-9 codes are widely used, data sets routinely include them and hence relevant data are available for analysis.

The weakness of the list-based approach is three-fold. The first involves problems in coding, which can be influenced by financial incentives and inconsistency across service settings. The second involves the relation between the presence of a condition and service use. If a child with a particular condition does not have a codable encounter with a health service provider in a particular year, then that child will not appear in the data base. Thus, the use of claims data bases to develop prevalence rates may be more defensible for complex or severe chronic health conditions than for milder chronic conditions because all children with more severe conditions are likely to have at least one encounter with a health provider in a year.

The third weakness relates to the problem of multiple conditions. Diagnostic-based approaches count *conditions* not *children*. Accounting for multiple conditions in a list-based approach is an important analytic problem to address (e.g., Do you include these children in several categories or have a separate category for those with multiple conditions? Should all combinations of conditions be included?).

Non-categorical approaches avoid this problem because they focus on the experiences of the child, regardless of whether those experiences are linked to one or more diagnostic labels.

CONCEPTS OF SEVERITY

The word "severity" is frequently used in clinical and research settings, but rarely defined with precision. What is meant by a severe condition? Some investigators might refer to biological processes. Children with "severe" hemophilia, for example, may have less of a critical clotting factor than children with "mild" hemophilia; children with a severe case of asthma may have lower peak flow rates than children with a mild case. Generally accepted measures of biological severity have been developed for some conditions but not others (Stein, Gortmaker, Perrin, Perrin, Pless et al., 1987).

The concept of severity is not restricted to biological levels; it also can refer to functional status. Some children with cerebral palsy (CP) may have limited range of motion in their legs, for example, while others have almost full range of motion. As noted below, functional status can be defined quite broadly to include physical, social, academic, and emotional functioning. Chronic conditions may have more or less of an impact on a child's capacity to perform age-appropriate activities, resulting in greater or lesser functional severity.

Finally, severity can refer to the degree of impact that a condition has on family or social resources. Health plan administrators typically consider chronic conditions to be severe when the child uses many services and incurs a great deal of expenses. Some children with a particular condition may require substantial resources from a family, while others with the same condition require relatively few. In the sense of resource utilization, chronic conditions will range from the mild to the severe both within and across diagnostic categories.

Distinguishing among the various means for defining severity is important for both research and policy purposes (Stein et al., 1987). For research purposes, making these distinctions is important because there may be little correlation among measures that would tap into these distinct dimensions. Children with conditions that are biologically severe might experience few functional limitations or use few resources in a particular year. Similarly, a child who has a biologically mild condition may nonetheless have poor functional capacity because of secondary emotional difficulties. Measures that distinguish among these levels of severity are likely to be conceptually and methodologically more precise than scales that mix items related to all of these dimensions.

ASSESSING HEALTH AND FUNCTIONAL STATUS

The consequences of a chronic condition can change in response to the medical course of the condition, treatment interventions, the child's development, and the family's experience in responding to the demands of care. For example, a child with leukemia who has finished treatment may have far fewer limitations than he or she did when receiving chemotherapy; the child still carries the diagnosis of leukemia, but the day-to-day consequences are quite different, and may have different implications for mental health status. Developmental transitions and physical growth spurts also will shape the meaning of a condition for the family and child. A school-aged child with diabetes, for example, may have a history of excellent adherence to dietary regimens and insulin injection schedules; as adolescence approaches, however, his or her adherence may erode, with a corresponding increase in mood swings or risk for ketoacidosis. Development, treatment efforts, and health status interact in complex ways.

These considerations have contributed to efforts to develop measures of health and functional status for this group of children. Again, some of these efforts have focused on specific conditions; other efforts have led to measures that are independent of particular diagnoses (e.g., Starfield et al., 1993; Stein & Jessop, 1990). Comprehensive reviews of issues related to assessing health status are available elsewhere (e.g., Lewis, Pantell, & Kieckerfer, 1989; Patrick & Deyo, 1989). For the purposes of this chapter, three general measures and two condition-specific measures are discussed to illustrate key issues.

The first example is a general measure of heath status termed the Child Health and Illness Profile — Adolescent Edition (CHIP-AE), which has been developed by Starfield and colleagues (Starfield, Bergner, Ensminger, Riley, Ryan et al., 1993; Starfield, Riley, Green, Ensminger, Ryan et al., 1995). The current form of this instrument has 20 subdomains grouped into 6 general domains: Discomfort, Disorders, Satisfaction with Health, Achievement in Social Roles, Risks, and Resilience. The scale includes 107 items plus 46 disease-specific or injury-related items. The subdomains include physical discomfort, emotional discomfort, and limitations of activity (which are grouped into the general domain of Discomfort); and family involvement, problem-solving, physical activity, and home safety and health (which are grouped under the general domain of Resilience). The validity and reliability estimates of this instrument are strong, especially at the subdomain level. The authors note (1995, p. 565), "Because the CHIP-AE detects differences in health that are predicted as a function of age, gender, and socioeconomic status (SES), we believe it is suitable for evaluations of the impact of community and health services interventions with populations or clinical groups".

A second example is Stein's measure of functional status, the FS II(R), a 43-item scale designed to assess health status of children with chronic health conditions, whether or not they have physical impairments (Stein & Jessop, 1990; Stein & Riessman, 1978). Scale items tap into "behavioral manifestations of illness that interfere with an individual's performance of the full range of age-appropriate activities" (Stein & Jessop, 1990, p. 1043). The FS II(R) places unique emphasis on determining whether difficulties in functioning are attributable to the presence of the child's health condition. The scale has excellent psychometric characteristics and distinguishes between groups of well and ill children.

The WeeFIM is a third example of a general measure of functional status (Msall, DiGaudio, Rogers, LaForest, Catanzo, et al., 1994). This scale is designed to measure functional severity of a disability and need for assistance in performing activities of daily living. Children between six months and 7 years of age are rated by parents or providers on a seven-point scale from complete dependence to complete independence in reference to six functional domains: self-care, sphincter control, transfers, locomotion, communication, and social cognition. The scale was constructed in order to assess change in function over time, and therefore can serve as a measure of treatment outcome. Early data suggest that the WeeFIM has strong psychometric characteristics and is a valid and reliable means for distinguishing children who have limitations in self-care, motor, and social interaction capabilities from those who do not (Ottenbacher, Taylor, Msall, Braun, Lane, et al. 1996). This scale is likely to be useful for assessing interventions for children with a wide range of physical and developmental disabilities, independent of the particular underlying diagnosis. The scale is not relevant for children with chronic illnesses, such as diabetes, sickle cell anemia, or hemophilia, who may not be restricted at all in these domains.

These three examples of general measures of health or functional status illustrate several points. First, some measures have been developed for children in general and then used with children who have chronic conditions; the CHIP illustrates this approach. In contrast, other measures (e.g., the FSII(R) and the WeeFIM) have been developed for children with chronic health conditions, rather than for children in general. These latter scales may be more sensitive than the former in detecting differences in the upper ranges of functional severity. The WeeFIM, for example, is likely to distinguish among children with different levels of activity limitation more effectively than the CHIP.

Second, these scales illustrate the point that "generalness" is relative. The CHIP is general by virtue of its applicability to broad populations; the WeeFIM is general in the sense that it is most applicable to children with physical disabilities, regardless of the underlying condition. The appropriate level of generality can be determined only in light of the goals and objectives of a particular study.

In contrast to studies on general methods of assessing functional or health status, other efforts have focused on developing condition-specific measures. For example, Sullivan and Olson (1995) developed a scale to assess the functional status and well-being of children with asthma. Their 56-item measure included seven domains: physical symptoms, the child's physical activity, the child's social activity, the family's social activity, emotional impact on the child, emotional impact on the family, and health care use. Response categories to some items (e.g., coughing, headaches) reflect number of occurrences; response categories to other items (e.g., school gym classes, being bothered by medical equipment at home) reflect intensity, such as "no limitation" or "not bothered" to "totally limited" or "bothered a great deal". The authors report that five of the seven scales had acceptable reliabilities, and that some of the scales differentiated children with mild asthma (as judged by physicians) from those with moderately severe asthma.

Another example of a self-report, condition-specific measure of functional status is the Juvenile Arthritis Functional Assessment Report for Children (Howe, Levinson, Shear, Hartner, McGirr et al., 1991). This 23-item scale was designed to measure "disability due to juvenile rheumatoid arthritis" in children from 7 to 18 years of age; both parent and child versions were developed. Items tap the physical capacity to perform daily functions, such as brushing teeth, walking up five steps, and cutting food with a knife and fork. The scale developers report excellent reliability and validity estimates and high correlation (.75) between parent and child versions. Although the scale is considered to be a "functional assessment", the items tap the single dimension of physical competence. This narrow focus may be of clinical utility in measuring effects of medication or physical therapy on the physical capacity of children with JRA, but it is less useful for assessing the overall functioning of the child.

Comparison between the asthma and the JRA studies illustrates different ways of approaching condition-specific functional assessment, and different conceptions of "functionality". On the one hand, a narrow conception of functionality will focus attention on dimensions that may be clinically relevant to a particular condition, but will fail to capture a comprehensive view of the child's overall experience. On the other hand, a broad definition of functionality includes the diverse dimensions of life that are important to child development; once these are included, however, items typically are cast at high levels of generality such that different condition names could be substituted, and they could be well used as general measures.

DEMOGRAPHIC DISTRIBUTION OF CHRONIC HEALTH CONDITIONS IN CHILDHOOD

AGE

Overall, the prevalence of chronic health conditions increases somewhat with age. Based on data from the 1989 National Health Interview Survey, Newacheck (1994) found 2.3 cases per 100 for children under 5; for children 5 to 11 and 12 to 17, the figures were 6.1 and 7.2, respectively. A review of studies on the prevalence of mental retardation indicated that in most studies that reported age-specific prevalence rates, the prevalence increased during childhood from 1 or 2 per 1,000 to 3 to 5 per 1,000 (Roeleveld, Zielhuis, & Gabreels, 1997). Moreover, the functional consequences of many chronic illnesses interact with age to produce complex patterns of disability and service use across developmental stages. For example, infants born at very low birth weight may need intensive medical treatments throughout their first year of life. As acute medical issues resolve, many of these children will require developmental interventions during their preschool years. Children with diabetes may maintain good control of insulin levels throughout middle school but may experience more difficulty in early adolescence as hormonal changes occur in conjunction with normal adolescent "acting out." These youth and their families will then need special support or counseling services to assist in negotiating new social challenges (Blum, 1984).

Improved survival patterns of children with many formerly fatal diseases raise complex new issues for the transition to adulthood.

Dramatic improvements in survival of children with cystic fibrosis, sickle cell anemia and other disorders have led to many questions about how these youths find employment, form intimate relationships, and make the transition to adult medical service systems (Ireys, Salkever, Kolodner, & Bijur, 1995).

Young adults with disabilities and chronic illnesses are at high risk for limited access to medical care and supportive services (Newacheck, McManus, & Gepart, 1992). This is a common problem in the United States. This problem usually results from age-based eligibility criteria for pediatric services or disruptions in insurance coverage, or both. Several anecdotal accounts (e.g., Knowles & Fernald, 1988; Schidlow & Fiel, 1990) indicate a dearth of carefully planned transition services. Few studies, however, have systematically addressed the process whereby older adolescents with chronic illnesses and disabilities leave pediatric health services and move into adult-oriented service systems (Blum, Garell, Hodgeman, Jorissen, Okinow et al., 1993). This transition is critical because disruptions in access to appropriate services may have particularly severe consequences for the continuity and quality of health care for this population of young persons and lead to preventable secondary health and mental health conditions (Kokkonen, Saukkonen, Timonen, Serlo, & Kinnunen, 1991).

GENDER

Overall, boys are reported to have more disabilities than girls; in one set of analyses, Newacheck (1994) found 6.3 cases per 100 boys and 4.3 cases per 100 girls. In these analyses, cases were determined based on limitations in activities as reported by parents. Sex-linked disorders are comparatively common in this population. Hemophilia, for example, rarely occurs in females. Survival rates for females with cystic fibrosis are lower than for males (Wielinski, Budd, & Warwick, 1990). Girls are far more likely to have juvenile chronic arthritis than boys (Manners & Diepeveen, 1996).

These gender differences raise interesting questions related to QL. For example, school age boys traditionally place a high premium on physical competence. Conditions that interfere with participation in sports may have quite different effects on boys than on girls. Moreover, the presence of a serious physical health condition may limit opportunities for certain types of employment that can differentially affect the genders.

POVERTY

Poverty and health status interact in complex ways to affect QL (Halfon & Newacheck, 1993). Poverty is associated with increased risk of disability and of hospitalization for problems related to chronic health conditions (e.g., Newacheck, 1989; Wissow, Gittelsohn, Szklo, Starfield, & Mussman, 1988). In a study using NHIS data from 1992 to 1994, Newacheck and Halfon (1998) found that rates of activity limitations in children living in poor families were significantly higher than rates for children in nonpoor families (96.2 vs 57.3 per 1,000, $p<.05$). Diminished access to service as a result of inadequate insurance coverage is considered to be a key factor in the relationship between socioeconomic status and disability.

RACE

Effects of race are difficult to disentangle from effects of poverty status. However, for certain conditions, race is a primary determinant of occurrence. In the United States, for example, sickle cell anemia occurs primarily in children of African descent; cystic fibrosis occurs primarily in children of European descent. From a national perspective white children are more likely to have at least one chronic condition than African-American or Hispanic children (Newacheck, Stoddard, & McManus, 1993). However, these latter two groups experience more limitation in their usual activities as a result of the condition and more days of restricted activity than white children. Absolute prevalence differences among races appear to result from higher prevalence of comparatively mild conditions (e.g., respiratory conditions, skin allergies) among white children. Minority children may experience more severe consequences of their conditions (Newacheck, Stoddard, & McManus, 1993; Weitzman, Gortmaker, & Sobol, 1990), although these differences may result in part from heightened exposure to social and economic impoverishment and associated deficits in access to health services.

Although recent publications have added considerably to knowledge about the associations between prevalence and both racial and income factors, much remains unknown about the relationships between health status of children with special needs and their ethnic or cultural background, especially when economic status is taken into account.

TRENDS IN PREVALENCE AND DISTRIBUTION

Changes in the prevalence of this population (the total number of cases of a given condition or disease at a given point in time) are determined by changes in (1) the size of overall birth cohorts, (2) incidence rates (the number of new cases in a given year per population unit), (3) survival rates, and (4) classification or diagnostic practices (e.g., adopting a noncategorical approach, more sensitive screening approaches, or new definitions of disease states). Since 1975, birth cohorts have been increasing but are expected to remain relatively stable for the next decade. There is little evidence that incidence rates in developed countries will change substantially for most of the major chronic illnesses with the possible exception of HIV infection (Gortmaker, 1985). Survival rates of children with chronic illnesses have increased substantially during the last 20 years (Gortmaker & Sappenfield, 1984; FitzSimmons, 1993), but further increases will probably contribute marginally to increased prevalence. Better reporting, more sensitive screening procedures, and changes in survey techniques have been seen as contributing to increased prevalence estimates (Newacheck, Budetti, & Halfon, 1986), but future effects of these factors are difficult to estimate.

Although a major increase in the prevalence of chronic illnesses is unlikely in the next decade, several critical service-delivery trends are emerging. First, continued advances in biomedical research are likely to increase the number of children living with severe medical conditions that require major emotional, family, and financial investment (Perrin, Shayne, & Bloom, 1993). Second, more children with complex medical needs will be cared for in the home as a result of health policies that emphasize rapid hospital discharge and greater use of home care services (Palfrey, Walker, Haynie, Singer, Porter, et al., 1991). This trend will increase the need for more specialized health and educational services at the community level. Third, deterioration in quality of the environment may contribute to increased rates of selected chronic conditions, such as cancer or asthma, which will require new approaches to preventive interventions and early detection. Fourth, in many Western societies, children with disabilities and chronic illnesses have become increasingly involved in mainstream activities — largely as a result of continued advocacy efforts on the part of families. Over the next decade, children with special health needs will play more active roles in community life as states implement policies to promote more comprehensive, community-based, family centered service systems (Ireys & Nelson, 1993). In turn, families will play increasingly collaborative roles in training of health care professionals, policy development, and program implementation (Jeppson & Thomas, 1995).

As a result of these trends, interest in the prevention of secondary health conditions is likely to increase, especially as societies work to limit growth in medical care expenditures. Many children with disabilities and chronic illnesses are at high risk for secondary health problems such as decubitus ulcers, obesity, contractures, respiratory insufficiency, and depression. Family members are at risk for a wide range of mental health problems (Perrin & MacLean, 1988). Despite this increased risk, preventive interventions to decrease the risk for secondary health conditions have been largely neglected (Institute of Medicine, 1991).

PATTERNS OF COST AND SERVICE UTILIZATION

At first glance, issues of financing of health services may seem distant from concerns with QL. Yet, knowledge of cost variation for children with chronic illnesses and disabilities is essential for purposes of program planning and for tracking changes in QL for this group of children. If a health plan decides to support only six visits per year to a physical therapist for children with cerebral palsy who need weekly physical therapy, the quality of the child's and family's life can be seriously threatened. Clinicians, administrators of managed care organizations, and leaders of advocacy organizations require cost-related information to allocate resources in a manner that will assure that these children have access to and receive needed services of high quality.

Children with chronic health conditions represent the high-cost segment of the childhood population (e.g., Hobbs, Perrin, & Ireys, 1985; Ireys, Anderson, Shaffer & Neff, 1997; Waitzman, Romano, & Scheffler, 1994). In broad public debates about heath care, a key question typically remains unspoken, but nevertheless influential: Why should a society spend so much money on specialty care for a few children with rare chronic illnesses when that money could be used to support primary care for many children? Most Western societies support strongly the ethical principle that government-subsidized care should be provided to children with serious health problems whose parents lack financial resources to pay for care directly. But the extent and manner of that care are matters of considerable debate in many countries.

Despite the need for a strong knowledge base regarding patterns of cost and financing of health and mental health care for this population, few studies have systematically examined this issue. A major challenge in estimating expenditures of care for this population involves accounting for the different types of expenditures, such as expenditures for hospitalization, physician services, ancillary therapies, medication, transportation and telephone charges, home modifications and other types of services. In the United States, families find coverage of these services through a wide array of sources including private insurance, public health programs, public education programs, charity, and their own financial resources. It is difficult to account for these diverse sources of expenditures and financing in systematic investigations, and even more difficult to relate different mixes of coverage to measures of QL for the child and family.

Another problem involves understanding expenditure variation between and within diagnostic categories. In any given year, for example, services for children with asthma are likely to cost on average less than most children with leukemia because of the clinical treatment protocols associated with the two conditions. In the same year, however, some children with asthma will require many services, with correspondingly high expenditures. Similarly, some children who have been treated for leukemia in previous years will be in remission; they may still carry the diagnosis but require relatively few follow-up services. Variation in service needs and expenditures is likely to be substantial both between *and* within diagnostic categories. Few data are currently available that can be used to compare annual cost and expenditure patterns for children with diverse chronic health conditions, or to compare these children with all children enrolled in a particular financing program.

However, one recent study estimated expenditures of care for American children with eight selected chronic illnesses who were enrolled in a state Medicaid program (Ireys et al., 1997). This study analyzed Medicaid claims data for 310,977 children aged 0 to 18 who were enrolled at any time in Fiscal Year 1993. Tracer conditions were used to examine expenditure variation within and between diagnostic groupings. A total of 18,233 children (5.9%) had at least one of the conditions. Expenditures were calculated based on payments made by the Medicaid program.

Children with one of the eight selected conditions incurred mean expenditures of $3,800, compared to $955 for all Medicaid-enrolled children. Mean payments associated with the selected conditions ranged from 2.5 times to 20 times more than payments to all children. About 10% of children accounted for about 70% of the payments in general and in each diagnostic grouping. Variation in mean, median, and total expenditures was extensive among the conditions. For most conditions, inpatient stays accounted for the greatest proportion of expenditures; for some conditions, durable equipment, home nursing, and medication-related services accounted for substantial proportions of total expenditures.

Extensive variation in mean and total expenditures between conditions suggests that different conditions will need to be kept distinct for purposes of establishing payment rates. In addition, the study indicates that children with certain conditions are vulnerable to restrictions in specific services, depending on what restrictions are imposed by a financing program (cf. Neff & Anderson, 1996).

IMPLICATIONS

Health is an important component of QL, and public policies that influence the availability of health services will influence a population's QL. This observation pertains with particular force to children and adolescents with disabilities and chronic illnesses, whose health status may be fragile. Failure to receive needed health services will threaten seriously the QL for this population of youth. Few Western societies have resources for access to unlimited health services for all; as a result, rationing is inevitable. Who will decide what is available for whom? At the present time, Western societies may embrace the principle of supporting care to those who have life-threatening or chronic illnesses, but support for this principle may waver if limited economic resources force citizens to choose between higher taxes for their own health care or more services to children who may need a lifetime of care. No government actively promotes denial of services to even the most impaired newborn, but most governments also recognize that unfettered access to sophisticated medical technology has serious financial implications that can threaten the well-being of all.

In the absence of a willingness to address these large ethical issues, the debate focuses on more narrow, technical questions: What subgroups of the population need what kinds of services? What services are "medically necessary"? Which show the best outcomes? What is the relationship between cost and outcome? How will services be paid for? Framed broadly, these questions are part of the quest for determining the QL for a country's citizens.

For children and youth with chronic illnesses, these questions raise many of the methodologic issues discussed in this chapter, and the concepts and methods of epidemiology and health services research are useful in seeking their answers. Clarifying who is part of this population, understanding the implications of categorical and non-categorical definitions, knowing the population distribution, and appreciating basic expenditure patterns are all central to the broad public debate about QL for this group of young persons.

The issues discussed throughout this chapter also suggest that method and outcome interact. How one defines and samples the population for a particular study, and whether one selects disease-specific or general approaches to measurement, will shape study results. The challenge is to be clear about the bias of one's choices. A public health approach to conceptualizing and designing a research project can help to identify these potential biases and to place research findings in a population-based context.

Children with chronic illnesses can be viewed as the "canaries in the mine". Problems in the health care system are most clearly evident among those who use many health services, and system-wide changes will be felt first by those whose lives depend most heavily on those services. In some Western societies, as governmental resources shrink, legislators view the health care system as a prime target for savings and may seek to reduce use of services by unleashing market forces. Unfortunately, the market is often unfriendly to young people who look different, who are dependent longer than what many would consider "normal", and who may provoke in others profound feelings of discomfort and unease. As scientists and health professionals concerned about these children, our long-term challenge must be to inform and participate in the ongoing debate about society's obligation to enhance the QL for these children and their parents.

References

Blum, R.W. (Ed.). (1984). *Chronic illness and disability in childhood and adolescence.* Orlando, FL: Grune and Stratton.

Blum, R., Garell, D., Hodgeman, C., Jorissen, T., Okinow, N., Orr, D., & Slap, G. (1993). Transition from child-centered to adult health-care systems for adolescents with chronic conditions. *Journal of Adolescent Health, 14,* 570–576.

Boyle, C.A., Decoufle, P., & Yeargin-Allsopp, M. (1994). Prevalence and health impact of developmental disabilities in US children. *Pediatrics, 93,* 399–403.

Cadman, D., Boyle, M., Szatmari, D., & Offord, D.R. (1987). Chronic illness, disability, and mental and social well-being: Findings of the Ontario Child Health Study. *Pediatrics, 79,* 805–813.

Drews, C., Yeargin-Allsopp, M., Decoufle, P., & Murphy, C. (1995). Variation in the influence of selected sociodemographic risk factors for mental retardation. *American Journal of Public Health, 85,* 329–334.

FitzSimmons, S. (1993). The changing epidemiology of cystic fibrosis. *Journal of Pediatrics, 122,* 1–9.

Gortmaker, S. (1985). Demography of chronic childhood diseases. In N. Hobbs & J.M. Perrin (Eds.), *Issues in the care of children with chronic illness: A sourcebook on problems, services, and policies.* San Francisco: Jossey-Bass.

Gortmaker, S.L., & Sappenfield, W. (1984). Chronic childhood disorders: Prevalence and impact. *Pediatric Clinics of North America, 31,* 3–18.

Gortmaker, S.L., Walker, D.K., Weitzman, M., & Sobol, A.M. (1990). Chronic conditions, socio-economic risks, and behavioral problems in children and adolescents. *Pediatrics, 85,* 267–276.

Halfon, N., & Newacheck, P. (1993). Childhood asthma and poverty: Differential impacts and utilization of health services. *Pediatrics, 91,* 56–61.

Haussler, M., Schafer, W., & Neugebaur, H. (1996). Multihandicapped blind and partially sighted children in South Germany I: Prevalence, impairments, and ophthalmological findings. *Developmental Medicine and Child Neurology, 38,* 1068–1075.

Hobbs, N., Perrin, J., & Ireys, H. (1985). *Chronically ill children and their families.* San Francisco, CA: Jossey-Bass.

Howe, S., Levinson, J., Shear, E., Hartner, S., McGirr, G., Schulte, M., & Lovell, D. (1991). Development of a disability measurement tool for juvenile rheumatoid arthritis: The Juvenile Arthritis Functional Assessment Report for children and their parents. *Arthritis and Rheumatism, 34,* 873–880.

Institute of Medicine. (1991). *Disability in America: Toward a national agenda for prevention.* Washington: National Academy Press.

Ireys, H., Anderson, G., Shaffer, T., & Neff, J. (1997). Expenditures for care of children with chronic illnesses enrolled in the Washington State Medicaid Program, Fiscal Year 1993. *Pediatrics, 100,* 197–204.

Ireys, H., Grason, H., & Guyer, B. (1996). Assuring quality of care for children with special health care needs in managed care organizations: Roles for pediatricians. *Pediatrics, 98,* 178–185.

Ireys, H. & Katz, S. (1996). The demography of disability and chronic illness in children. In R. Biehl, H. Wallace, J. MacQueen, & J. Blackman (Eds), *Children with disabilities and chronic illnesses: Challenges and solutions in community care.* Oakland, CA: Third Party Associates.

Ireys, H.T., & Nelson, R. (1992). New federal policy for children with special health care needs: Implications for pediatricians. *Pediatrics, 90,* 321–327.

Ireys, H., Salkever, D., Kolodner, K., & Bijur, P. (1996). Schooling employment, and idleness in young adults with chronic conditions. *Journal of Adolescent Health, 17,* 25–33.

Jeppson, E., & Thomas, J. (1995). *Essential allies: Families as advisors.* Bethesda, MD: Institute for Family-Centered Care.

Knowles, M., & Fernald, G. (1988). Diabetes and cystic fibrosis: New questions emerging from increased longevity. *Journal of Pediatrics, 112*, 415–416.

Kokkonen, J., Saukkonen, A.L., Timonen, E., Serlo, W., & Kinnunen, P. (1991). Social outcome of handicap children as adults. *Developmental Medicine and Child Neurology, 33*, 1095–1100.

Landgren, M., Pettersson, R., Kjellman, B., & Gillberg, C. (1996). ADHD, DAMP, and other neurodevelomental psychiatric disorders in 6-year-old children: Epidemiology and co-morbidity. *Developmental Medicine and Child Neurology, 38*, 891–906.

Lewis, C., Pantell, R., & Kieckhefer, G. (1989). Assessment of children's health status: Field test of new approaches. *Medical Care, 27*, S54–S70.

Manners, P., & Diepeveen, D. (1996). Prevalence of juvenile chronic arthritis in a population of 12-year-old children in urban Australia. *Pediatrics, 98*, 84–90.

Maternal and Child Health Bureau. (1997). *New definition of children with special health care needs.* Paper available from the MCH Bureau, Division of Integrated Services, Parklawn Building, 5600 Fishers Lane, Rockville, MD, 20857.

Moos, R., & Schaefer, J. (1984). The crisis of physical illness: An overview and conceptual approach. In R. Moos (Ed.), *Coping with physical illness 2: New perspectives.* New York: Plenum Press.

Msall, M., DiGaudio, K., Rogers, B., LaForest, S., Catanzo., N., Campbell, J., Wilczenski, F., & Duffey, L. (1994). The Functional Independence Measure for Children (WeeFIM). *Clinical Pediatrics*, 421–430.

Muldoon, J., Neff, J., & Gay, J. (1997). Profiling the health service needs of populations using diagnosis-based classification systems. *Journal of Ambulatory Care Management, 20 (3)*, 1–18.

Murphy, C., Yeargin-Allsopp, M., Decoufle, P., & Drews, C. (1995). The administrative prevalence of mental retardation in 10-year-old children in Metropolitan Atlanta, 1985 through 1987. *American Journal of Public Health, 85*, 319–323.

Neff, J. & Anderson, G. (1995). Protecting children with chronic illness in a competitive marketplace. *JAMA, 274*, 1866–1869.

Newacheck, P.W. (1989). Adolescents with special health needs: Prevalence, severity, and access to health services. *Pediatrics, 84*, 872–881.

Newacheck, P. (1994). Epidemiology of childhood chronic illnesses and disability. In H. Wallace, R. Nelson, & P. Sweeney (Eds.). *Maternal and child health practices, 4th edition*. Oakland, CA: Third Party Publishers.

Newacheck, P.W., Budetti, P.P., & Halfon, N. (1986). Trends in activity-limiting chronic conditions among children. *American Journal of Public Health, 76*, 179–184.

Newacheck, P., & Halfon, N. (1998). Prevalence and impact of disabling chronic conditions in childhood. *American Journal of Public Health, 88*, 610–617.

Newacheck, P., McManus, M., & Gepart, J. (1992). Health insurance coverage of adolescents: A current profile and assessment of trends. *Pediatrics, 90*, 589–596.

Newacheck, P.W., Stoddard, J.J., & McManus, M. (1993). Ethnocultural variations in the prevalence and impact of childhood chronic conditions. *Pediatrics, 91*, 1031–1039.

Newacheck, P.W., & Taylor, W.R. (1992). Childhood chronic illness: Prevalence, severity, and impact. *American Journal of Public Health, 82*, 364–371.

Office of Technology Assessment. (1987). *Technology-Dependent Children: Hospital v. Home Care — A Technical Memorandum.* Washington, DC: US Government Printing Office.

Ottenbacher, K., Taylor, E., Msall, M., Braun, S., Lane, S., Granger, C., Lyons, N., & Duffy, L. (1996). The stability and equivalence reliability of the functional independence measure for children (WeeFIM). *Developmental Medicine and Child Neurology, 38*, 907–916.

Palfrey, J.S., Walker, D.K., Haynie, M., Singer, J.D., Porter, S., Bushey, B., & Cooperman, P. (1991). Technology's children: Report of a statewide census of children dependent on medical supports. *Pediatrics, 87*, 611–618.

Palfrey, J.S., Haynie, M., Porter, S., Fenton, T., Cooperman-Vincent, P., Shaw, D., Johnson, B., Bierle, T., & Walker, D.K. (1994). Prevalence of medical technology assistance among children in Massachusetts in 1987 and 1990. *Public Health Reports, 109*, 226–233.

Patrick, D., & Deyo, R. (1989). Generic and disease-specific measures in assessing health status and quality of life. *Medical Care, 27*, S217–S232.

Perlin, E., Newacheck, P., Pless, I.B., Drotar, D., Gortmaker, S., Leventhal, J., Perrin, J., Stein, R., Walker, D., & Weitzman, M. (1993). Issues involved in the definition and classification of chronic health conditions. *Pediatrics, 91*, 787–793.

Perrin, J., Shayne, M., & Bloom, S. (1993). *Home and Community care for chronically ill children.* New York: Oxford University Press.

Perrin, J., & Stein, R. (1991). Reinterpreting disability: Changes in Supplemental Security Income for children. *Pediatrics, 88*, 1047–1051.

Pless, I., & Perrin, J. (1985). Issues common to a variety of illnesses. In N. Hobbs & J. Perrin (Eds.), *Issues in the care of children with chronic illnesses.* San Francisco: Jossey-Bass.

Pless, I., & Pinkerton, P. (1975). *Chronic childhood disorder: Promoting patterns of adjustment.* London: Henry Kimpton.

Roeleveld, N., Zielhuis, G., & Gabreels, F. (1997). The prevalence of mental retardation: A critical review of the literature. *Developmental Medicine and Child Neurology, 39*, 125–132.

Schidlow, D., & Fiel, S. (1990). Life beyond pediatrics: Transition of chronically ill adolescents from pediatric to adult health care systems. *Medical Clinics of North America, 74*, 1113–1120.

Starfield, B., Bergner, M., Ensminger, M., Riley, A., Ryan, S., Green, B., McGauhey, P., Skinner, A., & Kim S. (1993). Adolescent health status measurement: Development of the Child Health and Illness Profile. *Pediatrics, 91*, 430–435.

Starfield, B., Riley, A., Green, B., Ensminger, M., Ryan, S., Kelleher, K., Kim-Harris, S., Johnston, D., & Vogel, K. (1995). The adolescent Child Health and Illness Profile: A population-based measure of health. *Medical Care, 28*, 33, 553–566.

Stein, R., Coupey, S., Bauman, L., Westbrook, L., & Ireys, H. (1993). Framework for identifying children who have chronic conditions: The case for a new definition. *Journal of Pediatrics, 122*, 342–347.

Stein, R., Gortmaker, S., Perrin, E., Perrin, J., Pless, I., Walker, D., & Weitzman, M. (December 26, 1987). Severity of illness: Concepts and measurements. *Lancet*, 1506–1509.

Stein, R., & Jessop, D. (1982). A noncategorical approach to chronic childhood illness. *Public Health Reports, 97*, 354–362.

Stein, R., & Jessop, D. (1990). Functional Status II(R): A measure of child health status. *Medical Care, 28*, 1041–1055.

Stein, R., Westbrook, L., & Bauman, L. (1997). The questionnaire for identifying children with chronic conditions: A measure based on a noncategorical approach. *Pediatrics, 99*, 513–521.

Sullivan, S., & Olson, L. (1995). Developing condition-specific measures of functional status and well-being for children. *Clinical Performance and Quality Health Care, 3*, 132–139.

Waitzman, N., Romano, P., & Scheffler, R. (1994). Estimates of the economic expenditures of birth defects. *Inquiry, 33*, 188–205.

Wallander, J., Varni, J., Babani, L., Banis, H., & Wilcox, K. (1989). Family resources as resistance factors for psychological maladjustment in chronically ill and handicapped children. *Journal of Pediatric Psychology, 14*, 157–173.

Webb, E., Lobo., S., Hervas, A., Scourfield, J., & Fraser, W. (1997). The changing prevalence of autistic disorder in a Welsh health district. *Developmental Medicine and Child Neurology, 39*, 150–152.

Weitzman, M., Gortmaker, S., & Sobol, A. (1990). Racial, social, and environmental risks for childhood asthma. *American Journal of Diseases of Children, 144*, 1189–1194.

Westbrook, L., Silver, E., & Stein, R. (1998). Implications for estimates of disability in children: A comparison of definitional components. *Pediatrics, 101*, 1025–1030.

Wielinski, C., Budd, J., & Warwick, W. (1990). Measures of prognosis and survival for cystic fibrosis. *American Review of Respiratory Disease, 141*, A813–819.

Wissow, L., Gittelsohn, A., Szklo, M., Starfield, B., & Mussman, M. (1988). Poverty, race, and hospitalization for childhood asthma. *American Journal of Public Health, 78*, 777–782.

Yeargin-Allsopp, M., Drews, C., Decoufle, P., & Murphy, C. (1995). Mild mental retardation in black and white children in Metropolitan Atlanta: A case-control study. *American Journal of Public Health, 85*, 324–328.

Appendix A

THE NATIONAL HEALTH INTERVIEW (NHIS)
DISABILITY SUPPLEMENT

The 1994/95 National Health Interview (NHIS) Disability Supplement is the most comprehensive national survey on disability ever undertaken in the United States and the first ever to collect national population-based data on children with disabilities. The childhood component of the Disability Supplement is well suited for 1) identifying national prevalence rates for children with special needs, depending on the specific definition of "special needs", 2) identifying service needs and health outcomes for specific subgroups of this population, and 3) investigating links between disability and program participation. For these types of questions, these data are substantially more detailed than data from any other previous survey.

The NHIS Childhood Disability Supplement was administered in two phases. Phase I was administered at the same time as the NHIS core items to the 73,000 households in the total sample. It began in January 1994 and continued through December 1995. The Phase I instrument serves to identify children with special needs. For all children so identified, the core NHIS data are available. These data include condition onset, immunization status, health insurance, and basic demographic variables. There are a wide variety of disability-related survey items that could be used to identify children with disabilities and chronic illnesses, and so as a whole the data can be used to operationalize different conceptual definitions of the population.

Phase II was administered about 6 to 9 months after Phase I to 8,600 individuals under age 18 who were identified in Phase I as having a special need. It began in August 1994 and was completed in 1997. The Phase II instrument collects detailed data on family structure; home care; child care; use of medical and educational services, assistive devices, and related services; service coordination; impact of the illness on the family; child mental health; housing and transportation; physical activity limitations; and health insurance. The respondent for this survey was the parent or adult in the household who knew the most about the selected child's health.

The NHIS/CDS data has the potential to fill a major gap in knowledge about children with special needs. Previous data sets were limited by unrepresentative samples, narrow definitions of disability, severely limited number of variables, or combinations of these problems. It is important not to underestimate the value of the NHIS/CDS data set for families, program directors, and policy makers. The instruments used in both phases of the survey now are standards for the field because they were subjected to rigorous pre-testing and because they allow for multiple approaches to defining "special needs".

In addition, the extensive number of variables in Phase I and II instruments will yield estimates of prevalence, service use, and outcomes with levels of accuracy not previously possible. Weighted estimates of service use by subgroups of children with special needs can be calculated, such as home care services for school-aged children who require physical therapy. The number of questions related to national trends that can be addressed by the data will be limited more by a lack of awareness of what the data set contains than by any limitations within the data set or sampling frame itself.

The sampling frame used for the NHIS does not permit states to calculate state-specific rates of children with special needs. However, the data will allow for the calculation of rates within major racial and geographic subgroups, and states can use these rates to assist in adjusting national rates to gain estimates for specific states.

It is useful to understand the structure of the NHIS as a whole in order to locate potential items that are of relevance to particular purposes. The Phase I survey had a core section and five additional sections: The first core section includes the items used in previous NHIS surveys (with minor changes). These cover topics such as household composition, demographic data, the incidence of acute conditions, the prevalence of chronic conditions, restriction in activity due to chronic conditions, restriction in activity due to impairment or health problems, and utilization of health care services involving physician care and short-stay hospitalization. This is an important section because it provides critical background data, information on the specific conditions reported by the respondent, and, assessments of the limitations associated with the condition. Data from this section can be compared to previous years because the items are essentially the same as the NHIS core items used in prior years.

The five additional sections of the Phase I instrument are:

- immunizations
- Disability, with specific sections on

  - sensory, communication, and mobility
  - specific conditions
  - ADLs and IADLs
  - functional limitations
  - mental health
  - services and benefits
  - special health needs of children
  - early child development
  - special education services
  - respondent relationship to family members
  - perceived disability
  - etiology and duration of condition
- Family resources, with specific sections on
  - access to care
  - health care coverage
  - private plan coverage
  - income and assets
- Year 2000 objectives
- AIDS knowledge and attitudes

Chapter 6

QUALITY OF LIFE FROM A PATIENT GROUP PERSPECTIVE

Ulrike Ravens-Sieberer
Monika Bullinger

This chapter reviews applications of adult quality of life (QL) measures in clinical trials and how these may be applied to pediatric populations. It will begin with an overview of QL research given from a patient group perspective and then introduce the conceptual, methodological and practical problems of assessing QL in clinical trials. This will be followed by an overview of the available research on adult QL and concluded by a critical appraisal of the state of the art of QL research. The chapter then introduces pediatric QL research in a similar fashion, beginning with the current challenges, and proceeding to an overview of the research and lessons from pediatric oncology. The final discussion combines the areas of adult and pediatric research and gives recommendations for the further development of the field.

A BRIEF OVERVIEW OF THE QUALITY OF LIFE FIELD

In addition to changes in clinical symptomatology and the extension of the life span, the way in which chronically ill persons experience their health has gained importance as an outcome criterion for treatments in evaluations of the effect of medical interventions (Najman & Levine, 1981). The term quality of life (QL) brings this new approach to patient oriented outcomes to our attention. Although maintenance or improvement of QL in patients has traditionally been the goal of medical interventions, the attempt to explicitly include QL as a criterion in the choice and evaluation of treatments, rather than only implicitly considering it in the individual patient–physician contact, is new. The orientation towards QL as a concept reflects not only the prevalent skepticism concerning the relevance of classical clinical endpoints but is also a reflection of recent developments in the health care field. The increasing age of populations, for example, results in a larger proportion of potentially chronically ill patients needing long term treatment alongside a diminishing health care budget. Such changes in most of the health care systems world-wide and especially in the western industrialized nations, require a critical assessment of the state of the art of treatment in medial care (Patrick & Erickson, 1992).

Historically the QL concept was primarily used in political science as well as in the social science including sociology, politicology, anthropology, and psychology (Spilker, 1996). Relatively recently the term QL has been introduced into medicine. In contrast to sociological definitions, QL in medicine takes into account that medical interventions are specifically orientated at health-related aspects of human experience and behavior (Patrick & Erickson, 1992). The development of QL research in the medical area can be followed across the last few decades. The starting phase in the 1970s was characterized by philosophical publications concerning the question what QL is and whether it can be at all measured. In the 1980s, a more methodological approach to QL occurred with an increased effort to develop QL instruments. Since the beginning of the 1990s the third phase of QL research has been underway. A fourth phase of using QL data for quality assurance and health economic evaluation is just beginning. The development of health-related QL research in these years resulted in over 20,000 published articles on the conceptual basis, the methodological approaches of assessing QL and their application in different types of studies (Bullinger, 1997).

QUALITY OF LIFE RESEARCH FROM A PATIENT GROUP PERSPECTIVE

It is possible to distinguish four purposes for the use of QL research in medicine. The first purpose is to describe QL in specific populations in order to gain knowledge about these populations' well-being; results are relevant for health planners, epidemiologists, and developers of treatment strategies. The second purpose concerns the effects of treatments in comparative studies, especially in randomized controlled clinical trials; users are caregivers as well as health insurers. The third purpose concerns the use of QL indicators in health economics as related to prevention, treatment or rehabilitation; results are important for evaluations of health care systems. The fourth purpose concerns the establishment of medical outcome evaluation systems, in which several approaches to the measurement of clinical outcome, including QL, are implemented within routine care in order to exert online quality assurance regarding process and effect of health care.

The common denominator within these applications of QL research in medicine is that QL is viewed from a patient group perspective. The focus of the scientific attention is not on individual indicators for specific treatments from a QL perspective, nor the evaluation of treatment effects within the patient–physician interaction, nor a more structural evaluation of different care settings; it rather pertains to the question of how a specific patient group can be described in terms of treatment needs, treatment effects and treatment benefit so that recommendations for clinical care in these types of patient populations can be given (Furberg, 1985).

This is to be seen in conjunction with the new concept of so-called evidence based medicine. The term denotes the attempt to systematize published knowledge about the treatment in clinical conditions so that patient care is guided by empirically founded and scientifically sound treatment strategies which have been evaluated methodologically according to the state of the art. In order to be used for improved patient care, the evidence has to be accumulated from clinical trials.

THE CLINICAL TRIALS PHILOSOPHY

One of the main questions in the medical field is which treatment strategies are appropriate, or even optimal, for a given patient population. This is the objective of clinical studies, which can be ordered along a continuum of scientific merit. At the lower end are cross-sectional studies, in which comparison of a post treatment status of a patient group as compared to another is made to obtain information about a treatment effect. Obviously, even in cases in which the cohorts are matched according to main socio-demographic and clinical criteria, these evaluations do not allow us to relate group differences to underlying differences in treatment effects. More useful are longitudinal, observational studies, in which a population is assessed before and after treatment. However, time effects alone and not the treatment as such could affect the results, which is the reason why control groups are included in the study design. Unfortunately, if control groups and the experimental groups differ in certain character-istics (which have not been controlled for) the results are again questionable. Therefore the widely accepted and optimal approach to testing the effects of therapeutic interventions is a classical randomized controlled prospective clinical trial (in short "clinical trial" or RCT). Here, subjects are randomly allocated to different treatment arms from a basic cohort, with the option of so-called "blind" (patient does not know which medication she or he received) or "double-blind" settings (in which neither patient nor physician is informed about the type of treatment given). Approaches to quality assurance in clinical trials have reached an impressive sophistication within the past ten years and include standard operational procedures (SOP) explicitly formulated in study protocols, which guide the conduct and scientific analysis of the trials.

ASSESSING QUALITY OF LIFE IN ADULT CLINICAL STUDIES
THE CHALLENGE OF QUALITY OF LIFE RESEARCH IN ADULTS

Within adult QL research, several authors have addressed core questions which need to be answered as a prerequisite to the inclusion of QL measures in clinical trials (Aaronson, 1992). Basically these questions concern: the respondents (whom to ask), the dimensions (what to ask), the instruments (how to ask), the actual application (how to implement the measures), the statistical analyses (how to obtain results) and the interpretation of QL data (what it means). In relation to the respondents, the individual account of a subject's perceptions and evaluations is of utmost importance. Although there is an option of using external (expert) ratings of QL, these ratings are not identical to the person's self-report. Observer bias is a well known phenomenon in the social and behavioral sciences and the danger of such a bias is also present in external QL ratings. Basically, another person's perception in regard to the patient cannot be taken as a proxy, or equivalent information, but rather as a separate source of information about the patient's well-being. Several studies have shown that external assessments and internal assessments do differ. A clear preference towards using patient's self-report has been voiced in almost all relevant publications, however in cases in which self-report is difficult (e.g. in relation to psychiatric conditions or very young populations) it has been critically examined.

Dimensions of quality of life

There is a growing international consensus that QL is a multifactorial construct which should be assessed as such. It should at least encompass dimensions such as physical functioning, psychological well-being, social relations, and every day life functional capacity. Although a taxonomy of QL does not exist, these dimensions constitute the main body of QL assessments throughout the literature (Levine & Croog, 1984). The question of whether additional dimensions have to be added for specific purposes (such as sexuality, pain, or cognitive function) has been discussed and found to be a potentially useful addendum to the proposed standard measurements. The use of disease specific measurements has been advocated, especially for clinical trials, with the notion that such measurements are able to capture changes of well-being over time. However, generic measures have also been shown to pick up on such changes so that a combination of generic and disease specific measures in a modular fashion seems to be an appropriate way forward (Joyce, 1994).

Instruments

Over 800 QL instruments have been published in the literature, the majority of them concern QL in adults. Among them are measures such as the Nottingham Health Profile (Hunt et al., 1981), the WHOQOL questionnaire (Orley et al., 1994), the EUROQOL, and the SF-36 Health Survey, which have been translated, psychometrically tested and normed for representative populations over the years. The use of the SF-36 Health Survey (Stewart & Ware, 1992) has been widespread and established as a standard framework for QL research. Most of these generic questionnaires are internationally available (Bullinger et al., 1996). The SF-36 Health Survey assesses with 36 items eight dimensions of QL which can be reduced to two summary scores: mental health and physical health. A short form, the SF-12, is also available (Ware, 1990). In addition to well established generic questionnaires, disease specific questionnaires have been developed for various diseases and treatment settings which are also psychometrically tested and can be used in clinical trials (Bowling, 1991).

Application

As outlined by Koot (Chapter 1, this volume) each research question is associated with an optimal instrument type. From the patient group perspective and especially the clinical trials philosophy, it is important that instruments not only fulfill psychometric criteria, such as reliability and validity, but also fulfill the criterion of sensitivity to change or responsiveness. The likelihood of detecting changes and differences over time between treatment arms is dependent on the sensitivity of the instrument, which can be expressed as a form of criterion validity. Within psychometric testing procedures, most instruments have been tested for reliability and validity and increasingly are tested for sensitivity; a testing procedure which is dependent on longitudinal data, defined interventions and control groups. Basically, instruments should only be included in clinical trials if they have been tested for the psychometric criteria before and fulfill standard requirements.

In terms of design, it is recommended that QL be measured over time in clinical trials covering at least two points in time. It would be even more preferable for assessments to be made prior to the treatment phase as well as at follow-up after three, six and twelve months of treatment. It is important that both treatment and control groups receive identical QL questionnaires and that these are not biased in terms of their items for one or another treatment arm. Within the implementation it is important to address organizational matters such as making sure that the questionnaires are understood by the distributing staff, that patients are informed and motivated to participate in the study and that patient responses are closely measured. The problem here is that missing data cannot be included afterwards because patients cannot be relied on to recall their state of well-being during the prior time period. In addition to the above mentioned design considerations, such practical considerations are of utmost importance to ensure the proper collection of data (Walker & Rosser, 1991).

Statistical analysis of quality of life data

Descriptive statistics are often used to give a first overview over the QL data at the measure points. Depending on the nature of the trial, either analysis of variance techniques (MANOVA) or corresponding non parametric methods are used to analyze the data. Additional techniques include using QL information over a certain time period and calculating the time to, or the time spent in a certain QL state (survival analyses, Q-twist methods). A major problem with QL clinical trials data analysis is that periods of data may be missing due to censored observation or due to patient drop out. These require estimation procedures as well as that limitations of the measure points be included in the statistical analyses. There is a specific problem in relation to the statistical analyses of QL data in health economic data. Here, new methods can be used to obtain an index of QL which then can be used for weighing procedures in reference to survival or time to events (Gyatt et al., 1993).

Interpreting quality of life data

Interpretations of QL data include: comparisons with norm data (especially concerning age and gender matched reference populations), the change over time, improvement from before to after treatment, and the clinical meaning of QL data. Although statistical significance gives an insight into the robustness of QL results, this does not imply that statistically significant changes are also clinically meaningful (Lydick & Epstein, 1996). Few of the QL instruments include an interpretation guideline as to do personality tests or psychiatric symptomatology scales. The SF-36 Health Survey is one of the instruments in which a clinical interpretation according to the scale range from 0 to 100 is possible.

Another problem concerns the multidimensional nature of QL assessment. Contrary to endpoints in clinical trials, QL assessment necessitates the analysis of several indicators, which poses a statistical problem of multiple testing. Therefore QL endpoints are selected from a QL scale so that only one or two dimensions are considered relevant endpoints. These are also used for sample size estimation.

Ethics in quality of life research

Available QL approaches explicitly attempt to include the patient viewpoint in the evaluation of medical treatments. However, potential misuse of such data is possible in that indications for treatment might be unjustly tied to the QL level before treatment, e.g. in transplantation. In addition the QL concept is not value-neutral, it includes an implicit frame of reference in which subjective health is connected to reaching states of individually acceptable physical, psychological and social health. This might discriminate against populations with e.g. disabilities (Levine, 1996).

In general the QL clinical trials literature differs from the medical clinical trials literature. The willingness of the patients to actively participate in the study is important as is the continuous collection of data. Care has to be taken in the implementation and statistical analysis as well as interpretation of results, especially if they do not parallel clinical results.

The following paragraph deals with the clinical trials literature in the adult area developed so far and then proceeds to lessons from this literature.

A BRIEF OVERVIEW OF QUALITY OF LIFE RESEARCH IN ADULTS

A literature search regarding clinical studies published between 1991 and 1996 showed 154 listings of clinical studies including QL parameters (Bullinger, 1997). As compared to the first phases of QL research in which conceptual and principal methodological problems were in the foreground, this amount of clinical studies is remarkable. The papers can be classified according to the patient population or the therapeutic approaches chosen. In addition they also can be differentiated according to the study objectives and design, ranging from cross-sectional longitudinal studies evaluating the QL from before and after a treatment, to the randomized clinical trial in which two or more therapeutic trials are compared with each other. Most of the research in the adult clinical trial area has been performed in oncology and cardiology and more recently psychiatry. Other areas such as endocrinology or surgery are just beginning to include QL assessments. In addition to fundamental papers clinical trial groups have also devised guidelines and protocols on how to include QL assessments in clinical trial study protocols (e.g. Aaronson, 1992).

Oncology

Oncology has been one of the first disciplines to approach the topic of QL. This interest has been fueled by the question of whether an extension of life time for a few months by chemotherapeutic interventions in solid tumors is appropriate if the prognosis and expected therapeutic benefit are poor (Bullinger, 1991). From there, QL studies soon evolved around how to improve care for cancer patients. Most research has aimed at developing research instruments and their application in descriptive clinical studies. In this realm instruments such as the EORTC questionnaire (Aaronson et al., 1996), the FLIC questionnaire (Schipper & Clinch, 1996) and the FACT (Cella & Bonomi, 1996) are frequently used as well as the Rotterdam symptom-checklist (De Haes & van Knippenberg, 1987) and the QL in cancer care questionnaire (Padilla et al., 1996).

Initially, randomized clinical studies were primarily conducted by the large oncological clinical trials groups in North America as well as Europe (Huerny et al., 1992). In these study groups QL has been increasingly considered as an outcome parameter, e.g. in testing of chemotherapy regimens in patients with breast cancer (e.g. Kornblith et al., 1993), prostate cancer (e.g. Cleary et al., 1995) and lung cancer (e.g. Bleehen et al., 1993).

Cardiology

QL has also been quickly adopted in the study of cardiology (Bulpitt & Fletcher, 1994). In contrast to oncology where specific measurement instruments were developed, in cardiology existing instruments from public health research have been used. A classic study by Croog et al. (1986), in which a cohort of over 500 hypertensive men were treated with three different types of antihypertensive medications, has been widely discussed. A battery of measurement instruments derived from a multidimensional approach to QL assessment was used, showing the superiority of one medication in several of the documented QL areas.

Another major area featuring research in QL in clinical trials is that of coronary heart disease. A literature review shows that there are almost as many publications as in hypertension (Bulpitt & Fletcher, 1994). Specific new instruments have been developed (Brooks et al., 1994; Guyatt, 1993a) but also existing measures such as the Nottingham Health profile or the SF-36 Health Survey are widely used. Most clinical studies work with standardized generic measures, supplemented by a specific questionnaire (Wiklund et al., 1992; Guyatt, 1993a). For example, a placebo-controlled trial with 223 patients suffering from coronary heart disease showed an improvement of QL with the medication under study, but with no difference to the placebo group (Gundersen et al., 1995). One of the largest trials includes a study regarding left ventricular dysfunction in 5025 patients in which an improvement of QL due to Enalapril was reported (Rogers et al., 1994). In general the QL indicators for cardiovascular populations show that coronary heart disease is associated with a marked deterioration in QL which seems to be dependent on the NYHA classification and gender (Ekeberg et al., 1994).

Psychiatry and neurology

The topic of QL research is relatively recent in psychiatry, possibly due to a long-standing view that classical psychiatric instruments do already reflect the QL of patients. The focus however has mainly been on expert or external ratings of symptomatology; self-reported perceptions of patients have not been systematically included in psychiatric literature.

A recent review of assessment instruments in psychiatry relating to QL shows that a multitude of new inventories have been developed; however, these have mainly been constructed in the interview-form and are relatively time-consuming for the patients. New approaches to the assessment of QL from the patient-perspective are underway, e.g. in depression (Gregoire et al., 1994) or in schizophrenia (Naber et al., 1998). Studies into the QL of psychiatric patients during or after antidepressant treatment are few at present (Lonquist et al., 1994; Walker et al., 1995). QL assessment is also included as an outcome parameter in the behavioral treatment of anxiety and obsessive-compulsive behavior (Telch et al., 1995).

Several studies have addressed the QL of psychiatric patients descriptively. In one such study with 357 patients suffering from psychiatric disorders, a dramatic decrease in QL after disease onset in several relevant dimensions was reported (Massion et al., 1993). Spitzer et al. (1995), report a decrease in well-being as measured by the SF-36 in 1000 patients with affective and anxiety disorders as well as with alcoholism and eating disorders. In general, only a few QL oriented clinical trials are available in the psychiatric literature: the tendency to use patient interviews might be an obstacle for such studies.

In neurology, epilepsy as well as stroke have received much attention in terms of adult QL research. In epilepsy, development of specific measurement instruments has been performed (e.g. Wagner & Vickrey, 1995) including new developments such as the Epilepsy Scale (Wagner et al., 1995). Clinical studies in epilepsy, however, are rare and suggest that anti-epileptic medications with a better side effect profile are associated with better QL ratings (Dodrill et al., 1995).

Other conditions

Clinical studies have been reported in diabetology and in nephrology, especially in relation to the use of erythropoietin in dialysis patients (McMahon & Dawborn, 1992). Pain syndromes, especially headaches, have also been studied with regard to QL using the SF-36 Health Survey (e.g. Solomon et al., 1993). A recent study showed positive effects of sumatriptan treatment on headaches in terms of QL (Dahloef, 1995). In respiratory diseases, such as chronic obstructive pulmonary disease (COPD), progress has been made in terms of measurement development (Guyatt, 1993b) as well as clinical trials.

HIV-infection and AIDS is also a new area in which QL is assessed. Epidemiological studies show that in addition to severity of disease, unfavorable living conditions and financial problems contribute to a decreased QL in HIV-infected and AIDS patients (Cunningham et al., 1995). Instruments have been developed (Hays & Shapiro, 1992) and therapeutic studies have been conducted (Ganz et al., 1993). Gelber and colleagues (1992) for example, in a study of 700 patients comparing placebo to zidovudine, found increased adverse effects with the zidovudine group but also an improved QL and delayed disease progression. A consecutive study in 1338 patients supported these findings (Lenderking et al., 1994). Also erythropoietin showed positive effects on QL in 251 anemic patients with HIV-infection (Revicki et al., 1994).

In surgery, most studies relating to QL are available in gastrointestinal surgery, e.g. pouch reconstruction or hip replacement (Troidl et al., 1980, Cleary et al., 1993) as well as transplantation medicine (Rosenblum et al., 1993).

LESSONS FROM ADULT QUALITY OF LIFE RESEARCH

In these adult clinical areas, the QL studies have followed a certain pattern. First, theoretical and conceptual articles about QL assessment have been published followed by methodological work on the development of new assessment instruments or use of available ones. Cross-sectional and longitudinal clinical studies have followed to assess the QL impairments in specific patient populations, which as a recent literature review shows, is dramatic and also concerns a marked difference from the medical criteria. Clinical trials have only been conducted in several disease areas such as oncology, cardiovascular research and increasingly allergology and HIV-infection. Approaches in which multinational clinical study groups have joined efforts to produce state of the art study protocols to include QL assessment in clinical trials have been the most successfull.

To date, research cited in the area of adult QL shows that although trials have been conducted in oncology and especially in cardiovascular research, methods vary and study results are difficult to compare. Such diversity is disconcerting, especially since this has not been followed up in corresponding reviews of QL clinical trials in the adult area.

The work on adult QL highlights the importance for the pediatric area of developing appropriate instruments and recommendations for the implementation of QL outcomes within clinical trials, from the initial planning through to conducting and analyzing the study. Children's pediatric clinical trials will also benefit from additional recommendations on the issues of developmental change, the willingness of respondents to participate in a trial, and the ethical implications of research.

ASSESSING QUALITY OF LIFE IN CHILD CLINICAL STUDIES

While QL research on adults has progressed over the past years, health-related QL research on children is a recent field. As is the case in the adult area, but with a delay of about a decade, the development of child QL research has occurred in three phases. The first phase in the late 1980s was concerned with how to assess QL in children as a theoretical concept, especially with regard to differences from adult QL concepts. A second phase in the early 1990s, which is still going on, consists of constructing and developing QL measures for children. The third phase, which just recently began (about 1995) concerns the application of these measures in various clinical studies.

As in the adult area, the clinical research so far is centered around the description of quality of well-being in different populations of children, among them healthy children as well as children with oncological diseases, asthma, diabetes, epilepsy and other chronic conditions. Application of QL instruments in longitudinal studies to assess the effect of treatments is just beginning. Here the necessity emerges to re-evaluate psychometrically tested instruments, originally developed for descriptive studies, with attention to the measure's responsiveness as an instrument to be used in clinical trials. In terms of clinical trials, guidelines from the adult area have been used to address ways and modes for including QL assessments in pediatric clinical trials. Yet no clinical trial (to the knowledge of the authors) has been published in which the QL effects of interventions were tested and described. However, several study groups especially in oncology have begun to introduce QL assessment in their study protocols.

THE CHALLENGE OF QUALITY OF LIFE RESEARCH IN CHILDREN

As is the case for adult studies, the following areas need to be considered in relation to studies with children: respondents, dimensions, instruments, implementation, statistical analyses and interpretation of QL data (Landgraf & Abetz, 1997). On the issue of respondents, children's self-report is only possible from the age of six to eight years, or even later depending on the difficulty of the questions and answering modes. QL dimensions for children vary with the developmental stages and might, although in general the dimensions may be similar, be different in their operationalization across age. Much more work needs to be completed to identify relevant QL dimensions for children. In relation to QL instruments, several generic measures (especially from the Anglo-American literature) are available and disease specific instruments for children have been developed for asthma, oncology and other diseases. It is questionable whether instruments available for adults can be modified to correspond to children's needs. Innovative approaches are needed in terms of new assessment methods for children (such as "smileys" and "pictograms"; e.g. Christie et al., 1993), especially younger children. The assessment of parents is of special importance, however this should not be used as proxy but as additional information about the child's well-being. Such circular approaches to QL assessment as in asking parents how they think their children feel (as a measure of empathy) may be a way to operationalize children's QL and its change over time.

In terms of implementation in clinical trials, information from both patients and parents is necessary, and questions have to be formulated so that they are not regarded as intrusive.

A BRIEF OVERVIEW OF QUALITY OF LIFE RESEARCH IN CHILDREN

In a recent literature search incorporating over 20,000 articles on the QL topic from 1980 to 1994, 3050 articles relating to QL in children were found (Bullinger and Ravens-Sieberer, 1995a) which constitutes only thirteen percent of the QL publications for this time period. Using the search key "quality of life and child" resulted in 320 publications with a specific focus on QL in children as related to several medical areas. Of these 320 articles most publications regarded oncology or transplantation and fewer pertained to asthma, epilepsy, diabetes, rheumatism and other diseases. In terms of age, children in the age range from thirteen to eighteen years were most frequently studied, with children in the ages between six and twelve years and below being underrepresented. In terms of the type of study, most articles (52%) concerned theoretical and conceptual work, while empirical studies were less represented (33% disease specific, 6% generic) and 9% of the articles were devoted to developing and testing of instruments. Most of the instruments developed pertain to parent or external ratings of child well-being, whereas children's self-rating incorporates only 9% of the studies. In terms of assessment instruments, a wide variety of mostly English language questionnaires were identified, most of them generic in nature.

In these publications, 320 studies were identified in which at least one of three criteria were present: multi-dimensional assessment of the construct of health-related QL in children, randomized study with control group, and sample size over one hundred persons. Within these only five studies could be identified reflecting at least two of the above mentioned criteria, but no study which reflected all.

The literature search was repeated to include 1995 to 1997. In these years an increase was noted in articles relating to QL of children compared to the low percentage in the previous years. Over 50 articles have been published since 1995, some of which pertain to conceptual and theoretical issues in health-related QL assessment in children. The majority of articles however were on the development of disease specific instruments and the application of such instruments in clinical descriptive studies. In addition, the first reviews about the state of the art of QL assessment for children in asthma research and in oncology have been published.

Oncology

Pediatric oncology has achieved dramatic improvements in treatment, resulting in prolonged survival of children with cancer. The question of QL in oncological, pediatric populations is now being addressed and several pediatric oncology groups have assembled task forces for children's QL assessment in cancer.

One example of this is the "American Cancer Society workshop on QL in children's cancer and its implications for practice and research" (Reamann & Haase, 1996). This group stresses that QL assessment plays a vital part in the outcome of clinical trials in cancer; that QL relates to psychological, health and physical dimensions; that generic as well as disease specific measures should be used in trials; and that conceptual, methodological and practical efforts have to be made to bring forward QL assessment in pediatric oncology.

The QL research in the pediatric oncology group (POS) from 1991 to 1995 was reviewed by Bradlyn and Pollock (1996). Here the work group consisted of the pediatric co-operative groups (POG) and the children's cancer group (CCG) united to devise guidelines for a protocol driven treatment of the vast majority of children and adolescents in the United States diagnosed with a malignancy, and also including QL as an endpoint. For the children's cancer group (CCG), MacLean et al. (1996) have introduced three studies in which QL assessment will be incorporated in clinical trials, including bone marrow transplant in children with acute lymphatic leukemia and minimally invasive surgery in children with solid cancers.

In a review of QL assessment in pediatric oncology, Bradlyn et al. (1995) have analyzed seventy published reports of phase three clinical trials from the pediatric oncology group (1972–1991) and concluded that only 3% of these reports included QL data. The major finding was that there was a discrepancy in frequency between documentation of toxicity (75%) and that of QL (3%).

Most of the studies in oncology are cross-sectional. For example, one study included 25 patients under sixteen years who were treated for intracranial germ cell tumors and retrospectively questioned with regard to their QL. However in this cross-sectional study no established QL instrument was used (Kiltie et al., 1995). In a retrospective study, 67 children with CNS tumors were followed up and judged with regard to their QL, which was found to be low; however, again they did not use an established QL instrument (Slavc et al., 1994). In a long-term survival follow-up study of young children with medulla blastoma, 32 patients and their families were interviewed by telephone with regard to their QL. It was found that fewer psychological problems were prominent than before (Johnson et al., 1994).

More recently, an overview of measuring QL in pediatric oncology has been prepared by Eiser and Jenny (1996). One of the measures referred to is the comprehensive multi-attributive-system for classifying health states of survivors of childhood cancer developed by Feeny et al. (1992), which is an expert completed measure in the health economic tradition. Further work relates to the development and testing of such utility instruments as in the study by Glaser et al. (1997) in which 37 children, parents, doctors and physiotherapists completed health utility measures at home and in the clinic. There was no difference between the children's health state based on home and clinic assessment, however, there was high agreement between parent and patient and less agreement between doctors and physicians on subjective attributes. In a cross-sectional study, the QL of 168 survivors of childhood malignancy aged 16 to 35 years was compared to that of 129 matched normal controls using a health economic measure (Apajasalo et al., 1996). The survivors reported significantly higher levels of vitality and lower levels of distress, depression, discomfort, and sleeping problems than the controls.

In two longitudinal studies, children's and families' QL ratings were found to be high after pediatric liver transplantation (Stone et al., 1997). Another article referring to liver transplant patients QL in Japan also stresses the relatively high QL in this group (Kita et al., 1996).

Allergology

Although literature about the psychological sequelae of asthma is available, only few QL studies have been published. In a review article, Bender (1996) critically assesses the measurement of QL in pediatric asthma clinical trials. Using a MEDLINE-search, he identified nine measures of QL in asthma, only four of which referred to self-report. Stressing specific problems such as developmental changes, reading ability, adult assistance and differences in mothers' versus fathers' external ratings, recommendations to assess QL in asthma clinical trials are given. One of the more prominent measures is Christie's child centered disease specific questionnaire for living with asthma (Christie et al., 1993), which has been developed for different age spans, consists of 48 items and has been tested in 242 children with asthma as compared to a none asthma group of 214 age and gender matched control children. A second measure to assess QL in asthma is the pediatric asthma QL questionnaire by Juniper et al. (1996), containing 23 items which was tested in a longitudinal study involving asthmatic children in the age range of seven to seventeen years.

A descriptive study was carried out investigating 100 patients with moderate asthma, plus one parent for each patient, to determine the impact of the disease on day to day life. Using an interview method to cover respiratory symptoms and emotional function as well as activity limitations, the study found that pediatric populations find respiratory symptoms troublesome but do not consider asthma as the major disruption of their lives. For the parents, worry and concern about the disease and medications as well as inability to relieve the child's symptoms are a source of distress (Townsend et al., 1991).

Measuring QL for young children with asthma and their families was described by Usmann and Silberman (1996). Here eight measures to assess QL in asthmatic children are introduced, including one for the younger age range of four to seven years. The fact that existing health-related QL scales have not been used in intervention studies is stressed and problems of interpreting changes in QL data which may be changing independently from the clinical changes are critically discussed.

Another article relating to measures of QL in asthma (Richards & Hemstreet, 1994) discusses measurement issues in the adult area and goes on to describe QL measurement in children referring to generic measures (such as QWB, SF-36 Health Survey), functional measures, impact on family scales as well as several asthma specific measures for children. In the recommendations the authors stress that researchers should strive for samples that are representative of asthma in the general community and should take into account the possibility that the impact of the disease and asthma treatment on QL may be small. Methodo-logical problems are considered substantial and the development of measures separately for adults, adolescents and children is recommended.

An epidemiological study in which asthma knowledge, attitudes and QL were researched in a community survey of high school students (n = 4161) and their teachers (n = 1112), found that in 23% of the students suffering from asthma, moderate QL impairment was noticed especially in conjunction with strenuous exercise (Gibson et al., 1995).

Neurology and psychiatry

New questionnaires are being developed for QL assessment, such as the 17-D measure which is appropriate for children aged eight to eleven years and has been tested in healthy children and children with a chronic condition such as epilepsy (Apajasalo et al., 1996). Similar methodological developments include an 88-item instrument tested on 174 adolescents with spine deformities ranging in age from ten to twenty years (Climent et al., 1995).

Recently, descriptive studies have been reported on the QL of children with epilepsy (Wildrick et al., 1996). A QL assessment study was conducted on 25 families where children had undergone neurosurgery for epilepsy, using questionnaires and interviews for both parents and patients. Results indicated that QL dimensions improved after the intervention in terms of self-care, family life and school performance; these issues are also associated with higher life satisfaction (Yang et al., 1996). However this study was not controlled and did not use established QL instruments.

Studies with regard to child/adolescent psychiatric disorders have addressed post traumatic stress disorders (PTSD) and their effects on QL. In a cross-sectional study, involving 540 adolescents aged eighteen to twenty years were recruited from clinical and community samples and characterized according to the prevalent psychiatric disorders. It was found that PTSD had significant adverse effects on psychological, physical and social well-being especially as compared to major depression and alcohol abuse, which also affected negatively QL albeit in a different pattern (Clark et al., 1996).

In a longitudinal study on 64 adolescent headache sufferers, Langeveld et al. (1997) reported that changes in headache intensity and frequency were related to proportional changes in self-reported QL within all the QL domains of a newly developed questionnaire.

Other conditions

Within the published QL literature on children, pain, mental retardation, short stature, diabetes, spina bifida and urological incontinence have all been addressed. A generic QL questionnaire has been developed for adolescents between 12 and 18 years and was previously tested in two studies involving over 350 patients with good psychometric results

(Langeveld et al., 1996). For rhinoconjunctivitis a study in 83 patients suffering from the condition aged 12 to 17 years was conducted with regard to their actual symptoms which led to development of a condition-specific questionnaire (Juniper et al., 1994).

One of the first studies relating to QL in children with Crohn's gastrointestinal disease investigated 16 children aged 8 to 17 years using a newly developed questionnaire which describes the areas of impairment in terms of lack of energy and presence of stoma in the children (Rabett et al., 1996). Pediatric cochlear implant surgery has been the focus of a longitudinal study by Kelsay & Tyler, 1996, where parents reported post implantation benefits such as improved sound perception, speech perception and speech production. Three years later these effects remained stable and were assessed using a newly developed questionnaire.

Other chronic conditions that have been studied include; low birth weight infants (Harrison et al., 1996; Tyson & Broyles, 1996); children with mental retardation (Durkin, 1996; Raphael et al., 1996), and children in intensive care units (Schwerdt, 1996). In gastrointestinal disorders a surgical procedure was performed for children born with gastrointestinal dysfunction and found to be beneficial to QL, however this study used ad hoc assessments (Ellsworth et al., 1996).

An exploratory study investigated the QL of 51 Finnish adolescent diabetes patients between 13 and 17 years in an open interview study (Kyngas & Barlow, 1995).

A longitudinal study was published on the treatment of 96 short stature children (Pilpel et al., 1995). One of the first studies addressing liver transplantation in children that has been published is more exploratory in nature (Sokal, 1995).

LESSONS FROM PEDIATRIC QUALITY OF LIFE RESEARCH

Recent overviews of health-related QL measures for pediatric patients have appeared from Bullinger and Ravens-Sieberer (1996), Marra et al. (1996), Spieth and Harris (1996), Landgraf and Abetz (1997), Rosenbaum and Saigal (1996). These overviews focus on the instruments that are currently available for assessing QL and few have reviewed research results. This reflects the fact that instrument development (which is indeed much needed) has priority for original articles over that of clinical study. Most studies in the pediatric QL field have been cross-sectional, but there have also been a few longitudinal cohort studies.

To date, theoretical considerations in assessing the topic of QL in children have been confined to basic questions such as: the relevance of the QL concept for children, the dimensional equivalence of QL dimensions in adults and children, and developmental aspects and reliability of child self-report. In addition, the ability to reflect the role of external (proxy) ratings has to be critically examined (Landgraf, Ravens-Sieberer, & Bullinger, 1997).

Despite the increasing attention paid to research in pediatric QL assessment, few well validated instruments have been developed. Most instruments have been adapted from use with adults to use with children and where there are new instruments, these have been developed for specific clinical conditions.

The instruments available are often too long and not specific to age-group, disease entity, or cultural background and are not applicable to small children and infants. When developing QL instruments for small children under five years, emphasis should be placed on physical and developmental stages, temperament, and health related risk factors as well as parents' well-being. Assessment in children over five years should encompass functional capacity and well-being, as well as general health perception (Abetz 1997, personal communication).

The World Health Organization has stressed that measures should be child centered, self-reported, age-dependent and cross-culturally comparable (Gerhaz, Ravens-Sieberer, & Eiser 1998). The recommendation encourages coverage of the health enhancing aspects of QL and the use of a modular design for assessing core and supplemental disease specific dimensions of well-being and function. In general, the inclusion of children's cognitive concepts about health and illness, which is dependent on development and cultural settings, is important.

Factors that may hinder the development of child-specific measures are the assumption that children are relatively healthy anyway and the lack of consensus about normal behavior in children. The difficulty of integrating self- and external reports, as well as developmental changes over time, may also have impeded questionnaire construction. An ideal QL instrument should include generic scales in addition to specific modules depending on the type of chronic or acute disease, as well as different forms and numbers of items for different age levels according to the developmental stage. The inclusion of parent, physician and child perspectives is recommended, as well as setting considerations (e.g. in-patient, out-patient). For example one measure, the QL questionnaire for children (KINDL) was developed in an attempt to take into account these considerations. It is a 40-item child reported questionnaire which is now available in forms for different ages which can be completed by children, parents, or physicians. These external ratings are not developed as proxy measures but as a measure of empathy of, for example, a parent's empathy for their child's function and well-being (Ravens-Sieberer et al., 1998). Descriptive empirical research on QL in children using different measures, e.g. the KINDL, shows that QL dimensions in children are highly correlated and that ratings of QL in children are positive. Chronically ill children do not necessarily differ from healthy children and psychosocial factors explain a high proportion of QL variance. Results also suggest that younger children respond to QL questions in an 'all or none' fashion and that adaptation of adult instruments is possible only from the age of 14 years onward.

The literature overview also shows that the methodological quality of the clinical studies is still preliminary and sub-optimal. One reason for this is the small sample sizes, which are often the basis of comparative studies, such as comparing QL of children with asthma versus epilepsy. Research questions can also be limited in sophistication and this is reflected in the corresponding research design. No clinical trial result referring to children's QL has yet been published, although personal contact with researchers in the area has verified that there are several studies planned and ongoing. The results of QL research relevant to clinical problems are scarce and increased research efforts are needed to give a comprehensive overview.

DISCUSSION

In spite of the large number of articles dealing with QL research, especially in the adult area, very few examples of the inclusion of QL measures in clinical trials are available. Given the history of discussion of QL in the medical field and the increase in publication activity since 1974, the number of published studies which refer to inclusion of QL measures in adult clinical trials is disappointing. Although single reports are available from, for example, oncology, cardiology and surgery, these studies are very often limited by a small sample size, by the use of different instruments to assess QL and by poor study design. Furthermore, these few studies have not been subjected to review, nor are meta-analytical results available which would help to evaluate the methodological quality and the outcome of the QL concept in clinical trials. This is astonishing, since in adult oncology, for example, and especially in breast cancer, the efforts of the national oncological study groups which have in part included QL in their trial protocols should be available. In the area of research on adults, guidelines have been produced for the inclusion of QL measures in clinical trials, however, these do not seem to have been followed in practice. These guidelines originate from consensus conferences on the specific methodology to be used in terms of planning, conducting and statistically analysing of trials.

Recommendations on how to include QL measures in clinical trials differ from general guidelines on how to conduct clinical trials in their specific focus on the choice of assessment methodology, the time points of assessment and the self-report nature of the measure. The formulation of a priori research hypotheses is also important in order that sample sizes can be calculated and statistical analysis performed. Compared with the general guidelines on conducting clinical trials, the QL guidelines consider the fact that the patients' response is of utmost importance. Practical problems of including QL assessments in clinical trials include: the willingness of respondents to participate in the study, the willingness of physicians to distribute the forms (the most prevalent organizational problem as patient response is usually more favorable than anticipated), and problems with dropouts and missing data. In addition, statistical considerations of how to analyze QL data in relation to the clinical data collected, or in relation to the survival times, have been addressed. Here, recommendations for weighing the survival time with the QL have been proposed in relation to the so-called Qualy (Quality Adjusted Life Years) concept. Use of QL assessment in clinical trials to evaluate the health economic effect of an intervention has only recently begun.

Compared with the adult area, the children's QL field is still in the first phase of selecting and developing instruments for use in pediatric QL research. QL measures have been included in clinical studies, however studies are mainly oriented towards a description of the QL of certain populations before or after treatment using a cross-sectional approach. Thus, from a patient group perspective the pediatric QL work so far primarily consists of basic studies to describe dimensions of well-being and functioning in different populations, usually with a relatively small sample size. Cohort studies or longitudinal studies into the effects of intervention on children are beginning to be published, but to date there have been no clinical trials in the child pediatric area.

Recent reviews have addressed the current state of instrument development as well as the results of preliminary descriptive studies.

However, publications regarding the way to implement QL instruments in clinical pediatric trials are available. With the exception of the need to consider the developmental stage of the respondents and the problem of self-report, these do not differ widely from what has been recommended for adult areas. This, however, might reflect the fact that specific demands of QL assessment in pediatric clinical trials have not been appropriately anticipated. For example, the problem of motivating children especially to use self-report measures, as well as the question of how to analyze data from children's, and parents' self-report, or even to include the medical staff perspective, have not been described. Further clarification is also needed on the comparability of measures across different developmental states.

There are problems in implementing QL research that are specific to the instruments themselves. There are only a few self-report instruments available. In clinical trials it has been recommended that adult measures be included for the parents' assessment of their own QL, as well as for assessment of the children's QL. The use of proxy measures has been intensively discussed and criticized because of the disparity between self-report and external ratings which is known from the adult literature. However, it has been suggested that a measure be developed in which the parents do not give their perspective of the child's well-being but try to express how they think the child feels (a more emphatic or circular way of describing the child). One of the main concerns of QL research in children is the comparability of measures taken over developmental phases and also between child and parent assessments. Without such comparability, it will be difficult to include QL measures in clinical trials because age span or respondent choice would severely influence the results. Further research is needed into the changes of QL over different ages, and the corresponding measures accommodating those changes in terms of internal validity, as well as the correspondence between parental and children's QL as a form of external validity.

Another problem, not only specific to pediatric clinical trials, is the willingness of children and parents to participate in such studies. In the pediatric area, randomization is an especially sensitive issue because the parents have to make a choice whether or not the child should be taking part in a clinical trial in which the likelihood that is does not receive the medication which parents feel to be helpful is 50%. This leads to the ethics of QL assessment in children and the problem of randomization in general. Ethical issues pertain not only to the recruitment into clinical trials but also to the analysis and interpretation of that data. A further point concerns the sample sizes. Since several childhood diseases, especially childhood leukemia in the oncological area, represent rare clinical conditions, multi-center studies have to be performed in order to obtain the sample size necessary for data analysis. Such multi-center trials in the pediatric area involve even more organizational ground work than in the adult area because not only the children but also their parents have to be introduced to the procedures and cared for during the trial. The acceptance of QL measures, especially in these cases, is of the utmost importance and needs to be more clearly addressed and researched.

In terms of health economic uses of QL data, some of the utility based approaches maybe problematic in their use in childhood. It seems necessary to establish a way to derive indices from psychometrically based QL instruments rather than asking for preferences which, especially in children's self-report, might be a cognitively difficult task for children and an emotionally difficult task for the parents. The literature in the adult clinical trials area has produced methodological recommendations and results from clinical studies, however, these can only be principally used as guidelines for research in pediatric clinical trials. The next necessary step is the development of appropriate instruments and guidelines for implementation of these instruments in clinical trials in the pediatric area. Emphasis should be given to devising instruments of a modular structure which reflect developmental changes as well as patients' and parents' reports.

The most important things to learn from the research on adult QL when developing work on QL in children are the need for theory-based work, the need to methodologically evaluate (especially psychometric properties), and the need to develop appropriate instruments. Much of these aspects have been developed in the adult area and can be implemented in pediatric trials. Education of medical personnel and information from parents and children about the quality of medical personnel are necessary steps in the process. For the conceptual, methodological and practical work on QL assessment in clinical trials, more research efforts are needed along with adequate sponsoring of such studies.

QL is now considered an important endpoint in clinical trials and it may soon be considered the main relevant endpoint, therefore QL researchers as well as pediatricians need to cooperate to address this challenge.

References

Aaronson, N.K. (1992). Assessing the quality of life of patients in cancer clinical trials: Common problems and common sense solutions. *European Journal of Cancer, 28A*, 1304–1307.

Apajasalo, M., Rautonen, J., Holmberg, C. et al. (1996). Quality of life in pre-adolescence: A 17-dimensional health-related measure (17D). *Quality of Life Research, 5*, 532–538.

Apajasalo, M., Sintonen, H., Siimes, M.A., Hovi, L., Holmberg, C., Boyd, H., Makela, A., & Rautonen, J. (1996). Health-related quality of life of adults surviving malignancies in childhood. *European Journal of Cancer, 32A*, 1354–1358.

Bender, B.G. (1996). Measurement of quality of life in pediatric asthma clinical trials. *Annals of Allergy, Asthma, and Immunology, 77*, 438–447.

Bleehen, N.M., Girling, D.J., Machin, D., & Stephens, R.J. (1993). A randomised trial of three or six courses of etoposide cyclophosphamide methotrexate and vincristine or six courses of etoposide and ifosfamide in small cell lung cancer. II: Quality of life medical research council lung cancer working group. *British Journal of Cancer, 68*, 1157–1166.

Bowling, A. (1991). *Measuring health: A review of quality of life measurement scales.* Philadelphia: Open University Press.

Bradlyn, A.S., Harris, C.V., & Spieth, L.E. (1995). Quality of life assessment in pediatric oncology: A retrospective review of phase III reports. *Social Science and Medicine, 41*, 1463–1465.

Bradlyn, A.S., & Pollock, B.H. (1996). Quality of life research in the pediatric oncology group: 1991–1995. *Journal of the National Cancer Institute Monography, 20*, 49–53.

Bradlyn, A.S., Ritchey, A.K., Harris, C.V., Moore, I.M., O'Brien, R.T., Parsons, S.K., Patterson, K., & Pollock, B.H. (1996). Quality of life research in pediatric oncology: Research methods and barriers. *Cancer, 78*, 1333–1339.

Brooks, M.N., Gorkin, L., Schron, E.B., Wiklund, I., Campion, J., & Ledingham, R.B. (1994). Moricizine and quality of life in the cardiac arrhythmia suppression trials II (CAST II). *Controlled Clinical Trials, 15*, 437–449.

Bullinger, M. (1991). Quality of life — definition, conceptualization and implications: A methodologist's view. *Theoretical Surgery, 6*, 143–148.

Bullinger, M., Power, M.J., Aaronson, N.K., Cella, D.F., & Anderson, R.T. (1996). Creating and evaluating cross-cultural instruments. In B. Spilker (Ed.), *Quality of life and pharmacoeconomics in clinical trials* (pp. 659–668). Philadelphia: Lippincott-Raven.

Bullinger, M. (1997). Gesundheitsbezogene lebensqualität und subjektive gesundheit [Health-related quality of life and subjective health]. *Psychotherapie, Psychosomatik, Medicinische Psychologie, 47*, 76–91.

Bullinger, M., & Ravens-Sieberer, U. (1995). Health-related quality of life assessment in children: A review of the literature. *European Review of Applied Psychology, 45*, 245–254.

Bullinger, M., & Ravens-Sieberer, U. (1995). General principles, methods and areas of application of quality of life research in children. *Praxis der Kinderpsychologie und Kinderpsychiatrie, 44*, 391–399.

Bulpitt, C.J., & Fletcher, A.E. (1994). Quality of life and the heart: Evaluation of therapeutic alternatives. *British Journal of Clinical Practice*, Suppl. 73, 18–22.

Cella, D.F., & Bonomi, A.E. (1996). The functional assessment of cancer therapy (FACT) and functional assessment of HIV infection (FAHI) quality of life measurement system. In B. Spilker (Ed.), *Quality of life and pharmacoeconomics in clinical trials* (pp. 203–214). Philadelphia: Lippincott-Raven.

Christie, M.J., French, D.J., Sowden, A., & West, A. (1993). Development of child-centered disease-specific questionnaires for living with asthma. *Psychosomatic Medicine, 55*, 541–548.

Clark, D.B., & Kirisci, L. (1996). Posttraumatic stress disorder, depression, alcohol use disorders and quality of life in adolescents. *Anxiety, 2*, 226–233.

Cleary, P.D., Morrissey, G., & Oster, G. (1995). Health-related quality of life in patients with advanced prostate cancer: A multinational perspective. *Quality of Life Research, 4*, 207–220.

Cleary, P.D., Reilly, D.T., Greenfield, S., Mulley, A.G., Wexler, L., Frankel, F., & McNeil, B.J. (1993). Using patient reports to assess health-related quality of life after total hip replacement. *Quality of Life Research, 2*, 3–11.

Climent, J.M., Reig, A., Sanchez, J., & Roda, C. (1995). Construction and validation of a specific quality of life instrument for adolescents with spine deformities. *Spine, 20*, 2006–2011.

Cowley A.J., & Skene, A.M. (1994). Treatment of severe heart failure: Quantity or quality of life? A trial of enoximone. *British Heart Journal, 72*, 226–230.

Croog, S.H., Levine, S., & Testa, M.A. (1986). The effect of antihypertensive therapy on the quality of life. *New England Journal of Medicine, 314*, 1657–1664.

Cunningham, W.E., Hays, R.D., Williams, K.W., Beck, K.C., Dixon, W.J., & Shapiro, M.F. (1995). Access to medical care and health-related quality of life for low-income persons with symptomatic human immunodeficiency virus. *Medical Care, 33*, 739–754.

Dahloef, C.G. (1995). Health-related quality of life under six month treatment of migraine: An open clinic-based longitudinal study. *Cephalalgia, 15*, 414–422.

De Haes, I., & van Knippenberg, F. (1987). Quality of life of cancer patients: Review of literature. In N.K. Aaronson, & J.H. Beckman (Eds.), *The quality of life of cancer patients* (pp. 176–183). New York: Raven Press.

Dodrill, C.B., Arnett, J.L., Sommerville, K.W., & Sussman, N.M. (1995). Effects of differing dosages of vigabatrin (Sabril) on cognitive abilities and qualities of life in epilepsy. *Epilepsia, 36*, 164–173.

Durkin, M.S. (1996). Beyond mortality: Residential placement and quality of life among children with mental retardation. *American Journal of Public Health, 86*, 1359–1361.

Eiser, C., & Jenney, M.E. (1996). Measuring symptomatic benefit and quality of life in paediatric oncology. *British Journal of Cancer, 73*, 1313–1316.

Ekeberg, O., Klemsdal, T.O., & Kjeldsen, S.E. (1994). Quality of life on enalapril after acute myocardial infarction. *European Heart Journal, 15*, 1135–1139.

Ellsworth, P.I., Webb, H.W., Crump, J.M., Barraza, M.A., Stevens, P.S., & Mesrobian, H.G. (1996). The malone antegrade colonic enema enhances the quality of life in children undergoing urological incontinence procedures. *Journal of Urology, 155*, 1416–1418.

Feeny, D., Furlong, W., Barr, RD., Torrance, G.W., Rosenbaum, P. & Weitzman S. (1992). A comprehensive multiattribute system for classifying the health status of survivors of childhood cancer. *Journal of Clinical Oncology, 10*, 923–928.

Furberg, C.D. (1985). Assessment of quality of life. In L. Friedman, C. Furberg, & D. Demets (Eds.), *Fundamentals of clinical trials*. Littletown: PSG Publishing.

Ganz, P.A., Coscarelli Schag, C.A., Kahn, B., Petersen, L., & Hirji, K. (1993). Describing the health-related quality of life impact of HIV infection: Findings from a study using the HIV overview of problems — evaluation system (HOPES). *Quality of Life Research, 2*, 109–119.

Gelber, R.D., Lenderking, W.R., Cotton, D.J., Cole, B.F., Fischl, M.A., Goldhirsch, A., & Testa, M.A. (1992). Quality of life-evaluation in a clinical trial of zidovudine therapy in patients with mildly symptomatic HIV infection. The AIDS Clinical Trials Group. *Annals of Internal Medicine, 116*, 961–966.

Gerharz, E.W., Ravens-Sieberer, U., & Eiser, C. (1997). Kann man lebensqualität bei kindern messen? [Can you measure quality of life in children?] *Zeitschrift für Aktuelle Urologie, 28*, 355–363.

Gibson, P.G., Henry, R.L., Vimpani, G.V., & Halliday, J. (1995). Asthma knowledge, attitudes, and quality of life in adolescents. *Archives of Diseases in Childhood, 73*, 321–326.

Glaser, A.W., Davies, K., Walker, D., & Brazier, D. (1997). Influence of proxy respondents and mode of administration on health status assessment following central nervous system tumours in childhood. *Quality of Life Research, 6*, 43–53.

Gregoire, J., de Leval, N., Mesters, P., & Czarka, M. (1994). Validation of the quality of life in depression scale in a population of adult depressive patients aged 60 and above. *Quality of Life Research, 3*, 13–19.

Gundersen, T., Wiklund, I., Swedberg, K., Amtorp, O., Remes, J., & Nilsson, B. (1995). Effects of 12 weeks of ramipril treatment on the quality of life in patients with moderate congestive heart failure: Results of a placebo-controlled trial. Ramipril Study Group. *Cardiovascular Drugs Therapy, 9*, 589–594.

Guyatt, G.H. (1993a). Measurement of health-related quality of life in heart failure. *Journal of the American College of Cardiology, 22* , 185A–191A.

Guyatt, G.H. (1993b). Measurement of health-related quality of life in chronic airflow limitation. *Monaldi Archives of Chest Disease, 48*, 554–557.

Guyatt, G.H., Feeny, D.H., & Patrick, D.L. (1993). Measuring health-related quality of life. *Annals of Internal Medicine, 118*, 622–629.

Harrison, H. (1996). Extremely low-birth-weight infants at adolescence: Health status and quality of life. *JAMA, 276*, 1722–1723.

Hays, R.D., & Shapiro, M.F. (1992). An overview of generic health-related quality of life measures for HIV research. *Quality of Life Research, 1*, 91–97.

Huerny, C., Bernhard, J., Joss, R., Willems,Y., Cavalli, F., Kiser, J., Brunner, K., Favre, S., Alberto, P., Glaus, A., et al. (1992). Feasibility of quality of life assessment in a randomized phase III trial of small cell lung cancer: A lesson from the real world — The Swiss Group for Clinical Cancer Research SAKK. *Annals of Oncology, 3*, 825–831.

Hunt, S.M., McEwen, J., McKenna, S.P., Williams, J., & Papp, E. (1981). The Nottingham Health Profile: Subjective health status and medical consultations. *Social Science and Medicine, 15A*, 221–229.

Johnson, D.L., McCabe, M.A., Nicholson, H.S., Joseph, A.L., Getson, P.R., Byrne, J., Brasseux, C., Packer, R.J., & Reaman, G. (1994). Quality of long-term survival in young children with medulloblastoma. *Journal of Neurosurgery, 80*, 1004–1010.

Joyce, C.R. (1994). Health status or quality of life: Which matters to the patient? *Journal of Cardiovascular Pharmacology, 23*, S26–S33.

Juniper, E.F., Guyatt, G.H., & Dolovich, J. (1994). Assessment of quality of life in adolescents with allergic rhinoconjunctivitis: Development and testing of a questionnaire for clinical trials. *Journal of Allergy and Clinical Immunology, 93*, 413–423.

Juniper, E.F., Guyatt, G.H., Feeny, D.H., Ferrie, P.J., Griffith, L.E., & Townsend, M. (1996). Measuring quality of life in children with asthma. *Quality of Life Research, 5*, 35–46.

Kelsay, D.M., & Tyler, R.S. (1996). Advantages and disadvantages expected and realized by pediatric cochlear implant recipients as reported by their parents. *American Journal of Otology, 17*, 866–873.

Kiltie, A.E., & Gattamaneni, H.R. (1995). Survival and quality of life of paediatric intracranial germ cell tumour patients treated at the Christie Hospital, 1972–1993. *Medical Pediatric Oncology, 25*, 450–456.

Kita, Y., Ishimaru, Y., Sugimoto, N., Gotoh, M., Sakon, M., & Monden, M. (1996). Quality of life in children undergoing liver transplants overseas or in Japan. *Transplant Procedures, 28*, 2406–2408.

Kornblith, A.B., Hollis, D.R., Zuckerman, E., Lyss, A.P., Canellosd, G.P., Cooper, M.R., Herndon, J.E., Phillips, C.A., Abrams, J., Aisner, J. et al. (1993). Effect of megestrol acetate on quality of life in a dose-response trial in women with advanced breast cancer — The Cancer and Leukemia Group. *British Journal of Clinical Oncology, 11*, 2081–2089.

Kyngas, H., & Barlow, J. (1995). Diabetes: An adolescent's perspective. *Journal of Advanced Nursing, 22*, 941–947.

Landgraf, I., Abetz, L., & Ware, I. (1997). *Child health questionaire (CHQ): A user's manual.* Boston: The Health Institute Press.

Landgraf, J., Ravens-Sieberer, U., & Bullinger, M. (1997). Quality of life research in children. *Dialogues in Pediatric Urology, 20 (11).*

Langeveld, J.H., Koot, H.M., Loonen, M.C., Hazebroek-Kampschreur, A.A., & Passchier, J. (1996). A quality of life instrument for adolescents with chronic headache. *Cephalalgia, 16*, 183–196.

Langeveld, J.H., Koot, H.M., & Passchier, J. (1997). Headache intensity and quality of life in adolescents: How are changes in headache intensity in adolescents related to changes in experienced quality of life? *Headache, 37*, 37–42.

Lenderking, W.R., Gelber, R.D., Cotton, D.J., Cole, B.F., Goldhirsch, A., & Volberding, P.A. (1994). Asymptomatic human immodeficiency virus infection. The AIDS clinical trials group. *New England Journal of Medicine, 330*, 738–743.

Levine, R.J. (1996). Quality of life assessments in clinical trials: An ethical perspective. In B. Spilker (Ed.), *Quality of life and pharmacoeconomics in clinical trials* (pp. 489–496). Philadelphia: Lippincott-Raven.

Levine, S., & Croog, S.H. (1984). What constitutes quality of life? A conceptualization of the dimension of life quality in healthy populations and patients with cadiovascular disease. In N. Wenger, M. Mattson, C. Furberg, & J. Ellison (Eds.), *Assessment of quality of life in clinical trials of cardiovascular therapies* (pp. 44–66). New York: Le Jacq.

Lonqvist, J., Sintonen, H., Syvaelahti, E., Appelberg, B., Koskinen, T., Mannikko, T., Methonen, O.P., Naarala, M., Sihvo, S., Auvinen, J. et al. (1994). Antidepressant efficacy and quality of life in depression: A double-blind study with moclobemide and fluoxetine. *Acta Psychiatrica Scandinavia, 89*, 363–369.

Lydick, E.G., & Epstein, R.S. (1993). Interpretation of quality of life changes. *Quality of Life Research, 2*, 221–226.

Lydick, E.G., & Epstein, R.S. (1996). Clinical significance of quality of life data. In B. Spilker (Ed.), *Quality of life and pharmacoeconomics in clinical trials* (pp. 461–466). Philadelphia: Lippincott-Raven.

MacLean, W.E. Jr. (1996). Children's cancer group (CCG). *Journal of the National Cancer Institute Monography, 20*, 87–88.

Marra, C.A., Levine, M., McKerrow, R., & Carleton, B.C. (1996). Overview of health-related quality-of-life measures for pediatric patients: application in the assessment of pharmacotherapeutic and pharmacoeconomic outcomes. *Pharmacotherapy, 16*, 879–888.

Massion, A.O., Warshaw, M.G., & Keller, M.B. (1993). Quality of life and psychiatric morbidity in panic disorder and generalized anxiety disorder. *American Journal of Psychiatry, 150*, 600–607.

McMahon, L.P., & Dawborn, J.K. (1992). Subjective quality of life assessment in hemodialysis patients at different levels of hemoglobin following use of recombinant human erythropoietin. *American Journal of Nephrology, 12*, 162–169.

Naber, D. (1998). Subjective experiences of schizophrenic patients treated with antipsychotic medication. *International Clinical Psychopharmacology, 13*, 41–45.

Najman, J.M., & Levine, S. (1981). Evaluating the impact of medical care and technology on quality of life: A review and critique. *Social Science and Medicine, 15*, 107–115.

Orley, J. and the WHOQOL-Group (1994). The development of the WHO quality of life assessment instruments (The WHOQOL). In J. Orley, & W. Kuyken (Eds.), *Quality of life assessment: International perspectives* (pp. 41–57). Berlin: Springer Verlag.

Padilla, G.V., Grant, M.M., Ferrell, B.R., & Pressant, C.A. (1996). Quality of life — cancer. In B. Spilker (Ed.), *Quality of life and pharmacoeconomics in clinical trials* (pp. 301–308). Philadelphia: Lippincott-Raven.

Patrick, D.L., & Erickson, P. (1992). Health status and health policy. New York: Oxford University Press.

Pilpel, D., Leiberman, E., Zadik, Z., & Carel, C.A. (1995). Effect of growth hormone treatment on quality of life of short-stature children. *Hormone Research, 44*, 1–5.

Rabbett, H., Elbadri, A., Thwaites, R., Northover, H., Dady, I., Firth, D., Hillier, V.F., Miller, V., & Thomas, A.G. (1996). Quality of life in children with Crohn's disease. *Journal of Pediatric Gastroenterology and Nutrition, 23*, 528–533.

Raphael, D., Brown, I., Rukholm, E., & Hill-Bailey, P. (1996). Adolescent health: Moving from prevention to promotion through a quality of life approach. *Canadian Journal of Public Health, 87*, 81–83.

Ravens-Sieberer, U., & Bullinger, M. (1998). Assessing the health related quality of life in chronically ill children with the German KINDL: First psychometric and content analytical results. *Quality of Life Research, 7*, 399–407.

Reaman, G.H., & Haase, G.M. (1996). Quality of life research in childhood cancer. The time is now. *Cancer, 78*, 1330–1332.

Revicki, D.A., Brown, R.E., Henry, D.H., McNeill, M.V., Rios, A., & Watson, T. (1994). Recombinant human erythropoietin and health-related quality of life of AIDS patients with anemia. *Journal of AIDS, 7*, 474–484.

Richards, J., & Hemstreet, M.P. (1994). Measures of life quality, role performance, and functional status in asthma research. *American Journal of Respiratory and Critical Care Medicine, 149,* S31–S39.

Rogers, W.J., Johnstone, D.E., Yusuf, S., Weiner, S.H., Gallagher, P., Bittner, V.A., Ahn, S., Schron, E., Shumaker, S.A., & Sheffield, L.T. (1994). Quality of life among 5025 patients with left ventricular dysfunction randomized between placebo and enalapril: The studies of left ventricular dysfunction. The SOLVD Investigators. *Journal of the American College of Cardiology, 23,* 393–400.

Rosenbaum, L.P., & Saigal, S. (1996). Measuring health-related quality of life in pediatric populations: Conceptual issues. In B. Spilker (Ed.), *Quality of life and pharmacoeconomics in clinical trials* (pp. 793–802). Philadelphia: Lippincott-Raven.

Rosenblum, D.S., Rosen, M.L., Pine, Z.M., Rosen, S.H., & Borg-Stein, J. (1993). Health status and quality of life following cardiac transplantation. *Archives of Physical Medicine Rehabilitation, 74,* 490–493.

Schipper, H., Clinch, J.J., & Olweny, Ch.L.M. (1996). Quality of life studies: Definition and conceptual issues. In B. Spilker (Ed.), *Quality of life and pharmacoeconomics in clinical trials* (pp. 11–24). Philadelphia: Lippincott-Raven.

Schwerdt, M. (1996). Growing up on the intensive care unit: Results of a survey on quality of life of long-term ventilated children on intensive care units. *Medizinische Klinik, 91,* 53–55.

Slavc, I., Salchegger, C., Hauer, C., Urban, C., Oberbauer, R., Pakisch, B., Ebner, F., Schwinger, W., Mokry, M., Ranner, G., et al. (1994). Follow-up and quality of survival of 67 consecutive children with CNS tumors. *Children's Nervous System, 10,* 433–443.

Sokal, E.M. (1995). Quality of life after orthotopic liver transplantation in children: An overview of physical, psychological and social outcome. *European Journal of Pediatrics, 154,* 171–175.

Solomon, G.D., Skobieranda, F.G., & Gragg, L.A. (1993). Quality of life and wellbeing of headache patients: Measurement by the medical outcomes study instrument. *Headache, 33,* 351–358.

Spieth, L.E., & Harris, C.V. (1996). Assessment of health-related quality of life in children and adolescents: An integrative review. *Journal of Pediatric Psychology, 21,* 175–193.

Spilker, B. (1996). *Quality of life assessment in clinical trials.* New York: Raven Press.

Spitzer, R.L., Kroenke, K., Linzer, M., Hahn, S.R., Williams, J.B., deGruy, F.V., Brody, D., & Davies, M. (1995). Health-related quality of life in primary care patients with mental disorders. Results from the PRIME-MD 1000 Study. *JAMA, 274,* 1511–1517.

Stewart, A.L., & Ware, J. (1992). *Measuring function and wellbeing.* Durham, NC: Duke University Press.

Stone, R.D., Beasley, P.J., Treacy, S.J., Twente, A.W., & Vacanti, J.P. (1997). Children and families can achieve normal psychological adjustment and a good quality of life following pediatric liver transplantation: A long-term study. *Transplant Proceedings, 29,* 1571–1572.

Telch, M.J., Schmidt, N.B., Jaimez, T.L., Jacquin, K.M., & Harrington, P.J. (1995). Impact of cognitive-behavioral treatment on quality of life in panic disorder patients. *Journal of Consulting Clinical Psychology, 63,* 823–830.

Townsend, M., Feeny, D.H., Guyatt, G.H., Furlong, W.J., Seip, A.E., & Dolovich, J. (1991). Evaluation of the burden of illness for pediatric asthmatic patients and their parents. *Annals of Allergy, 67,* 403–408.

Troidl, H., Wood-Dauphinee, S., & Williams, I. (1980). *Endpoints in surgical trials.* New York: Thieme.

Tyson, J.E., & Broyles, R.S. (1996). Progress in assessing the long-term outcome of extremely low-birth-weight infants. *JAMA, 276,* 492–493.

Wagner, A.K., Keller, S.D., Kosinski, M., Baker, G.A., Jacoby, A., Hsu, M.A., Chadwick, D.W., & Ware, J.E. (1995). Advances in methods for assessing the impact of epilepsy and antiepileptic drug therapy on patients' health-related quality of life. *Quality of Life Research, 4,* 115–134.

Wagner, A.K., & Vickrey, B.G. (1995). The routine use of health-related quality of life measures in the care of patients with epilepsy: Rationale and research agenda. *Quality of Life Research, 4,* 169–177.

Walker, S.R., & Rosser, R.M. (1991). *Quality of life assessment and application.* Lancaster: MTP Press.

Walker, V., Streiner, D.L., Novosel, S., Rocchi, A., Levine, M.A., & Dean, D.M. (1995). Health-related quality of life in patients with major depression who are treated with moclobemide. *Journal of Clinical Psychopharmacology, 15*, 60S–67S.

Ware, J.E. (1996). The SF-36 health survey. In B. Spilker (Ed.), *Quality of life and pharmacoeconomics in clinical trials* (pp. 337–346). Philadelphia: Lippincott-Raven.

WHOQOL Group. (1994). The development of the WHO quality of life assessment instruments (WHOQOL). In I. Orley & W. Kuykyen (Eds.), *Quality of life assessment: International perspectives* (pp. 33–40). Berlin: Springer.

Wiklund, I., Gorkin, L., Pawitan, Y., Schron, E., Schoenberger, J., Jared, L.L., & Shumaker, S. (1992). Methods for assessing quality of life in the cardiac arrhythmia suppression trial (CAST). *Quality of Life Research, 1*, 187–201.

Wildrick, D., Parker-Fisher, S., & Morales, A. (1996). Quality of life in children with well-controlled epilepsy. *Journal of Neuroscience Nursing, 28*, 192–198.

Yang, T.F., Wong, T.T., Kwan, S.Y., Chang, K.P., Lee, Y.C., & Hsu, T.C. (1996). Quality of life and life satisfaction in families after a child has undergone corpus callostomy. *Epilepsia, 37*, 76–80.

Chapter 7

QUALITY OF LIFE IN FAMILIES OF YOUTHS WITH CHRONIC CONDITIONS

Cindy L. Hanson

A childhood chronic condition is a term that encompasses chronic illnesses, impairments, and disabilities (Robert Wood Johnson Foundation, 1996). Approximately 14% of children from birth to 17 years of age live with a chronic condition (Robert Wood Johnson Foundation, 1996). Children with a chronic condition are at risk for lowered quality of life (QL) because of the additional demands and stressors the condition places on children and families. The presence of a chronic condition also increases the risk of psychosocial difficulties for children and families (Gortmaker, Walker, Weitzman, & Sobol, 1990).

QL can be differentiated from "health-related QL" in that health-related QL focuses on the person's perceptions of leading a fulfilling life given the impact of the chronic health condition (Bullinger, Anderson, Cella, & Aaronson, 1993). QL encompasses a broader perception of overall well-being that cuts across developmental, social, mental, spiritual, emotional, economic, and physical dimensions. The World Health Organization taps aspects of QL by defining health as "complete physical, mental, and social well-being, not merely the absence of disease or infirmity." In the US, the *Healthy People 2000: National Health Promotion and Disease Prevention Objectives* (1990) defines healthy life as "a vital, creative, and productive citizenry contributing to thriving communities and a thriving nation." This latter definition has expanded the concept of individually-oriented views of health to include the interconnections of individuals and families to their broader communities, which is an important aspect of QL. In support of a more broad-based conceptualization of QL versus health-related QL, the pediatric literature suggests that it is the psychosocial and emotional aspects associated with the chronic conditions rather than the condition-specific parameters (e.g., illness severity) that most affect the QL of a child (e.g., Kazak & Barakat, 1997; Wallander & Thompson, 1995). For children with chronic health conditions, the family plays a pivotal role in their adaptation to their disease and in their QL. The "QL of the child" and the "QL of the family" are therefore interdependent, and both of these aspects of QL are discussed in this chapter.

The chapter first highlights some of the conceptual models and issues related to examining the QL of the family, and then a brief overview is provided of our current knowledge about how children and families are affected by a childhood chronic condition. Next, the most salient correlates of QL are addressed, such as beliefs and attitudes, coping styles, social support, and stress, followed by suggestions for future directions in the area of QL in families with children who have chronic conditions.

DEFINING QUALITY OF LIFE

Definitions of QL in the literature have not been uniform. Gill and Feinstein (1994) found that half of the 579 referenced articles in a QL bibliography did not use the term QL, and many investigators used health status as an indicator of QL. When researchers have attempted to define QL across childhood chronic conditions, multiple types of data across various contexts have been used (Spieth & Harris, 1996).

Although there is controversy as to the measurement of QL, there is general agreement among QL researchers regarding the broad concepts that define QL and the nature of QL. Cross-cultural studies, for example, indicate considerable universality in the concepts that compose QL, including concepts such as satisfaction, relationships, economic security, and health (Keith, Heal, & Schalock, 1996). There is also general consensus that QL first refers to a person's "perceptions" of well-being rather than to an objective assessment of health status. Historically, many researchers have assessed adults' perceptions of children's QL, as well as overall adjustment (Spieth & Harris, 1996). Children's views of their own adjustment and QL differ from others' views (e.g., teachers, parents, health care professionals). Listening to the children's different perceptions of their own QL across various settings, as well as the perceptions of the adults with whom the children interact in these settings will increase our understanding of the multiple factors that enrich the QL for these children and their families (Perrin, Ayoub, & Willett, 1993).

QL is also a multidimensional construct (Kuyken, Orley, Hudelson, & Sartorius, 1994; Gill & Feinstein, 1994). Kuyken et al. (1994) define various components of QL, including the physical, psychological, social, and spiritual domains. The *physical* domain includes the child's view of his or her physical state relative to the norms of the culture. Kuyken et al. distinguish between *disease* (organic problems) and *illness* (perceptions of disease). The authors describe how European and North American cultures are largely concerned with treatment of disease, whereas many indigenous cultures are geared primarily toward healing illness. A child's appraisal of his or her *illness*, as well as the impact of the type and severity of the *disease* on the child are both pertinent to QL (Wallander & Thompson, 1995).

The *psychological* domain refers to the child's perceptions of his or her cognitive and affective abilities and experiences relative to the self and others. These perceptions are shaped by the environment, by experiences within the various settings in which the child is embedded (e.g., family, school, neighborhood, and peer environments), and the values of the culture. In some cultures, the value of the "self" is more closely aligned with the sense of connection to the *social* domain compared with other cultures that emphasize independence, such as in Europe and the United States.

The *social* domain involves the child's perceptions and satisfaction with his or her social relationships (e.g., friends, family, extended family, school network). Within different cultures and across varying socioeconomic levels, the social domain is differentially related to QL. For example, in situations where the youth shares crowded living space, the social domain may have more of an impact on QL than do certain illness- or condition-specific parameters.

The *spiritual* domain is less easily defined, but involves the child's perceptions of his or her own sense of significance and beliefs about the meaning of his or her life. The spiritual domain is often influenced by the religious beliefs of the child. Spirituality has been traditionally defined in ways that involve abstract types of reasoning (e.g., perceptions of the "meaning of life") that are not consistent with the cognitive developmental levels of children. The spiritual domain can be more broadly expressed through a child's perceptions of his or her aspirations and dreams; creative, artistic, musical, and imaginative expressions; religious beliefs, experiences, and practices; and faith, hope, and love.

In addition to being multidimensional, QL is a *fluid* concept that changes as the child, family, culture, and circumstances change. The child and family are by their nature evolving, changing organisms that interact with the broader environment. This broader cultural environment is also dynamic, as evidenced most recently by the technological advances in communication, which are revolutionizing lives. Some of the changes and differences *within* cultures, such as socioeconomic levels or urban and rural differences are even more pronounced than intercultural differences (Kuyken et al., 1994). Thus, the QL of the child and the family at one point in time depends on multiple interrelating factors. Extrapolating from the developmental and psychological literatures, QL is a highly fluid concept, especially during certain developmental periods, such as early adolescence when multiple changes are occurring physically, cognitively, emotionally, and socially.

FAMILY QUALITY OF LIFE AND FAMILY FUNCTIONING
CONCEPTUAL MODELS

The QL of children with chronic conditions depends heavily on the QL of the family. Several theoretical orientations delineate how family members develop and maintain patterns of interaction (e.g., Kerns, 1995; Thompson & Gustafson, 1996). Early family research from both psychological and sociological perspectives studied *individuals* within families. Theories were then expanded to evaluate the dyadic influences of the parent–child relationships (Kreppner & Lerner, 1989; Schnee-wind, 1989). Initially, the perspective was guided by a linear approach to parent–child functioning (e.g., unidirectional parental influences on the child), which then changed to a reciprocal framework. Dyadic relationships became viewed as bi-directional, wherein each family member affected other family members to produce concurrent changes in the individual family members, dyads or subgroups, as well as the family system as a whole.

An example of synergy whereby family members' responses to each other's behaviors affect the entire family climate can be found in the Chaney et al. (1997) investigation of family processes in childhood adaptation to diabetes. The researchers found that as the adjustment of fathers declined over time, mothers exhibited better adjustment. As Chaney et al. (1997) discuss, "the inverse relationship observed in spousal adjustment may indicate that as one parent's distress increases, the other parent actually collects his/her intrapersonal resources to equalize or neutralize the level of distress in the family" (p. 240). Most pediatric research studies have focused on cross-sectional views of individual family members. Further research is needed to evaluate how individual family members' views are interdependent on the feelings, perceptions, behaviors, and QL of other family members over time.

Conceptual and empirical models have now evolved into an examination of multiple systems that interact with and affect the adaptation and QL of individual family members and the family (Kazak, Segal-Andrews, & Johnson, 1995). Examples of the social ecology of children that are important in understanding the QL of children and families include: peer relations, social support, sibling interactions, extended family members, the parental workplaces, life stressors, school systems, neighborhoods, financial and coping resources, cultural factors, community and religious resources, and both access to and the quality of the health care received (Kazak, 1997). Developmental psychologists, such as Bronfenbrenner (1979), and Ford and Lerner (1992), have provided some illustrations of the multiple levels of interrelating systems that are linked to the development and well-being of the child and family.

In the pediatric psychology literature, systems-based or biopsychosocial models that incorporate the family within the broader environmental context have been proposed and tested (e.g., Hanson, 1992; Hanson, De Guire, Schinkel, & Kolterman, 1995; Kazak, 1992; Kazak et al., 1995; Mullins, Gillman, & Harbeck, 1992; Wallander, Varni, Babani, Banis, & Wilcox, 1989). Thompson and Gustafson (1996) describe several models of adaptation to childhood chronic conditions that are based on social learning theory and social ecological systems theories. Most of these models also take an interactive and family perspective. For example, the chronic condition of the child affects family routines, but family routines affect the nature and course of the chronic condition. Separating these two paths of influence is helpful when communicating and developing models of influence, but each path affects the other in ways that change both. These biopsychosocial models view chronic conditions as potential stressors and seek to identify the processes that place youths and their families at increased risk of poor QL, as well as those resources that enhance adaptation and QL. The roles of the parents and the family climate remain critically important in child adaptation and QL, but there is an increasing recognition of the significance of other ecological systems.

CONCEPTUAL ISSUES

Defining quality of life of the family vs family members

Researchers have quantified family functioning along several dimensions that affect QL, such as; family conflict, cohesion, adaptability, organization (e.g. Moos et al., 1985; Olson & Moos, 1981). Much of the research on family relations categorizes families using these broad concepts. This type of conceptualization is based on general systems theoretical underpinnings suggesting that the "whole is more than the sum of its parts" (e.g., see Weiss, Marvin, & Pianta, 1997). That is, family members' behaviors and interactions synchronize to form the family "climate." Social ecological systems models, as described earlier, evaluate these whole-family variables and their interrelations within the broader environment (Mash & Dozois, 1996).

Other research suggests that defining the family as a whole masks important differences between family members (Ambert, 1997). Research shows that siblings from the same family may view their parents' behaviors as differently as children from nonrelated families (e.g., Dunn, 1983; Dunn & Stocker, 1989). For example, siblings perceive parental behavior differently because parents act differently toward each of their children, and because siblings' interpretations of parental behavior differ. Parents treat siblings differently for many reasons. For example, the developmental age of the child, the developmental stage of the family, the fit or compatibility between the parent and child, and the characteristics and behaviors of the siblings result in differential parent–child interaction. In addition, changes in external circumstances (e.g, life stressors, divorce, financial changes) and in the parents' own QL and health also affect parental behaviors and sibling perceptions.

Extrapolating from this research, youths with chronic conditions may have very different perceptions of the quality of family life compared with their healthy siblings. In part, this is because children with chronic conditions have treatment demands that may require differential parental treatment or different parenting behaviors. Siblings may feel that their sibling with the chronic condition is receiving preferential treatment or too much parental attention. On the other hand, the child with the chronic condition may perceive differences in parental behavior as a result of specialized treatment demands as unfair. These self-perceptions affect how the children view their QL, chronic condition, and their family. This in turn affects how they behave, and how other family members behave toward them. Youths who feel worse about themselves may be more difficult to parent, and as a result, may feel less parental warmth because of the strain on the parents. Children may also perceive less parental warmth because of low self-esteem, rather than because parents are showing less support or nurturing behaviors. In either situation, the QL of the child is compromised.

The perceptions of parents are also qualitatively different from their children and often from each other. The responsibilities associated with maintaining the emotional well-being of the family and the instrumental tasks required of the chronic condition (e.g., clinic visits, treatment demands) are handled differently by each parent. Although more data are needed because fathers have been infrequently studied, most research suggests that mothers are more involved than fathers in handling the emotional and instrumental demands of care-taking responsibilities (Gallant, Coons, & Morokoff, 1994). Even as research participants, fathers' involvement has been less than mothers long-itudinally (Janus & Goldberg, 1997). Sargent et al. (1995) has suggested that this parental gender difference may begin during adolescence. The researchers found that older male siblings felt that they handled treatment effects least well (e.g., seeing sibling after surgery, negative feelings when sibling is vomiting). Differences in parental coping behaviors, among families with a child who has a chronic condition compared those without, have been more strongly related to gender differences than to between-group differences (Holmbeck et al., 1997). Gender and role differences within the family affect each member's perceptions of their QL, as well as the quality of family life as a whole.

In summary, as a result of a chronic condition in the family, each family member will experience different changes that affect the family climate as a whole, and the QL of each member uniquely. Broad-based terms used to describe the family climate capture some of these important changes in family routines and interactions. For example, changes in the level of structure in the family to accommodate a treatment regimen can be captured by the flexibility or rigidity of family rules and routines. As one example, longitudinal research suggests that families of children with diabetes become less flexible and more structured as a response to the demands of the illness (Northam, Anderson, Adler, Werther, & Warne, 1996). In addition to the family climate, the different roles and unique perspectives of each family member can also result in considerable differences in the perceptions of family life and in the QL of family members. Evaluation of individual perceptions across settings and time, and within various contexts, will help in our understanding of intrapersonal and interpersonal variations in QL across chronic childhood conditions. Current research strategies that examine distinct patterns or trajectories are providing valuable data on individualized adaptation to chronic conditions (Frank et al., 1998; Weiss et al., 1997).

Noncategorical vs condition-specific assessments

Noncategorical and condition-specific assessments of family and child functioning are both important (Hanson, De Guire, Schinkel, Henggeler, & Burghen, 1992; Holden, Chmielewski, Nelson, Kager, & Foltz, 1997). Hanson et al. (1992) tested whether illness-specific and general family relations represented independent aspects of family functioning, and secondly, whether one type of assessment related most strongly to the child's adjustment. Both types of family relations covaried and both uniquely related to important outcomes in unexpected ways. For example, *general* family relations uniquely predicted the youths' dietary adherence (an illness-specific outcome), and *illness-specific* family relations uniquely predicted the youths' general psychosocial adaptation.

The findings of Holden and colleagues (1997) also support the important role of both general family variables and disease-related factors. Holden et al. found that "... general family stress variables and disease-related factors that can be conceptualized across chronic illnesses such as asthma and diabetes are more salient predictors of adjustment outcomes than individual illness categories. Investigations that do not control for these more general factors may find effects attributable to individual disease states that may actually be accounted for by these more generic variables" (pp. 24–25). Research studies that evaluate correlates of QL outcomes need to include those that take a categorical and noncategorical approach, as well as those that compare condition-specific and general family and child functioning. Drotar (1997) has identified the need for further testing of these various theoretical models, and across different chronic conditions.

EFFECTS OF A CHILDHOOD CHRONIC CONDITION ON CHILDREN AND FAMILIES

Most family researchers agree that a combination of individual, family, and extrafamilial variables are needed to understand the development of family members and the family system as a whole. It is also recognized that the linkages between the family and external systems, such as social and peer influences, can either foster or inhibit adaptation at the individual or family level (Kreppner & Lerner, 1989). The presence of a chronic condition in a child undoubtedly creates additional stress; however, many other experiences and events in the life of a family are stressful as well. Parental or family functioning in families with chronic conditions is different than in families without chronic conditions, but pathological functioning is not the norm in these families. Higher levels of anxiety, distress, and/or depression have been found in some parents with children who have chronic conditions; overall, parental adjustment has been consistently correlated with the levels of support and stress in the family (Thompson & Gustafson, 1996). Recent findings in this area suggest that parental adaptation over time is associated with the course of the disease (Frank et al., 1998). The abilities and resources available to families in order for them to obtain the support they need to moderate the stressors associated with the chronic condition needs further evaluation. For mothers, however, a larger support network can also add stress if it increases the demands on her time and care-taking burdens.

CHILD EFFECTS

Children's adjustment to their condition depends on many variables, such as developmental factors (e.g., lower intelligence relates to higher risk; the age of the children at diagnosis has differential implications on their QL), condition-related factors (e.g., the visibility of the disease impacts QL; children with neurological diseases and those with unpredictable courses are at higher risk for adjustment problems), and other contextual factors (e.g., the availability of family support and resources may buffer the impact of the additional stressors and improve QL). In addition to condition-specific risk factors, the risk factors for poor QL for children with chronic conditions also include all the risk factors for children without chronic conditions (Gortmaker et al., 1990).

A study with approximately 11,700 youths aged 4 to 17 years suggests that the presence of a chronic condition places a child at a 55% increased risk for psychosocial problems (Gortmaker et al., 1990). Importantly, 62% of the children and adolescents with chronic conditions who need help (e.g., behavioral scores in the top 10th percentile) have not received mental health services. There have been several reviews of the hundreds of studies on the adjustment of children with chronic conditions. Wallander and Thompson (1995), Thompson and Gustafson (1996), and Drotar (1997) discuss the epidemiological studies and meta analyses that have been conducted (e.g., Lavigne & Faier-Routman, 1992, 1993). In general, the conclusion is that there is a wide range of responses to childhood chronic conditions, and multiple factors relate to child adjustment. Overall, Wallander and Thompson (1995) state, "although major psychiatric disturbance is not common among children with chronic conditions, this population is at increased risk for mental health and adjustment problems" (p. 128). Based on the meta-analysis with more than 700 studies reviewed (Lavigne & Faier-Routman, 1992), Thompson and Gustafson (1996) summarized that children with chronic physical illness were (a) more likely to exhibit internalizing than externalizing problems, but (b) were *not* likely to show lowered levels of self-esteem compared with matched healthy control groups and normative data.

One issue that has not been addressed is the possibility that internalizing problems might predispose certain children to develop physical illness. Cohen and Williamson (1991) cite studies that suggest that introversion relates to a higher susceptibility to illness and more severe illness. They suggest that people who are more introverted might be less able to draw support from their social networks. Whether children who are more introverted or anxious have more difficulty obtaining the benefits of support *prior* to the onset of the illness, or the internalizing behaviors occur as a *result* of the condition, inadequate support and a lowered sense of social competence impedes QL and adjustment. Research is needed to evaluate whether higher levels of internalizing problems in children with chronic illness has in fact placed them at higher risk for the development of chronic illness, rather than viewing it solely as an outcome of having a chronic condition.

Family functioning is one of the strongest contributors to adjustment in children with chronic health conditions (Drotar, 1997; Hamlett, Pellegrini, & Katz, 1992), as well as in healthy children. This is not to infer that genetics, intrapersonal, or extrafamilial contexts are not important, such as individual differences in ability levels, peer relations, or contacts with the health care system. Nor does it suggest that family relations universally predict child outcomes. Drotar (1997) points out that in almost every study reviewed, there were non-significant findings related to family/parental functioning and child psychological out-comes. In addition, the amount of variance accounted for in children's psychological outcomes was low overall, estimated by Drotar (1997) as approximately 10–15%. Over-attributing child outcomes to family functioning can create unnecessary feelings of blame and guilt in parents and children who already have additional stressors that can impede QL.

Nonetheless, the ability of the family to remain flexible and cohesive in the face of changing demands, albeit difficult, is particularly important for a child who has the additional burdens associated with a chronic health condition. Research suggests that high family cohesion and low family conflict consistently predict better adjustment in youths with chronic illness (Drotar, 1997; Perrin et al., 1993). For example, family flexibility was a significant predictor of perceived social acceptance and scholastic competence in youths with cancer, which are two significant stressors facing youths with cancer (Kazak & Meadows, 1989). Youths with cancer are often absent from school because of treatment demands, which places them at risk for poor academic functioning. Peer teasing and the physical changes that can occur as a result of the cancer treatment, such as loss of hair, scars, weight changes, amputation, are strong illness-related stressors reported by adolescents (Anholt, Fritz, & Keener, 1993; Madan-Swain et al., 1994; Varni, Katz, Colegrove, & Dolgin, 1995).

Summarizing the findings from numerous studies, Drotar (1997) found that family cohesiveness "predicted fewer behavioral problems and more competent psychological functioning (e.g., self-esteem)" (p. 151). Examples include families with children who have diabetes and those who have cancer. Family cohesiveness has been shown to be important throughout adolescence in predicting health outcomes in youths with diabetes (Hanson et al., 1989a, 1989b, 1995). Family cohesiveness has also been associated with less parental depression following the diagnosis of cancer in children (Manne et al., 1995). Parents have the tasks of balancing their concerns about the treatment demands and relapse, with the developmental needs for independence in youths with cancer, diabetes, and other chronic childhood conditions. Both family flexibility and cohesiveness have been shown to be key factors in balancing treatment and general life concerns for both the children and family members.

Family flexibility and cohesiveness may also serve as mediators or moderators of illness-specific outcomes. For example, flexible family relations were found to covary with positive health outcomes early in the course of the diabetes (Hanson et al., 1995, 1989b). Positive family relations may also help to buffer or impede the development of poor coping strategies in response to these stressors. Family flexibility buffered the expression of maladaptive coping behaviors in youths with diabetes of long duration (Hanson et al., 1989a). Youths with long illness duration used ventilation and avoidance coping less frequently when families demonstrated flexible relations. In contrast, youths in rigid families frequently coped by ventilating feelings, such as yelling, blaming others, avoiding people, and/or engaging in drug use. Other coping behaviors are more fully discussed later in the chapter.

SIBLING EFFECTS

Thompson and Gustafson (1995) reviewed the studies of siblings with chronic conditions and concluded that although they were at increased risk of adjustment difficulties, positive adjustment was possible. The authors also noted the wide variability and the individual differences that were apparent in adaptation. For example, Sargent et al. (1995) found that siblings of children with cancer (N = 254) report distress about "family separations and disruptions, lack of attention to them and focus of the family on caring for the ill child, negative feelings in themselves and other family members, changes in the ill child's behavior, cancer treatment and adverse side effects, and possible death of the ill child" (p. 161). The researchers also reported positive perceptions from siblings. Siblings reported that "they had become more compassionate and caring, family members were closer to each other, they had experiences they otherwise would not have had, and they felt they had been helpful to the ill children and to their families" (p. 162). More studies, particularly longitudinal studies, are needed to identify the factors that relate to QL and adaptation of siblings with chronic conditions.

Few studies have examined the associations between sibling relations and the health of the child with the chronic condition (Thompson & Gustafson, 1995). In one of the few studies, Hanson et al. (Hanson et al., 1992b) sought to identify whether sibling relations contributed a unique source of variance above and beyond the effects of general family relations and demographic factors on the youths' illness-specific and general adaptation. Hanson et al. found that sibling interactions, especially sibling conflict, predicted the youths' acceptance of their illness, self-esteem, and behavioral adjustment above and beyond the effects of the general family climate. Interestingly, certain aspects of the youths' adjustment were more strongly mediated by the sibling relations than by the family climate and marital relationship.

Researchers have documented the relationships between marital conflict and behavioral problems in children, but have not examined the relative importance of sibling relations. Hanson et al. (1992a) found that the youths' adjustment was more strongly mediated by siblings relations than by the marital relationship. For example, the findings indicated that low marital satisfaction predicted sibling conflict (perhaps through marital conflict), but it was sibling conflict rather than marital satisfaction that predicted the youths' adjustment (e.g., acceptance of illness, self-esteem, externalizing behaviors). Internalizing behaviors were predicted by high family life stress and high status/power in the sibling relationship.

Although highly speculative, if internalizing behaviors predispose children to develop serious health problems, it could be that high levels of chronic stress contribute both to internalizing difficulties and to the development of serious conditions. Again, this is a hypothesis that would need to be tested longitudinally. In any case, evaluating the QL and adjustment of siblings and youths are best done within a biopsychosocial or contextual framework in order to identify potential mediators or moderators of these outcomes (Peyrot, 1996).

FAMILY CORRELATES OF QUALITY OF LIFE

In this section, the correlates of adaptation are discussed across four areas that are most salient to QL: attitudes and beliefs, coping styles, social support, and life stress.

FAMILY BELIEFS AND ATTITUDES

Preliminary studies indicate that certain personal beliefs, such as self-blame, or blaming the medical staff or God, relate to poor adjustment and coping with cancer and treatment (Bearison, Sadow, Granowetter, & Winkel, 1993). Most of the parents (70%) and half of youths held specific beliefs regarding the causes of their cancer, even when physicians had told families that the etiology of the cancer was unknown (Bearison et al., 1993). Few empirical studies have examined this potent area, especially in youths and their parents.

Current beliefs in many parts of the world still view chronic illnesses and disabilities as deficits, punishments, or weaknesses of the spirit (Klonoff & Landrine, 1994; Wellenkamp, 1995; Young & Zane, 1995). The youth may feel that the chronic condition *itself* somehow represents a "failure." In addition, the youth may feel that he or she is a failure, and has failed by burdening the family. The youth may question why he or she was the one in the family to become ill, and what he or she did to deserve such a fate. The wide-scale public health campaigns about the links between lifestyles and health outcomes in industrialized nations can lead to an overemphasis on one's personal control over health. These misinterpretations and oversimplifications of scientific findings can result in a "blame-the-victim" attitude by others as well (Whalen & Kliewer, 1994).

The interpretation of the causality of the condition (e.g., poor self-care behaviors, an act of God) and beliefs regarding the consequences of the condition (e.g., long-term medical complications, premature death) clearly affect the quality of family life. For example, if the youth and family believe that the youth's condition resulted from his or her unhealthy thoughts or unsafe behaviors, the youth will feel personal inadequacy and the pressure of family disapproval. Beliefs about what causes improvements in the condition may serve to buffer or worsen QL depending on the veracity of the beliefs and whether the behaviors are doable and manageable. If the family believes that the youth has control over the severity of the disease symptomatology, for example, unreasonable expectations will create stress for the youth and family.

Youths can be particularly vulnerable to misinterpreting the causes of their illness and their ability to exert control over their illness or condition because of their developmental level (Thompson & Gustafson, 1995). In addition to developmental levels, unrealistic perceptions of control over one's health are also likely to reflect the human desire to perceive a sense of control over one's life. Perceptions of control can instill a sense of optimism versus helplessness when facing life's challenges. People's beliefs and expectations are powerful in affecting QL, as are the benefits of positive thinking and the ability to control choices in one's life. If these beliefs are taken to an extreme, however, youths or parents can erroneously infer that the youths (a) have control over whether or not they get ill, and (b) have the ability to cure themselves with "positive thinking." These types of beliefs place a tremendous burden and undeserved guilt on the youths with chronic conditions and their families. The youths can be singled out as deficient in some way, and the parents can be stigmatized as not providing an appropriate environment for their children. It is helpful for families to understand that psychological processes are only one part of the much broader context of contributors (e.g., genetics, biological factors, physical susceptibility, environmental factors, nutrition, supportive resources, knowledge, self-care behaviors, stress, unknown factors) that impinge on health outcomes and QL.

Spiritual understanding and beliefs are another aspect of QL, and until recently have been less frequently discussed in the professional psychological literature, but nonetheless have influenced current thinking related to QL and health outcomes. Religious beliefs can improve QL by providing a more positive and adaptive appraisal of the situation, comfort and emotional support, and positive social connections (Jenkins & Pargament, 1995; Spiegel, 1995; Wagner, Armstrong, & Laughlin, 1995). For example, the stress of a particular condition or treatment is likely buffered if the youth believes strongly that a supreme or higher power is supporting and guiding him or her. Many adolescents with cancer report that having a personal faith in a higher power provides them with a sense of security that is otherwise unavailable (Tebbi, Mallon, Richards, & Bigler, 1987). In addition, many youths felt that their faith allowed them to maintain a sense of control over their lives, and gave them a better understanding of and ability to accept the events in their lives. Religious faith may also function as a protective factor in coping with illness, though the empirical research is scant (Jenkins & Pargament, 1995). In a group of adults facing serious health risk, Oxman, Freeman, and Manheimer (1995) found that the lack of strength and comfort from religion and the lack of participation in groups were strong independent risk factors for death within six months after open heart surgery in a large group of adults.

The significance that the family places on the condition, that is, whether the treatment for the condition fits easily into daily routines, or whether it is accepted as a part of family life affects the QL and stress of all family members. Family members who experience difficulties accepting differences among family members, whether they be opinions, likes and dislikes, or the motivational levels of various family members, will experience more stress when treatment demands require that changes be made in family routines. Likewise, cultural and societal attitudes and responses to families and youths with chronic conditions that are inflexible, derogatory, or discriminatory hinder positive QL. Some of the attitudes, beliefs, and behaviors of family members that affect QL can also be captured in the coping styles that they employ in facing these types of stressors.

COPING STYLES

With the loss of health or the onset of a chronic condition in a child, the sense of vulnerability and perceived loss of control are natural feelings that occur (Goleman, 1995). Questions arise as to "why?, why now?, why ever? why my child?" The answers provided by the youngsters, families, and friends to these types of questions and to the condition itself have a profound impact on the QL of the youths and families. Coping responses that are most helpful are those that help to change the perception of uncontrollability accompanying the severe stress to manageability (Goleman, 1995). These include:

- engaging others for emotional support,
- promoting an active reframing of the situation into an examination of alternatives and options to pursue, and
- building a sense of trust in self, others, and/or a higher power to effectively handle the new daily challenges.

Certain coping styles are more disruptive to the illness-specific outcomes and QL of youths. Behavioral disengagement, avoidance coping, and venting emotions have been found to be maladaptive for parents and youths (Hanson et al., 1989a; Holmbeck et al., 1997). For example, ventilation and avoidance coping behaviors predicted poor illness-specific self-care behaviors by youths with diabetes (Hanson et al., 1989a). Although poor adherence to treatment is often attributed to the youths' age (e.g., "typical behavior during adolescence"), it was the maladaptive coping styles rather than the youths' developmental age that predicted poor adherence to treatment. Ventilation and avoidance coping styles, such as the youths' blaming and avoidance behavior, likely exacerbate family difficulties and stress. On the other hand, distant parent–youth relations coupled with high levels of stress could perpetuate this style of coping in youths. Positive changes in the family climate, such as more cohesion or flexibility in family relations, reduced levels of life stress, or more adaptive coping styles, would improve the QL for the youth and family.

Coping behaviors are nested within certain family and social contexts, and these *contexts* may be more important in predicting QL and adaptation, than are the individual characteristics of the youths (e.g., behavioral repertoires, ability levels) or their chronic condition (e.g., type, severity). For example, social and family contexts, such as parental coping, family support, and lack of family stress, rather than the individual characteristics of children with cancer distinguished "good" copers from "bad" copers (Kupst, 1992; Kupst & Schulman, 1988). Another example is families with the lowest coping and social resources found intensified home-based treatments more beneficial than families of youths with the most medically burdensome diseases (Jessop & Stein, 1991). QL may be more strongly linked with the available "resources" to meet the needs of children and families rather than risk factors. Health care professionals can help families determine what specific personal, interpersonal, and community resources are needed that will enable families and youths with chronic conditions to improve their QL.

Positive *parental* coping is also an important aspect of family functioning related to children's adjustment to chronic conditions (Sanger, Copeland, & Davidson, 1991). Negative parental emotional responses, such as depression, relate to poor adjustment in children with cancer, as well as in healthy children (Mulhern, Fairclough, Smith, & Douglas, 1992). Many problems that parents of youths with serious or chronic conditions experience, however, might not be revealed by traditional testing methods (Kazak, Christaskis, Alderfer, & Coiro, 1994; Kazak & Nachman, 1991; Van Dongen-Melman et al., 1995). In an innovative study, Van Dongen-Melman et al. (1995) found that 84% of the parents of children who survived cancer reported loneliness and continued uncertainty. Further, approximately 50% of the parents were experiencing problems above the 75th percentile ranking in one or more areas, such as loneliness and uncertainty. Procedures for cancer treatment, such as lumbar punctures and bone marrow aspirations, cause serious distress for both parents and youths throughout active treatment, and memories can be upsetting for many years (Kazak, Boyer, Brophy, Johnson, & Scher, 1995). Further research studies are needed to evaluate the specific areas of parental stress; and how parental coping affects QL in these areas.

Further research studies are needed to identify the specific coping styles that may act as protective factors during certain stages in the particular illness or condition. Identification of the contextual factors that predict these coping styles can then be used to develop clinical interventions. In addition, some research suggests that cognitive coping styles, such as hopefulness versus hopelessness, optimism versus pessimism, and certain religious beliefs may be stronger predictors of adjustment than specific coping behaviors, and possibly relate more strongly to QL (Pargament et al., 1990; Parle & Maguire, 1995; Scheier & Carver, 1992; Spiegel, 1995).

SOCIAL SUPPORT

Family and social support are key determinants of QL. Based on the early work of social support researchers (Berkman, 1984; Cobb, 1976; Cohen & Syme, 1985), Amick and Ockene (1994) define support as involving the following beliefs:

- "That one is cared for and loved and has an opportunity for shared intimacy (emotional support)
- That one is esteemed and valued (sense of personal worth)

- That one shares mutual obligations, communication, and companion-ship with others (sense of belonging)
- That one has access to information, advice, appraisal, and guidance from others (informational support)
- That one has access to material or physical assistance (instrumental support)"

Both families and children need these types of support for positive QL. For example, Weiss et al. (1997) found that high levels of extended family support to care for children with cerebral palsy were associated with the lowest levels of parenting stress. Innovative ways to provide support to families have also been tried successfully with multi-family groups (Satin et al., 1989). Enlisting community resources (e.g., religious institutions) to help provide many of the types of support that are useful to these families is highly needed.

Encouragement and social support can reduce the emotional distress associated with a chronic condition and can promote youths' positive adaptation to the condition (e.g., see Blanchard, Albrecht, Ruckdeschel, Grant, & Hemmick, 1995; Hanson et al., 1992a; Hockenberry-Eaton, Kemp, & Dilorio, 1994). Supportive resources for children and adolescents with serious or chronic conditions include the family environment and health care professionals, as well as others, such as relatives, friends, pets, teachers, community leaders and groups, coaches, and a personal faith in a higher power. Children with serious illnesses, such as cancer, have a higher need for emotional support in patient–provider interactions, and frequently these needs are unmet (Rose, 1993). Youths who feel a high sense of worth and support are better able to cope with the demands of their condition, and many adapt in a positive fashion despite the severity of the condition. This is not universally true however. For example, even though some children with cancer have positive self-worth and a desire to be with other children, they can still report feelings of loneliness and may play less with children their age (Spirito et al., 1990).

For youths with chronic illness, support from family and friends is essential in carrying out treatment regimens and in maintaining a sense of belonging and self-worth. In our research with a relatively large sample of youths who have diabetes (N = 157; Hanson et al., 1995), we were surprised to find that parents and adolescents reported significantly lower levels of family cohesiveness and a sense of belonging than normative controls. In fact, over a third of the families (36.3%) fell in the disengaged range of cohesiveness compared with 18.6% of normative families, and a much smaller percentage fell in the very connected or enmeshed range (4.9% compared to normative data of 14.7%). This is of concern because feeling a sense of cohesion and belonging is highly important to the youths' QL and health. Psychosocial treatment programs can be useful in providing supportive services to facilitate QL and supportive interpersonal relations for the child and family.

In addition to the beneficial effects of support on QL, there are negative sides to support. Youths may not feel supported by their families in ways that are beneficial to them. Sometimes family and friends inadvertently engage in a kind of "miscarried helping" of the youngster with the chronic disease, which can affect their QL (Anderson, 1996; Anderson & Coyne, 1993). In these cases, the support and help are excessive or inappropriate. Miscarried helping can actually make the youth feel less supported because it can undermine his or her sense of independence and competency. This places the youth in a stressful situation because he or she wants support from the family member or friend, but the situation causes frustration or irritation. In some cases, miscarried helping is tapping problematic interactional patterns that are maintained by the needs of the parent and/or child. The parent might not be allowing the youth enough independence because of his or her own fears, which may or may not be realistic, related to the management of the condition.

Generally, miscarried helping reflects inadequate knowledge about the condition, misjudging the youth's needs or desires, and/or concern by the parent about the health of the youth (in addition to the genuine desire of the parent to be helpful). During some developmental periods, such as adolescence, a pattern of miscarried helping can develop because of the parent–adolescent sensitivities, struggles, and problem-solving associated with normative issues related to emancipation and adolescent independence–dependence. In some situations and in some chronic conditions, vigilance and close scrutiny is appropriate and needed. Redirecting miscarried helping, however, is necessary so that QL is not compromised, and other problems do not develop. Anticipatory guidance and support by health care professionals are important to prevent miscarried helping, and for any problems that may arise that would impede the QL and normal development of the youth and family across a wide range of functioning.

Supportive resources and social activities can also be stressful at times for the youngster and family. As mentioned earlier, the QL of children is in part dependent on the coping abilities of their parents to life stressors. Parents of children who are busy with multiple responsibilities at work and home may find it stressful to engage in extensive social support activities. For example, the mother who brings her child with cancer to several weekly physician appointments has multiple additional stressors added to her life in addition to the emotional upheaval related to prognostic concerns. She may have taken primary responsibility for handling her child's discomfort with the treatment and side effects. Undoubtedly, she needs to make changes in her daily routine in order to accommodate to the treatment schedule, such as taking extended time off work. She may find her social support network weakened by not having supportive interactions within the work environment, or as much leisure time at home. She may feel saddened about less time for her other children or for her husband. On the positive side, support from close friends might increase to help ease the burden. Although social support is generally healthy and improves QL, too many social activities and expectations can be stressful for both parents and children.

STRESS

Stress responses are idiosyncratic and not necessarily predictable. The link between high stress and poor health is complex, involving immune, endocrine, and psychological processes. Indirect pathways between stress and poor health outcomes often occur concurrently with direct associations. The associations that have been evaluated most frequently in pediatric psychology involve the indirect links between stress and health outcomes through self-care behaviors; that is, high stress relates to unhealthy eating and exercise patterns, and/or less frequent contact with health care professionals, which then causes poor health. Most of the studies examining the link between stress and health outcomes have been with adults rather than children (Andersen, Kiecolt-Glaser, & Glaser, 1994; Cohen et al., 1998; Cohen & Herbert, 1996; Kiecolt-Glaser & Glaser, 1992).

In youths with diabetes, family life stress has been related directly and indirectly to poor health outcomes (Hanson, 1992). For example, under high stress, family relations were more likely to deteriorate, which was then linked to poor self-care behaviors in youths with diabetes (Hanson et al., 1995). Stress was also associated directly with poor health outcomes, such as poor metabolic control (Hanson, Henggeler, & Burghen, 1987; Hanson et al., 1995), as well as with less cohesive and more conflictual family relations. The levels of stress in these youths and families were lower than would be expected based on normative data; however, even at these lower levels, stress was linked both directly and indirectly to poor health outcomes. This raises several concerns, particularly because the disease itself can be a stressor, and poor control of the disease heightens the physical and psychological levels of stress.

Perceptions of a low QL predicted poor metabolic control in youths with diabetes as well. Youths' perceptions of a high negative impact of diabetes on their lives, such as being embarrassed in public when having to deal with their diabetes, having to miss school, or feeling that diabetes interfered with their social activities, significantly predicted poor metabolic control, and marginally predicted self-care behaviors (Hanson, Steltenkamp, Schinkel, De Guire, & Harris, 1997). The youths also had significant illness-specific social and vocational concerns related to current and future functioning. Almost half were worried about whether they would be able to pay for future doctors' bills, and other illness-related expenses.

Given the multiple associations between stress and poor QL and/or physical health outcomes (Cohen & Park, 1992; Kiecolt-Glaser & Glaser, 1992), it is a priority to identify the buffers or moderators of stress in the lives of these youths and families. As one example, high social competence buffered the link between high stress and poor metabolic control in youths with diabetes (Hanson et al., 1987). Under conditions of stress, youths with low social competence evidenced poor metabolic control in contrast to youths with high social competence. High social competence involves many of the following factors that can improve QL and help protect youths from the negative effects of stress. Whether the stress disrupts self-care behaviors or is more direct through endocrine and nervous system responses, the factors that would likely buffer the negative effects of stress are:

- a sense of personal competence
- a sense of belonging
- social support
- effective coping
- a sense of control over one's life
- faith in a higher power

Further research is needed to explore the links longitudinally between QL, stress, and health outcomes in pediatric conditions.

FUTURE DIRECTIONS

The following 12 recommendations are provided to stimulate directions for future research in the area of QL in childhood chronic conditions.

1. Because QL is a relatively new concept in childhood chronic illness, further research is clearly needed in defining and measuring the concept in children and their families. Issues related to this challenge have been highlighted in this chapter. QL is a multi-dimensional and fluid concept as it relates to children's perceptions of their world. Although QL includes an appraisal of functioning across several areas, further distinction is necessary when defining QL, adjustment, and adaptation. In general, researchers have documented that children with chronic conditions are for the most part resilient in the ways that they adapt to the additional stressors associated with their conditions. We have yet to tap, however, the perceptions, beliefs, and experiences that these children and families embrace, as well as overcome, to improve their QL. When researchers define "subclinical" levels of distress they are beginning to tap the areas that impede QL in the lives of these children and families.

2. Historically, researchers have relied on others' perceptions of the adjustment and QL of children, which at best, gives us an incomplete understanding of the feelings and beliefs of children as they relate to QL. As a starting point, researchers need to begin to evaluate the children's views of their QL. Evaluating the similarities and differences in QL between family members will then give us a better understanding of what promotes a positive QL, as well as the chronic burdens that need to be addressed to improve QL.

3. Evaluation of individual perceptions across settings and time, and within various contexts, is necessary to help in our understanding of intrapersonal and interpersonal variations in QL across chronic childhood conditions.

4. Research strategies that examine distinct patterns or trajectories can provide valuable data on individualized patterns of adaptation, and identify those patterns that lead to the best QL outcomes.

5. Children's QL is one aspect of a complex, interwoven, social ecological context. The assessment of QL will be guided and advanced by the theoretical models of adaptation that are proposed. Researchers will need to develop theoretical models of QL that can be tested. Theoretical and empirical models of

adaptation that were discussed in the chapter can be further refined to focus on issues related to QL in children and their families.

6. A better understanding of children's QL is dependent on the ways in which researchers explore family life. As discussed in the chapter, evaluating the "family climate" as well as the individual differences in family members' perceptions of the quality of family life are necessary. Research documents that are both condition-specific and general family functioning provide unique roles in the adaptation of children, and both types of functioning need to be evaluated in QL research as well.

7. Very few studies have examined how sibling relationships affect the child with the chronic condition, and a limited number of studies have examined the effects of having a sibling with a chronic condition. As discussed in this chapter, initial research suggests that sibling relations relate uniquely to the adaptation of children with chronic conditions above and beyond the effects of general family relations. Evaluating sibling relationships and their impact on QL is a potent and critical area that has not been studied.

8. Children who live with chronic conditions and their families, especially those conditions that are serious and life-threatening, face questions that are spiritual in nature. There is a paucity of research evaluating the perceptions and experiences of spirituality in children. As such, how spiritual beliefs, attitudes, and experiences affect QL has been largely unexplored.

9. Longitudinal research is needed to more clearly delineate the relationships between the stressors of the condition and child outcomes. Whether some of the predominant psychosocial outcomes of childhood chronic conditions (e.g., internalizing behaviors) are a function of the condition, or alternatively, have placed the child at risk for the development of the condition is a hypothesis that needs empirical testing.

10. Evaluating whether QL is more strongly linked to social and family "resources" than to "risk" factors is an empirical question that needs further study. Health care professionals can determine the specific resources that are most needed at the individual family level, as well as those that are needed to be advocated at the public policy level.

11. Further research is needed on the specific coping patterns, as well as the global styles of coping (e.g., hopefulness), that act as protective factors during certain stages of the chronic illness or condition for optimal QL.

12. Exploration of innovative ways to provide additional sources of support and resources to these children and their families via community action is also needed.

SUMMARY

This chapter presented a framework for understanding the interconnectedness between the family and being a child or adolescent with a chronic condition. QL was discussed from a family perspective, within the context of the broader cultural and social environment. In addition to the importance of the family environment, findings related to the links between QL and beliefs and attitudes, coping, social support, and stress were discussed in childhood chronic conditions. Research from several sources of literature were integrated to provide an entry into this emerging field.

References

Ambert, A.M. (1997). *Parents, children, and adolescents: Interactive relationships and development in context.* New York, NY: Haworth Press.

Amick, T.L., & Ockene, J.K. (1994). The role of social support in the modification of risk factors for cardiovascular disease. In S.A. Shumaker & S.M. Czajkowski (Eds.), *Social support and cardiovascular disease* (pp. 21–40). New York, NY: Plenum.

Andersen, B.L., Kiecolt-Glaser, J.K., & Glaser, R. (1994). A biobehavioral model of cancer stress and disease course. *American Psychologist, 5,* 389–404.

Anderson, B.J. (1996). Involving family members in diabetes treatment. In B.J. Anderson & R.R. Rubin (Eds.), *Practical psychology for diabetes clinicians: How to deal with the key behavioral issues faced by patients and health-care teams* (pp. 43–50). Alexandria, VA: American Diabetes Association.

Anderson, B.J., & Coyne, J.C. (1993). Family context and compliance behavior in chronically ill children. In N.A. Krasnegor, L. Epstein, S.B. Johnson, & S.J. Yaffe (Eds.), *Developmental aspects of compliance behavior* (pp. 77–89). Hillsdale, NJ: Erlbaum.

Anholt, U.V., Fritz, G.K., & Kenner, M. (1993). Self-concept in survivors of childhood and adolescent cancer. *Journal of Psychosocial Oncology, 11,* 1–16.

Baum, A., Grunberg, N.E., & Singer, J.E. (1982). The use of psychological and neuroendocrinological measurements in the study of stress. *Health Psychology, 1,* 217–236.

Bearison, D.J., Sadow, A.I., Granowetter, L., & Winkel, G. (1993). Patients' and parents' causal attributions for childhood cancer. *Journal of Psychosocial Oncology, 11,* 47–61.

Berkman, L.F. (1984). Assessing the physical health effects of social networks and social support. *Annual Review of Public Health, 5,* 413–432.

Blanchard, C.G., Albrecht, T.L., Ruckdeschel, J.C., Grant, C.H., & Hemmick, R.M. (1995). The role of social support in adaptation to cancer and to survival. *Journal of Psychosocial Oncology, 13,* 75–95.

Bronfenbrenner, U. (1979). *The ecology of human development.* Cambridge, MA: Harvard University.

Bullinger, M., Anderson, R., Cella, D., & Aaronson, N. (1993). Developing and evaluating cross-cultural instruments from minimum requirements to optimal models. *Quality of Life Research, 2,* 451–459.

Chaney, J.M., Mullins, L.L., Frank, R.G., Peterson, L., Mace, L.D., Kashani, J.H., & Goldstein, D.L. (1997). Transactional patterns of child, mother, and father adjustment in insulin-dependent diabetes mellitus: A prospective study. *Journal of Pediatric Psychology, 22,* 229–244.

Cobb, S. (1976). Social support as a moderator of life stress—presidential address. *Psychosomatic Medicine, 38,* 300–314.

Cohen, L.H., & Park, C. (1992). Life stress in children and adolescents: An overview of conceptual and methodological issues. In A.M. La Greca, L.J. Siegel, J.L. Wallander, & C.E. Walker (Eds.), *Advances in pediatric psychology: Stress and coping with pediatric conditions* (pp. 25–43). New York, NY: Guilford.

Cohen, S., Frank, E., Doyle, W.J., Skoner, D.P., Rabin, B.S., & Gwaltney, Jr., J.M. (1998). Types of stressors that increase susceptibility to the common cold in healthy adults. *Health Psychology, 17,* 214–223.

Cohen, S., & Herbert, T.B. (1996). Health psychology: Psychological factors and physical disease from the perspective of human psychoneuroimmunology. *Annual Reviews in Psychology, 47,* 113–142.

Cohen, S., & Syme, S.L. (Eds.) (1985). *Social support and health.* New York: Academic Press.

Cohen, S., & Williamson, G.M. (1991). Stress and infectious disease in humans. *Psychological Bulletin, 109,* 5–24.

Drotar, D. (1997). Relating parent and family functioning to the psychological adjustment of children with chronic health conditions: What have we learned? What do we need to know? *Journal of Pediatric Psychology, 22,* 149–165.

Dunn, J. (1983). Sibling relationships in early childhood. *Child Development, 54*, 787–811.

Dunn, J., & Stocker, C. (1989). The significance of differences in siblings' experiences within the family. In K. Kreppner & R.M. Lerner (Eds.), *Family systems and life-span development* (pp. 289–301). Hillsdale, NJ: Erlbaum.

Ford, D.H., & Lerner, R.M. (1992). *Developmental systems theory: An integrative approach.* Newbury Park: Sage.

Frank, R.G., Thayer, J.F., Hagglund, K.J., Vieth, A.Z., Schopp, L.H., Beck, N.C., Kashani, J.H., Goldstein, D.E., Cassidy, J.T., Clay, D.L., Chaney, J.M., Hewett, J.E., & Johnson, J.C. (1998). Trajectories of adaptation in pediatric chronic illness: The importance of the individual. *Journal of Consulting and Clinical Psychology, 66*, 521–532.

Gallant, S.J., Coons, H.L., & Morokoff, P.J. (1994). Psychology of women's health: Some reflections and future directions. In V.J. Adesso, D.M. Reddy, R. Fleming (Eds.), *Psychology perspectives on women's health.* Washington, DC: Taylor & Francis.

Gill, T.M., & Feinstein, A.R. (1994). A critical appraisal of the quality of quality-of-life measurements. *JAMA, 272*, 619–626.

Goleman, D. (1995). *Emotional intelligence: Why it can matter more than IQ.* New York: Bantam Books.

Gortmaker, S.L., Walker, D.K., Weitzman, M., & Sobol, A.M. (1990). Chronic conditions, socioeconomic risks, and behavioral problems in children and adolescents. *Pediatrics, 85*, 267–276.

Hamlett, K.W., Pellegrini, D.S., & Katz, K.S. (1992). Childhood chronic illness as a family stressor. *Journal of Pediatric Psychology, 17*, 33–47.

Hanson, C.L. (1992). Developing systemic models of the adaptation of youths with diabetes. In A.M. La Greca, L.J. Siegel, J.L. Wallander, & C.E. Walker (Eds.), *Advances in pediatric psychology: Stress and coins with pediatric conditions* (pp. 212–241). NY: Guilford.

Hanson, C.L., Cigrang, J.A., Harris, M.A., Carle, D.L., Relyea, G., & Burghen, G.A. (1989a), Coping styles in youths with insulin-dependent diabetes mellitus. *Journal of Consulting and Clinical Psychology, 57*, 644–651.

Hanson, C.L., De Guire, M.J., Schinkel, A.M., Henggeler, S.W., & Burghen, G.A. (1992a). Comparing social learning and family systems correlates of adaptation in youths with IDDM. *Journal of Pediatric Psychology, 17*, 555–572.

Hanson, C.L., De Guire, M.J., Schinkel, A.M., & Kolterman, O.G. (1995). Empirical validation for a family-centered model of care. *Diabetes Care, 18*, 1347–1356.

Hanson, C.L., Henggeler, S.W., & Burghen, G.A. (1987). Social competence and parental support as mediators of the link between stress and metabolic control in adolescents with insulin-dependent diabetes mellitus. *Journal of Consulting and Clinical Psychology, 55*, 529–533.

Hanson C.L., Henggeler, S.W., Harris, M.A., Burghen, G.A., & Moore, M. (1989b). Family system variables and the health status of adolescents with insulin-dependent diabetes mellitus. *Health Psychology, 8*, 239–253.

Hanson C.L., Henggeler, S.W., Harris, M.A., Burghen, G.A., Cigrang, J.A., Schinkel, A.M., Rodrigue, J.R., & Klesges, R.C. (1992b). Contributions of sibling relations to the adaptation of youths with insulin-dependent diabetes mellitus. *Journal of Consulting and Clinical Psychology, 60*, 104–112.

Hanson, C.L., Steltenkamp, T.L., Schinkel, A.M., De Guire, M.J., & Harris, M.A. (1997). *Quality of life in youths with diabetes.* Presented at the Southeastern Psychological Association meeting, Atlanta, GA.

Healthy People 2000: National Health Promotion and Disease Prevention Objectives (1990). U.S. Department of Health and Human Services, DHHS Publication No. (PHS) 91–50512. Washington, D.C.: U.S. Government Printing Office.

Hockenberry-Eaton, M., Kemp, V., & Dilorio, C. (1994). Cancer stressors and protective factors: Predictors of stress experienced during treatment for childhood cancer. *Research in Nursing Health, 17*, 351–361.

Holden, E.W., Chmielewski, D., Nelson, C.C., Kager, V.A., & Foltz, L. (1997). Controlling for general and disease-specific effects in child and family adjustment to chronic childhood illness. *Journal of Pediatric Psychology, 22*, 15–28.

Holmbeck, G.N., Gorey-Ferguson, L., Hudson, T., Seefeldt, T., Shapera, W., Turner, T., & Uhler, J. (1997). Maternal, paternal, and marital functioning in families of preadolescents with spina bifida. *Journal of Pediatric Psychology, 22,* 167–182.

Janus, M., & Goldberg, S. (1997). Factors influencing family participation in a longitudinal study: Comparison of pediatric and healthy samples. *Journal of Pediatric Psychology, 22,* 245–262.

Jenkins, R.A., & Pargament, K.I. (1995). Religion and spirituality as resources for coping with cancer. *Journal of Psychosocial Oncology, 13,* 51–74.

Jessop, D.J., & Stein, R.E.K. (1991). Who benefits from a pediatric home care program? *Pediatrics, 88,* 497–505.

Kazak, A.E. (1992). The social context of coping with childhood chronic illness: Family systems and social support. In A.M. La Greca, L.J. Siegel, J.L. Wallander, & C.E. Walker (Eds.), *Advances in pediatric psychology: Stress and coping with pediatric conditions* (pp. 262–278). NY: Guilford.

Kazak, A.E. (1997). A contextual family/systems approach to pediatric psychology: Introduction to the special issue. *Journal of Pediatric Psychology, 22,* 141–148.

Kazak, A.E., & Barakat, L.P. (1997). Brief report: Parenting stress and quality of life during treatment for childhood leukemia predicts child and parent adjustment after treatment ends. *Journal of Pediatric Psychology, 22,* 749–758.

Kazak, A.E., Boyer, B.A., Brophy, P., Johnson, K., & Scher, C.D. (1995). Parental perceptions of procedure-related distress and family adaptation in childhood leukemia. *Children's Health Care, 24,* 143–158.

Kazak, A.E., Christakis, D., Alderfer, M., & Coiro, M.J. (1994). Young adolescent cancer survivors and their parents: Adjustment, learning problems, and gender. *Journal of Family Psychology, 8,* 74–84.

Kazak, A.E., & Meadows, A.T. (1989). Families of young adolescents who have survived cancer: Social-emotional adjustment, adaptability, and social support. *Journal of Pediatric Psychology, 14,* 175–191.

Kazak, A.E., & Nachman, G.S. (1991). Family research on childhood chronic illness: Pediatric oncology as an example. *Journal of Family Psychology, 4,* 463–483.

Kazak, A.E., Segal-Andrews, A.M., & Johnson, K. (1995). Pediatric psychology research and practice: A family/systems approach. In Michael C. Roberts (Ed.), *Handbook of pediatric psychology* (2nd ed.) (pp. 84–104). New York, NY: Guilford.

Keith, K.D., Heal, L.W., & Schalock, R.L. (1996). Cross-cultural measurement of critical quality of life concepts. *Journal of Intellectual and Developmental Disability, 21,* 273–293.

Kerns, R.D. (1995). Family assessment and intervention. In P.M. Nicassio & T.W. Smith (Eds.), *Managing chronic illness: A biopsychosocial perspective* (pp. 207–244). Washington, DC: American Psychological Association.

Kiecolt-Glaser, J.K., & Glaser, R. (1992). Psychoneuroimmunology: Can psychological interventions modulate immunity? *Journal of Consulting and Clinical Psychology, 60,* 569–575.

Klonoff, E.A., & Landrine, H. (1994). Culture and gender diversity in commonsense beliefs about the causes of six illnesses. *Journal of Behavioral Medicine, 17,* 407–418.

Kreppner K., & Lerner, R.M. (1989). Family systems and life-span development: Issues and perspectives. In K. Kreppner & R.M. Lerner (Eds.), *Family systems and life-span development* (pp. 1–14). Hillsdale, NJ: Erlbaum.

Kupst, M.J. (1992). Long-term family coping with acute lymphoblastic leukemia in childhood. In A.M. La Greca, L.J. Siegel, J.L. Wallander, & C.E. Walker (Eds.), *Advances in pediatric psychology: Stress and coping with pediatric conditions* (pp. 242–261). New York, NY: Guilford.

Kupst, M.J., & Schulman, J.L. (1988). Long-term coping with pediatric leukemia: A six-year follow-up study. *Journal of Pediatric Psychology, 13,* 7–22.

Kuyken, W., Orley, J., Hudelson, P., & Sartorius, N. (1994). Quality of life assessment across cultures. *International Journal of Mental Health, 23,* 5–27.

Lavigne, J.V., & Faier-Routman, J. (1992). Psychological adjustment to pediatric physical disorders: A meta-analytic review. *Journal of Pediatric Psychology, 17,* 133–157.

Lavigne, J.V., & Faier-Routman, J. (1993). Correlates of psychological adjustment to pediatric physical disorders: A meta-analytic review and comparison with existing models. *Journal of Developmental and Behavioral Pediatrics, 14,* 117–123.

Madan-Swain, A., Brown, R.T., Sexson, S.B., Baldwin, K., Pais, R., & Ragab, A. (1994). Adolescent cancer survivors: Psychosocial and familial adaptation. *Psychosomatics, 35,* 453–459.

Manne, S.L., Lesanics, D., Meyers, P., Wollner, N., Steingherz, P., & Redd, W. (1995). Predictors of depressive symptomatology among parents of newly diagnosed children with cancer. *Journal of Pediatric Psychology, 20,* 491–510.

Mash, E.J., & Dozois, D.J.A. (1996). Child psychopathology: A developmental-systems perspective. In E.J. Mash & R.A. Barkley (Eds.), *Child psychopathology* (pp. 3–60). New York, NY: Guilford.

Moos, R.H., & Moos, B.S. (1981). *Family Environment Scale manual.* Palo Alto, CA: Consulting Psychologists.

Mulhern, R.K., Fairclough, D.L., Smith, B., & Douglas, S.M. (1992). Maternal depression, assessment methods, and physical symptoms affect estimates of depressive symptomatology among children with cancer. *Journal of Pediatric Psychology, 17,* 313–326.

Mullins, L.L., Gillman, J., & Harbeck, C. (1992). In A.M. La Greca, L.J. Siegel, J.L. Wallander, & C.E. Walker (Eds.), *Advances in pediatric psychology: Stress and coping with pediatric conditions* (pp. 377–399). NY: Guilford.

Noll, R.B., Bukowski, W.M., Davies, W.H., Koontz, K., & Kulkarni, R. (1991). Adjustment in the peer system of adolescents with cancer: A two-year study. *Journal of Pediatric Psychology, 18,* 351–364.

Northam, E., Anderson, P., Adler, R., Werther, G., & Warne, G. (1996). Psychosocial and family functioning in children with insulin-dependent diabetes at diagnosis and one year later. *Journal of Pediatric Psychology, 21,* 699–717.

Olson, D.H., McCubbin, H.I., Barnes, H.I., Larsen, A., Muxen, M., & Wilson, M. (1985). Family adaptability and cohesion evaluations scales. In D.H. Olson, H.I. McCubbin, H. Barnes, A. Larsen, M. Muxen, & M. Wilson (Eds.), *Family inventories: Inventories used in a national survey of families across the family life cycle* (2nd ed., pp. 1–46). St. Paul: Family Social Science, University of Minnesota.

Oxman, T.E., Freeman, D.H., & Manheimer, E.D. (1995). Lack of social participation or religious strength and comfort as risk factors for death after cardiac surgery in the elderly. *Psychosomatic Medicine, 57,* 5–15.

Pargament, K.I., Ensing, D.S., Falgout, K., Olsen, H., Reilly, B., Van Haitsma, K., & Warren, R. (1990). God help me: (I) Religious coping efforts as predictors of the outcomes to significant negative life events. *American Journal of Community Psychology, 18,* 793–824.

Parle, M., & Maguire, P. (1995). Exploring relationships between cancer, coping, and mental health. *Journal of Psychological Oncology, 13,* 27–50.

Perrin, E.C., Ayoub, C.C., & Willett, J.B. (1993). In the eyes of the beholder: Family and maternal influences on perceptions of adjustment of children with chronic illness. *Developmental and Behavioral Pediatrics, 14,* 94–105.

Peyrot, M. (1996). Causal analysis: Theory and application. *Journal of Pediatric Psychology, 21,* 3–24.

Robert Wood Johnson Foundation (1996). *Chronic care in America: A 21st century challenge.* Princeton, NJ: Robert Wood Johnson Foundation.

Rose, J.H. (1993). Interactions between patients and providers: An exploratory study of age differences in emotional support. *Journal of Psychological Oncology, 11,* 43–67.

Sanger, M.S., Copeland, D.R., & Davidson, E.R. (1991). Psychosocial adjustment among pediatric cancer patients: A multidimensional assessment. *Journal of Pediatric Psychology, 16,* 463–473.

Sargent, J.R., Sahler, O.J.Z., Roghmann, K.J., Mulhern, R.K., Barbarian, O.A., Carpenter, P.J., Copeland, D.R., Dolgin, M.J., & Zeltzer, L.K. (1995). Sibling adaptation to childhood cancer collaborative study: Siblings' perceptions of the cancer experience. *Journal of Pediatric Psychology, 20,* 151–164.

Satin, W., LaGreca, A.M., Zigo, M.A., & Skyler, J. (1989). Diabetes in adolescence: Effects of multifamily group intervention and parent simulation of diabetes. *Journal of Pediatric Psychology, 14,* 259–275.

Scheier, M.F., & Carver, C.S. (1992). Effects of optimism on psychological and physical well-being: Theoretical overview and empirical update. *Cognitive Therapy and Research, 16,* 210–228.

Schneewind, K.A. (1989). Contextual approaches to family systems research: The macro-micro puzzle. In K. Kreppner & R.M. Lerner (Eds.), *Family systems and life-span development* (pp. 197–221). Hillsdale, NJ: Erlbaum.

Spiegel, D. (1995). Commentary. *Journal of Psychosocial Oncology, 13*, 115–121.

Spieth, L.E., & Harris, C.V. (1996). Assessment of health-related quality of life in children and adolescents: An integrative review. *Journal of Pediatric Psychology, 21*, 175–193.

Spirito, A., Stark, L.J., Cobiella, C., Drigan, R., Androkites, A., & Hewett, K. (1990). Social adjustment of children successfully treated for cancer. *Journal of Pediatric Psychology, 15*, 359–371.

Tebbi, C.K., Mallon, J.C., Richards, M.E., & Bigler, L.R. (1987). Religiosity and locus of control of adolescent cancer patients. *Psychological Reports, 61*, 683–696.

Thompson, R.J., Jr., & Gustafson, K.E. (1996). *Adaptation to chronic childhood illness*. Washington, D.C.: American Psychological Association.

Uchino, B.N., Cacioppo, J.T., & Kiecolt-Glaser, J.K. (1996). The relationship between social support and physiological processes: A review with emphasis on underlying mechanisms and implications for health. *Psychological Bulletin, 119*, 488–531.

Van Dongen-Melman, J.E.W.M., Pruyn, J.F.A., De Groot, A., Koot, H.M., Hahlen, K., & Verhulst, F.C. (1995). Late psychosocial consequences for parents of children who survived cancer. *Journal of Pediatric Psychology, 20*, 567–587.

Varni, J.W., Katz, E.R., Colegrove, R., & Dolgin, M. (1995). Perceived physical appearance and adjustment of children with newly diagnosed cancer: A path analytic model. *Journal of Behavioral Medicine, 18*, 261–278.

Wagner, M.K., Armstrong, D., & Laughlin, J.E. (1995). Cognitive determinants of quality of life after onset of cancer. *Psychological Reports, 77*, 147–154.

Wallander, J.L., & Thompson, Jr., R.J. (1995). Psychosocial adjustment of children with chronic physical conditions. In Michael C. Roberts (Ed.), *Handbook of pediatric psychology* (2nd ed.) (pp. 124–141). New York, NY: Guilford.

Wallander, J.L., Varni, J.W., Babani, L., Banis, H.T., & Wilcox, K.T. (1989). Family resources as resistance factors for psychological maladjustment in chronically ill and handicapped children. *Journal of Pediatric Psychology, 14*, 371–387.

Weiss, K.L., Marvin, R.S., & Pianta, R.C. (1997). Ethnographic detection and description of family strategies for child care: Applications to the study of cerebral palsy. *Journal of Pediatric Psychology, 22*, 263–278.

Wellenkamp, J. (1995). Cultural similarities and differences regarding emotional disclosure: Some examples from Indonesia and the Pacific. In J. W. Pennebaker (Ed.), *Emotion, disclosure, & health* (pp. 293–311). Washington, DC: American Psychological Association.

Whalen, C.K., & Kliewer, W. (1994). Social influences on the development of cardiovascular risk during childhood and adolescence. In S.A. Shumaker & S.M. Czajkowski (Eds.), *Social support and cardiovascular disease* (pp. 223–257). New York: Plenum.

Young, K., & Zane, N. (1995). Ethnocultural influences in evaluation and management. In P.M. Nicassio & T.W. Smith (Eds.), *Managing chronic illness: A biopsychosocial perspective* (pp. 163–206). Washington, DC: American Psychological Association.

SPECIFIC CHRONIC CONDITIONS

Chapter 8

ABDOMINAL DISORDERS

Nico H. Bouman

Abdominal disorders consist of rather diverse disorders with equally diverse consequences for quality of life (QL). On the one hand there is recurrent abdominal pain (RAP), a common problem affecting some 10% of all children. Although RAP is a disorder with little organic pathology, it raises much concern with parents and it may influence the QL of a large proportion of children. On the other hand there are the inflammatory bowel diseases (IBD), which are rare diseases with severe morbidity affecting QL in several domains. The congenital abdominal anomalies fall somewhat outside the scope of the former conditions. They are not diseases in the strict sense, but may nonetheless have long-term consequences for the health and QL of children who were born with these anomalies.

Research on the QL of abdominal disorders in childhood and adolescence in the strict sense is scarce, although several studies have been performed focusing on the physical and psychological functioning of RAP, IBD, and congenital abdominal anomalies. Very few QL instruments have been developed for children and adolescent age groups. In this chapter QL is defined as a multidimensional construct including the physical, psychological, and social functioning domains (Aaronson, 1991; Spieth & Harris, 1996). The physical functioning domain generally includes disease state or symptomatology and functional status, i.e. the ability to perform age-appropriate daily activities (Spieth & Harris, 1996). There is no clarity about which aspects of psychological and social functioning should be included in QL measurement. Inclusion of overt behavioral problems in the psychological functioning domain is recommended by Spieth and Harris (1996). Other aspects of psychological functioning such as cognitive functioning and self-esteem will be described. In the social functioning domain relations with peers, with family members, and teachers are primarily identified as the most important aspects and will be discussed (Spieth & Harris, 1996).

This review will focus on what is known about the physical, as well as the psychological and social consequences in childhood and adolescence of these disorders. In the first part RAP will be described, in the second part IBD, and in the last part congenital abdominal anomalies. In each part the medical aspects of the disorder will be described, followed by the description of the physical functioning and the psychological and social functioning, and will end with a brief discussion of possible future QL research.

RECURRENT ABDOMINAL PAIN

Recurrent abdominal pain (RAP) is a common problem during childhood. It is defined as at least three episodes of abdominal pain affecting the activities of the child over a period of more than three months (Apley, 1959, 1975). The reported prevalence of RAP among school-aged children varies from 5% to 25% (Faull & Nicol, 1986; Stevenson, Simpson, & Bailey, 1988). Hyams, Burke, Davis, Rzepski, and Andrulonis (1996) found that 21% of a community based sample of 507 adolescents had weekly complaints of abdominal pain severe enough to interfere with activities.

Longitudinal research indicates that RAP is a chronic condition. In a follow-up study of their original groups of patients, Apley and Hale (1973) showed that abdominal pain is persistent into adulthood in one-third of cases. In a follow-up study of a cohort of 136 children from the age of 4 years up until the age of 10 years, Borge, Nordhagen, Moe, Botten, and Bakketeig (1994) found a strong relationship between the number of complaints at the age of 4 and at the age of 10. Fifty-five percent of children with frequent stomachaches at the age of 4 still had these complaints at the age of 10, while only 13% of children without stomachache at the age of 4 had frequent stomachaches at the age of 10. Finally, Walker, Garber, Van Slyke and Greene (1995) reported persistent high levels of abdominal pain in a group of 31 children with RAP 5 to 6 years after diagnosis.

An organic cause is only found in about 10% of cases with RAP (Apley, 1959). Based on a study of 106 children with chronic stomachache in which 42% of children had organic causes for their complaints, Van Der Meer (1993), argues that this is an under-estimation and that more efforts should be made to find an organic cause in children presenting with RAP. However, these results may be explained by the fact that this study concerned only clinically referred children, a proportion of whom were hospitalized, which may represent a more serious subgroup of children with RAP with a greater chance to find organic causes.

Treatment of RAP in the first instant consists of avoiding invasive medical procedures. Apley and Hale (1973) recommend explanation, reassurance, and discussion with the child and its parents by the treating physician. Finney, Lemanek, Cataldo, Katz, and Fuqua (1989) and Sanders, Shepherd, Cleghorn, and Woolford (1994) describe brief structured therapies primarily based on cognitive-behavioral techniques as successful treatment strategies.

PHYSICAL FUNCTIONING

By definition children with RAP suffer from frequent abdominal pains. Other common complaints are nausea, vomiting, and food intolerance (Van Der Meer, 1993; Hyams et al., 1996). Although, as included in the definition, pain should interfere with daily activities of the child, it is not clear in most studies to what extent children with RAP are limited in their activities. In the study by Hyams et al. (1996) 51% of adolescents with abdominal pain missed at least one school day in the previous year versus 39% of the adolescents without pain. However, there were no differences in significant school loss (6 days or more) between these two groups. Robinson, Alvarez, and Dodge (1990) reported in a study of 40 referred children with RAP, that children with RAP had four times as many school absences as a matched normal control group. In a study by Walker and Green (1989) 41 children with RAP scored much higher than control children on the Functional Disability Inventory, which measures difficulties of functioning in the domains of home, school, recreation, and social interaction. The scores of the children with RAP were comparable to those with organic causes for their abdominal pain. Walker et al. (1995) showed in their follow-up study of 31 children with RAP that these not only had persistent abdominal pain 5 to 6 years after diagnosis, but also continued to have more functional limitations and twice as many absences from school or work than controls. These results indicate that children with RAP suffer from pain and from limitations in their physical functioning, but further clarification is needed as to which aspects of physical functioning are most affected by RAP.

PSYCHOLOGICAL AND SOCIAL FUNCTIONING

The psychological functioning of children with RAP has been the focus of many studies since the pioneering study by Apley (1959). Apley found a clear relation between emotional disturbance and non-organic abdominal pain. Almost two-thirds of his series of children with RAP showed signs of emotional problems. Later studies approached this problem in a more specific way. Raymer, Weininger, and Hamilton (1984) found that the mean self-esteem scores of a group of 16 children with non-organic abdominal pain was lower than those of 30 controls. The mean depression score of children with RAP was almost twice as high as that of the control children. Faull and Nicol (1986) found psychiatric disturbance among the population of 6-year-olds with RAP using the Rutter A(2) questionnaire in an epidemiological study. Of the 48 cases with RAP 31 showed clear signs of psychiatric disturbance. In another study of 13 children with RAP using a standardized child psychiatric interview and several standardized questionnaires, all children met criteria for a psychiatric diagnosis (Garber, Zeman, & Walker, 1990). These were mainly internalizing disorders including depressive disorders and anxiety disorders. In this study, the children with RAP obtained scores on the internalizing subscale of the Child Behavior CheckList (CBCL) comparable to scores of psychiatrically referred children. The scores on the externalizing subscale of the CBCL of the children with RAP were not higher than those of normal controls. Walker and Green (1989) investigated a group of 41 children with RAP and compared these with 28 children with organic abdominal pain and 41 controls. They found that children with RAP scored higher on anxiety and depression self-report questionnaires than control children, but that they did not differ in these respects from children with organic abdominal pain. The mothers of the children with RAP, however, reported more internalizing problems on the CBCL for their children than mothers of children with organic abdominal pain and controls. In the follow-up study of these children it was found that a large proportion of children with RAP continued to have higher levels of emotional problems than controls 5 to 6 years after diagnosis (Walker et al., 1995). In the study by Van Der Meer (1993) only a few differences were found between the psychological functioning of RAP children compared to the general population. These results may be explained by the fact that the instruments used to assess psychological functioning in this study were mostly personality inventories used to investigate a possible etiological relation between RAP and psychological factors. Emotional problems such as depression and anxiety are not well detected by these instruments and may have been missed. Hyams et al. (1996) found more anxiety and depression using standardized questionnaires among a community based population of adolescents with recurrent abdominal pain.

Social functioning has been poorly studied in children with RAP. Apley (1959) reported that the level of school functioning of children with RAP was comparable to that of control children. Faull and Nicol (1986) reported that 6-year-old children with RAP tend to settle less in school and more frequently dislike school than control children.

Little is known of the parent–child relation and family functioning of children with RAP. Robinson et al. (1990) concluded that children with RAP were more dependent and needed more attention than children from non-RAP control groups. In their study of 13 children with RAP Garber et al. (1990) found that the mothers of children with RAP showed more symptoms of anxiety than mothers of children with organic abdominal pain and normal controls.

It can be concluded that a large proportion of children with RAP have problems in psychological functioning mainly of internalizing nature and that these problems appear to be persistent over time, while organic pathology is minor or absent over longer time periods. So, RAP should be regarded as a problem which can only be explained within a biopsychosocial model. Physical factors together with psychological, and possibly social factors play an important role in causing and maintaining the abdominal pain.

Future QL research should be aimed at identifying those aspects of a child's functioning which are most affected by RAP. More attention should be paid to limitations in functioning which are caused by RAP, such as limited participation in physical activities, in school attendance, and in social activities. Together with pain severity measures and measures of psychological functioning, more information could be yielded on the QL of these patients and in a broader sense than has been done until now. Eventually the aim should be to identify those children with RAP who are most limited in their physical, psychological, and social functioning and who might benefit from specified treatment strategies.

INFLAMMATORY BOWEL DISEASES

Inflammatory bowel diseases (IBD) are characterized by chronic inflammation of the small and/or large intestines of unknown origin. IBD is a collective heading for two diseases, Crohn's disease (CD) and ulcerative colitis (UC). The estimated incidence of CD is between 4 to 6 per 100,000 with 25% to 40% of cases under the age of 20 years, and the incidence of UC is 3 to 15 per 100,000 with 20% of cases beginning in childhood or adolescence (Herbst, 1992). So, a total of 1.6 to 5.4

children or adolescents per 100,000 present yearly in childhood or adolescence with IBD.

In CD inflammation of the intestines is limited to the small bowel in 30% to 35% of cases, to the large bowel in 10% to 15% of cases, and affecting the small and large bowel at the same time in 50% to 60% of cases (Hyams, 1996). Clinical features of CD are gastrointestinal as well as extraintestinal. Abdominal pain and bloody diarrhea are presenting symptoms in the majority of affected children. Abdominal pain is often severe and disturbing children's sleep. However, presentation may also be obscure with abdominal pain and depression as the only symptoms, so that the delay between onset of disease and diagnosis may be 2 years (Büller, 1997). Anorexia, nausea, and vomiting are common concomitant complaints. Growth retardation and late onset of puberty are frequent in CD probably caused by chronic malnutrition and chronic inflammation. Apart from these symptoms, there is a myriad of possible extraintestinal complaints affecting almost every tract (Hyams, 1996). Medical treatment is primarily aimed at reducing the inflammation process with anti-inflammatory agents such as 5-aminosalicilate and corticosteroids. Corticosteroids in particular have many side-effects including growth suppression, moon facies, and depression. Surgery, aimed at resection of the affected part of the intestine, is necessary in 50% to 70% of cases within 10 to 15 years after diagnosis (Hyams, 1996). Hyams, Grand, Colodny, Schuster, and Eraklis (1982) reported that in 42% of cases there was a relapse of inflammation within 5 years after colectomy requiring a second resection. None of these patients had more than one recurrence (Hyams et al., 1982).

UC shares many aspects of CD but localization in UC is limited to the large intestines. Clinical features are stools mixed with blood and mucus and lower abdominal cramping most intense during defecation. In children and adolescents UC tends to run a more complicated course than in adults and more frequently involves the entire colon (Kirschner, 1996). Delayed growth and sexual maturation are less frequent in UC than in CD. Arthralgia and arthritis are the most frequent extraintestinal complaints of children with UC (Kirschner, 1996). Medical and surgical treatment of UC is similar to that of CD. Recurrence of colitis after resection is reported to be much less frequent, i.e. 0% in the series of Hyams et al. (1982). In short, CD and UC are chronic conditions with severe and prolonged symptomatology affecting the gastrointestinal as well as other tracts necessitating intensive medical and surgical treatment with potentially harmful side-effects.

PHYSICAL FUNCTIONING

Adult populations

Several measures exist for measuring health status of adult IBD patients (see for reviews: Garret & Drossman, 1990; Drossman, 1996). These measures can be divided into disease activity measures and disease specific QL measures. Disease activity measures are completed by physicians and include patients' symptomatology, results of physical examinations, and laboratory measures. These measures are useful in clinical practice but have limited value in QL assessment. Disease activity appears to be weakly related to overall QL in IBD patients (Turnbull & Vallis, 1995). Several instruments have been developed to assess IBD related QL (Drossman, 1996). These measures are in most cases questionnaires to be completed by patients and mostly cover bowel symptoms, systemic symptoms, social and emotional functioning, and functional impairment. Based upon these studies it appears that in adults with IBD, QL is generally good, that patients with CD have greater disease severity and more impaired health related QL than patients with UC, and that impairment in the psychological and social dimensions are greater than in the physical dimension (Drossman, 1996). These instruments were all developed for adults and no comparable measures, neither as self-report nor as parent-report, are available yet for children with IBD.

Pediatric populations

The physical symptoms of IBD are well described. The four most frequent symptoms of children with both CD and UC are diarrhea, rectal bleeding, abdominal pain, and weight loss (Langholz, Munkholm, Krasilnikoff, & Binder, 1997). Physical functioning in pediatric populations has been studied far less than in adults. Langholz et al. (1997) studied disease activity of IBD in a geographically derived cohort of children. Comparing CD and UC, they found that 74% (UC) to 83% (CD) had moderate to high activity; however, functional impairment due to IBD symptoms was not described. Rabbett et al. (1996) assessed the QL of 16 children with CD using a questionnaire which was read to each child with questions concerning a wide range of topics from disease activity to emotional and social functioning, and views about the future. The most common symptoms were abdominal pain and lack of energy. Almost all children expressed concerns about the side-effects of medication. Although all children indicated that they were doing well at school, two-thirds thought that they would do better without CD. Nineteen percent to 44% of the children experienced limitations in participating in physical education lessons and sports. In a recent study on the development of a QL measure for children with IBD, Griffiths et al. (1999) identified several important aspects of physical functioning which may be of concern for these children. Bowel symptoms, being bothered by having to take medicines, worries about surgery, and concerns about height, specifically for children with CD, were important issues. It is clear that physical symptoms of IBD in children can lead to considerable limitations in functioning and, together with consequences of treatment procedures, may affect their psychological and social functioning.

PSYCHOLOGICAL AND SOCIAL FUNCTIONING

CD and UC were considered as classical "psychosomatic" diseases for which it was believed that psychological factors were a main cause. Personality was assumed to play a major role in the onset and course of these diseases (see for example Prugh, 1951). Finch and Hess (1962) proposed that children with UC should be considered as suffering from "severe psychopathology often close to psychosis". The main methodological flaw of these studies was that they were mostly concerned with psychiatrically referred patients. It must be stressed that the presence of a psychiatric disturbance or of emotional problems alongside a somatic disorder is no evidence that the somatic disorder is caused by the psychiatric disturbances. The studies by Helzer (Helzer, Stillings, Chammas, Norland, & Alpers, 1982; Helzer, Chammas, Norland, Stilling, & Alpers, 1984) did much to refute this psychosomatic hypothesis. They compared a consecutive series of patients with CD and UC with control subjects with chronic diseases. UC patients did not have a higher frequency of psychiatric disturbances, while CD patients did show more obsessive-compulsive disorder and more depression (50%) than controls. There was no evidence that a psychiatric disorder consistently preceded or caused the IBD.

Although the cause of CD and UC is unknown, there is a consensus over the fact that both diseases are immunologically mediated reactions triggered in a genetically determined susceptible host (Herbst, 1992). In this light, IBD should be regarded as chronic diseases with possible negative consequences for psychological and social functioning.

Several recent studies have assessed the psychological and social functioning of children with IBD. In these studies two approaches are taken. The first is to investigate the presence of psychiatric disorders using semistructured psychiatric interviews (Steinhausen & Kies, 1982; Burke et al., 1989a, 1989b; Engstrom & Lindquist, 1991). The second approach is to assess the amount of behavioral and emotional problems using standardized parent and child questionnaires (Steinhausen & Kies, 1982; Wood et al., 1987; Engstrom, 1992). An advantage of the last method is that the outcome of IBD children can be compared with normative data.

Steinhausen and Kies (1982), investigated a group of 17 children with IBD using a structured psychiatric interview and a behavior questionnaire. They found more than three times as many psychiatric disorders (60%), predominantly emotional disorders, among children with IBD compared to a normal control group (18%). Burke et al. (1989a, and 1989b) studied emotional problems in a consecutive series of children with IBD compared to children with cystic fibrosis (CF). The lifetime prevalence of depression was highest for CD compared to UC and CF, while children with UC had a higher lifetime prevalence for dysthymia and phobic disorder than CD and CF. The current prevalence of depressive disorders was higher in children with CD and UC than in children with CF. The highest rates for phobias, separation anxiety, and obsessive compulsive symptoms were found in UC. Engström and Lindquist (1991) found that psychiatric disorder, assessed using a reliable and well validated psychiatric interview, was four times as frequent in children with IBD (60%) compared to a group of healthy children (15%).

Steinhausen and Kies (1982) using the Children's Behavior Questionnaire found that children with IBD had more emotional problems but not more behavioral problems than normal controls. Wood et al. (1987) compared problem behavior in a group of children with CD, UC, and their siblings, with normative data. They found that children with IBD obtained significantly higher total problem scores and higher internalizing problem scores on the Child Behavior CheckList (CBCL) than their siblings and than children in the norm groups. Engström (1992) investigated the mental health and psychological functioning of a group of 20 children with IBD and compared them to children with chronic headache, diabetes mellitus, and healthy children. He assessed their functioning with a wide range of standardized instruments. Children with IBD and headache showed higher rates of total problems and internalizing problems on the CBCL than healthy children. Social competence of children with IBD was lowest among the three illness groups. According to the mothers, general well-being was worst for the children with headache, and according to their self-reports it was worst for the children with IBD. Low self-esteem and depression were more frequent for children with IBD and chronic headache than for children with diabetes or healthy children. It appeared that many children with IBD denied their emotional problems.

There are few data available relating psychosocial functioning to disease parameters. Wood et al. (1987) did not find a relation between disease severity and the amount of problem behavior. This is comparable to the results of Turnbull and Vallis (1995) who did not find a relation between disease activity and QL in an adult population with IBD. So it is not clear if there are specific aspects of IBD, such as short stature in CD or side-effects of medication, which negatively influence psychosocial functioning. Very little is known about the effect of medical interventions on psychosocial functioning. Most studies concern the effects of medical and surgical procedures on morbidity alone. Lask, Jenkins, Nabarro, and Booth (1987) compared the different aspects of functioning of 12 children with a stoma with 13 children who had been operated on but had no stoma and 13 children who were treated medically. They found no differences in QL, psychosocial functioning, or self-esteem between these groups of children.

Family functioning of children with IBD has been poorly studied. Only one study presents some reliable data in this respect. Engström (1991a) compared family functioning of 20 children with IBD, healthy controls and children with diabetes. He concluded that families with a child with IBD showed more dysfunction than the other families. However, he concludes that these results should be interpreted with some caution because the validity of the questionnaire was not fully presented. He also found that parents, especially mothers, of children with IBD experienced more distress and less social support compared to parents of a group of normal controls (Engström, 1991b). No relations were detected between these social parameters and disease activity; however, mothers with low social support, reported higher degrees of problem behavior for their children.

It may be concluded that QL in children with IBD is clearly reduced in the physical as well as in the psychological and social functioning domains. Physical symptoms are often serious and embarrassing, and the side-effects of treatment are often a matter of concern. Limitations in social functioning due to the disease is considerable and emotional problems are frequent. Most studies do not find a correlation between objective measures of disease activity and QL. Although the ancient "psychosomatic" hypothesis of IBD has been refuted, it has become clear that there is a complicated interplay between IBD, its effects on psychosocial functioning and relations within the family. Many aspects are still unclear and need further investigation. For example, the fact that children with IBD show predominantly emotional problems and few behavioral disorders is still insufficiently explained.

There is a need for future QL research in IBD. Efforts should be made to develop QL measures for children and adolescents with IBD. Next to more objective measures of disease activity it will be necessary to include measures taking into account the subjective appraisal of disease severity and of the burden of treatment by the child. It will be necessary to assess those domains of functioning (school, peers, sports) in which a child is mostly limited by the disease or its treatment. The effort by Griffiths et al. (1999) to adapt the IBD QL questionnaire for child and adolescent populations seems to be an important step in this direction. However, to these disease specific measures, generic measures of psychological and social functioning must be added. It will be necessary to study the QL of children with IBD not only in a cross-sectional design, but also to perform prospective longitudinal studies. In this way it will be possible to make a more funded balance of the positive and negative consequences of the disease and its treatment, and physicians, patients, and parents can be guided in the choice of treatment strategies.

CONGENITAL ABDOMINAL ANOMALIES

Congenital abdominal anomalies are in most cases life-threatening anomalies necessitating acute and sometimes lengthy hospitalization of the newborn and intensive surgical and medical treatment. As a consequence, the early physical development of children with these conditions is problematic. However, the impact of congenital abdominal disorders is not limited to the neonatal period. Prolonged morbidity may negatively influence future QL of these children. The overall incidence of congenital abdominal anomalies can be estimated at 1 to 1.5 per 1,000 live births. As such they are rare disorders but they form a large proportion of children in neonatal surgical intensive care units. Because congenital abdominal conditions are very different in initial presentation and subsequent physical problems, and because research on QL in these condition differs considerably, they will be treated separately.

CONGENITAL DIAPHRAGMATIC HERNIA

Congenital Diaphragmatic Hernia (CDH) is characterized by a defect in the diaphragm leading to herniation of the gut into the pleural cavity thereby compressing the lung. A hypoplasia of the lung on the contralateral side is also seen, and it is likely that a primary abnormality in the developing lungs exists. The infant with CDH has respiratory difficulties immediately after birth and begins to swallow air. Consequently, the gastrointestinal tract is gradually filled with air compressing the lungs, which further worsens the respiratory functioning. The condition of the infant deteriorates rapidly and immediate hospitalization in a specialized centre is necessary. Up to ten to fifteen years ago, the infant with CDH was operated on immediately to repair the defect in the diaphragm, but nowadays management has changed to delayed surgery. The infant is first hospitalized in a surgical intensive care unit and operation is delayed until the condition of the child has been stabilized. Despite several developments in treatment procedures such as artificial ventilation and vaso-active medication, the mortality of CDH is still high. Only between 35% and 45% of children with CDH survive (Langham et al., 1996). The incidence of CDH is estimated between 0.24 to 0.36 per 1,000 live births (Langham et al., 1996). Some 20 years ago Extra Corporeal Membrane Oxygenation (ECMO) was introduced in the treatment of CDH. ECMO is an intensive and costly treatment procedure for infants with respiratory distress. Although at first the outlook of survival for children with CDH treated with ECMO seemed more favorable this has recently been questioned (Langham et al., 1996).

Physical functioning

CDH is a disorder which primarily affects pulmonary and gastro-intestinal functioning. Several authors report some residual defects in pulmonary functioning in children and adolescents with CDH (Chatrath, El Shafie, & Jones, 1971; Reid & Hutcherson, 1976; Wohl et al., 1977; Delepoulle et al., 1991; IJsselstijn, Tibboel, & Hop; 1997). In other studies no reduction in lung functioning is reported (Kerr, 1977; Freyschuss, Lännergren, & Frenken, 1984; Falconer, Brown, Helms, Gordon, & Baron, 1990; Wischermann, Holschneider, & Hubner, 1995). Although these reports seem contradictory, the overall view is that long-term pulmonary dysfunction of children with CDH during childhood is mostly minor and does not lead to severe functional impairment. Pulmonary dysfunction may become more pronounced in adulthood. Vanamo, Rintala et al. (1996) described ventilatory impairment in half of the adult survivors of CDH. This outcome may be related to chest-wall deformities and scoliosis which are common among adults with CDH (Vanamo, Peltonen et al., 1996). Gastro-intestinal symptoms are described by several authors; gastroesophageal reflux with symptoms such as heartburn and regurgitation is especially common in patients with CDH (Kieffer et al., 1995; Vanamo, Rintala, Lindahl, & Louhimo, 1996). Although these symptoms are frequent, they are seldom disabling. Therefore, despite the fact that CDH is a very serious condition with extensive physical problems in the newborn period, long-term morbidity and physical limitations are limited.

Psychological and social functioning

Literature on long-term psychological and social functioning of children with CDH is very scarce. The introduction of ECMO, which is costly but expected to enhance survival of children with a very poor outcome, more attention has been paid to follow-up. Several studies have shown that more children than expected who had CDH and were treated with ECMO had light to moderate cognitive developmental delays (Van Meurs et al., 1993; Lund et al., 1994; D'Agostino et al., 1995; Stolar, Crisafi, & Driscoll, 1995). These studies mainly looked at young to very young children, and longer follow-up periods are needed to appraise the significance of these findings. Only two studies have reported on the cognitive development of children with CDH not treated with ECMO (Davenport, Rivlin, D'Souza, & Bianchi, 1992; Nobuhara, Lund, Mitchell, Kharasch, & Wilson, 1996). Davenport et al. (1992) reported that none of 23 children with CDH aged 18 to 94 months, not treated with ECMO but with delayed surgery, had developmental delays on the Griffiths' mental developmental scales. Based upon the results of non-specified developmental examinations Nobuhara et al. (1996) con-cluded that children with CDH treated with ECMO much more often had developmental delays than CDH children not treated with ECMO. In a recent follow-up study of 11 children with CDH, Bouman, Koot, Tibboel, and Hazebroek (2000) found that the mean IQ of these children was 15 points below the norm of 100, indicating a significant delay in cognitive functioning. None of these children had been treated with ECMO.

In the same study Bouman et al. (2000) found that children with CDH, compared to normative samples, showed more emotional and behavioral problems as reported by parents and teachers, and more depressive problems as reported by the children themselves. No other follow-up studies on the psychosocial functioning of children with CDH are available. However, the conclusion seems justified that children with CDH, not only those treated with ECMO, are at risk for cognitive as well as psychosocial problems and that further studies will be necessary to evaluate these aspects of the QL of children with CDH.

Esophageal atresia (EA) is a congenital malformation of the esophagus which can have several forms. Incidence for all forms of atresia is estimated at 0.22 per 1,000 live births. In the most common form (85% of the cases), the proximal part of the esophagus ends as a blind sac while the distal part is as a fistula connected to the trachea. In other cases there is only an interruption between the two parts of the esophagus. The earliest sign of EA is regurgitation of saliva. The first feed is followed by choking, coughing, and regurgitation therefore diagnosis is mostly made during the first days of life. Operation can be immediate or delayed depending on the type of anomaly, the condition of the infant, and the presence of other serious congenital anomalies. Due to narrowing of the constructed esophagus, frequent dilatations under general anaesthesia may be required until 2 to 3 years of age. Half of the infants born with EA have other congenital anomalies. Cardiovascular, urogenital, and anorectal anomalies are especially common. Mortality rates vary from 0% for children with normal birth-weights and absence of pneumonia to 43% for children with low birth-weight, severe pneumonia, or other serious congenital anomalies. Overall survival is about 83%.

Physical functioning

Feeding problems are common among patients with EA. As the constructed esophagus never functions normally, mainly due to the absence of peristaltic movements, patients with EA frequently complain of delayed passage of foods, the food being stuck in the esophagus with complaints of breathlessness, and heartburn due to reflux esophagitis (Anderson, Noblett, Belsey, & Randolph, 1992; Biller, Allen, Schuster, Treves, & Winter, 1987; Chetcuti & Phelan, 1993; Lindahl, Rintala, & Sariola, 1993; Puntis, Ritson, Holden, & Buick, 1990; Robertson, Mobaireek, Davis, & Coates, 1995; Saeki, Tsuchida, Ogata, Nakano, & Akiyama, 1988; Ure et al., 1994). In early childhood up to one-third of parents report severe feeding problems, but these tend to ameliorate in later childhood (Puntis et al., 1990). Although feeding problems persist into adulthood, they are seldom severe (Biller et al., 1987; Chetcuti & Phelan, 1993; Ure et al., 1994). Pulmonary problems, consisting of lower airway disease, increased respiratory symptoms, and reduced pulmonary function are reported in up to 40% of patients (Chetcuti, Phelan, & Greenwood, 1992; Robertson et al., 1995). Overall, 90% of patients with EA have good to excellent outcome with no or minor gastrointestinal or pulmonary dysfunction. Between 19% and 35% of patients with EA have skeletal anomalies of the spine and thorax (Chetcuti, Dickens, & Phelan, 1989; Chetcuti, Myers, Phelan, Beasley, & Dickens, 1989) and these may contribute to the pulmonal problems, which may become more pronounced with increasing age as is the case in CDH. Children with EA may be small and relatively light probably due to prolonged feeding problems. Growth retardation is described in several studies (Ahmed & Spitz, 1986; Anderson et al., 1992; Puntis et al., 1990).

In summary, EA is a condition causing long-term gastro-intestinal and pulmonary morbidity with, however, limited functional impairment in about 10% of cases.

Psychological and social functioning

Very few studies have focused on the psychological and social consequences of EA. The earliest study was by Dera, Mies, and Martinus (1980), who assessed the psychosocial functioning of 10 children with EA with a mean age of 4.3 years. They found a mean IQ of almost 10 points below the norm of 100 and frequent symptoms of anxiety, regression, and disturbances of contact. Lehner (1984) sent a questionnaire to parents of children with EA who were members of a patient organisation for congenital abdominal anomalies. One hundred and twenty-two parents responded with children aged 0 to 19 years. They reported that the mental and physical development of most patients was normal and that most children visited normal schools. No further specifications were given by the author. Chetcuti, Myers, Phelan, and Beasley (1988) followed 125 children with EA into adulthood. They reported that almost all enjoyed a normal lifestyle. Employment and marital status were in the normal range. Ure et al. (1994) investigated the outcome in adulthood of 8 patients with EA after colon interposition. Two patients were slightly mentally disabled and 7 patients reported unimpaired QL on the Spitzer index. Bouman, Koot, and Hazebroek (1999a) studied the psychological and social functioning of 36 children with EA using interviews and standardized assessment procedures. The mean IQ of these children was almost 10 points lower than the norm of 100. Children with major associated congenital anomalies who had been artificially ventilated in the newborn period (n = 8) even had a mean IQ more than 20 points below the norm. More than twice as many children (30 to 35%) as in the general population (15%) showed elevated rates of emotional and behavioral problems as reported by parents and teachers. The children themselves did not report more negative self-esteem or more depressive symptoms than children in the general population.

EA appears to have only slight negative consequences for adults, but younger children with EA seem to suffer more from emotional and developmental difficulties. These may be related to the long period of separation from the parents when they were infants and the frequent feeding difficulties (Dera et al., 1980) or to other risk-factors such as the presence of other associated congenital anomalies and artificial ventilation in the newborn period (Bouman et al., 1999a).

ABDOMINAL WALL DEFECTS

Children with abdominal wall defects (AWD) are born with a large abdominal mass protruding through a defect of the abdominal wall without (gastroschizis) or with (omphalocele), a covering amniotic membrane. Mortality was high before the introduction of total parenteral nutrition. Operation is performed after stabilizing the infant. Mortality is nowadays between 10 and 20% (Halsband & Von Schwabe, 1989).

Physical functioning

The earliest report on the long-term functioning of children with AWD was by Touloukian and Spackman (1971). They found normal growth in all and normal gastrointestinal function in five of six patients. Generally, good health, few gastrointestinal problems, and the absence of physical limitations were reported for children and adolescents with AWD (Daum, 1984; Halsband & Von Schwabe, 1989; Larsson & Kullendorf, 1990; Lindham, 1984; Swartz, Harrison, Campbell, & Campbell, 1986; Tunell, Puffinbarger, Tuggle, Taylor, & Mantor, 1995). The absence of a navel or a disfiguring abdominal scar was reported to be a point of embarrassment for 20 to 25% of the patients, especially for girls (Lindham, 1984; Halsband & Von Schwabe, 1989; Tunell et al., 1995).

Psychological and social functioning

Very few data are available on the psychological and social aspects of the QL of children with AWD. Swartz et al. (1986) reported satisfactory academic performance for 25 school-aged children. In a follow-up study by Tarnowski, King, Green, and Ginn-Pease (1991) including 22 children with AWD, intelligence, reading and mathematical abilities were tested. The mean scores on these academic measures were all within normal limits. The same study assessed the level of problem behavior and social competence using the CBCL. The children with AWD showed more emotional and behavioral problems than could be expected based upon the normative data. About 18% of the children obtained total problem scores in the clinical range (versus the norm of 10%) and they showed as much emotional problems (28% internalizing scores in the clinical range) as behavioral problems (25% externalizing scores in the clinical range) (Tarnowski et al., 1991). The children with AWD obtained lower social competence scores than in the norm group (23% in the clinical range). In the same study children with anorectal anomalies (ARM) were included. No differences were found between children with AWD or with ARM on any of the outcome measures. This is counterintuitive because children with ARM were expected to have worse psychological functioning caused by their life long physical problems especially incontinence, while children with AWD are relatively free of physical problems after the neonatal period. It can be hypothesized that the embarrassment about the absence of a navel and the abdominal scar, which are both clearly visible defects, may have a negative influence on self-esteem and hence contribute to behavioral problems. There is, therefore, reason to perform further studies on the QL of children with AWD.

HIRSCHSPRUNG'S DISEASE AND ANORECTAL MALFORMATIONS

Although Hirschsprung's disease (HD) and anorectal malformations (ARM) are different anomalies they share many characteristics especially concerning long-term functioning. This is why they will be described together. The nature of HD is the absence of ganglion cells in the distal intestine; this aganglionosis not only can involve the lower rectum, but can extend higher into the colon and even into the small intestine. The absence of ganglion cells causes abnormalities of the intestinal peristaltic movements and accounts for a functional obstruction. This obstruction causes a widening, megacolon, proximal to the aganglionotic segment. The presenting symptomatology is variable from complete obstruction at birth with vomiting and abdominal distention to a long-standing mild constipation. Final diagnosis is made by radiological examinations, a rectal biopsy, and rectal manometry, but may be delayed several years in some cases due to mild symptomatology. Treatment consists of resecting the aganglionotic bowel and connecting normal bowel to the distal rectum. The incidence of HD is about 1 in 5,000 live births. Mortality is around 5% mainly due to ischemic enterocolitis in the neonatal period (Rescorla, Morrison, Engles, West, & Grosfeld, 1992).

In ARM the anus ends in a blind loop with often a fistula between the blind anal canal and the urethra in men and the genital region in women. In some cases there is an anus visible from the outside and in other cases the normal anal opening is covered with skin. Not only does the anus end in a blind loop but also the innervation and musculature of the pelvis and anorectum are partly or completely absent. Depending on the anatomical level of the anomaly ARM is divided into high and low ARM. Due to its localisation, high ARM is the most surgically complicated. Presenting symptoms of ARM are the absence of an anus or signs of fistulation on inspection of the neonate and absence or abnormal passage of meconium, the infant's first stools. Treatment is surgical in the vast majority of cases. In some cases when there is only a narrowing of the anal canal progressive dilatation will be sufficient. In low ARM the surgical procedure is less complicated. However, after repair, daily dilatations of the anus are necessary for several months to a year. In high ARM surgical procedures are often very difficult due to the localisation and the concomitant vesico-urinary anomalies. A staged procedure with a colostomy is sometimes necessary. Incidence of ARM is around 1 in 5000 live births. ARM often is associated with other serious congenital anomalies such as genito-urinary, cardiovascular, or central nervous system anomalies, which may be the primary cause of death.

Physical functioning

The most problematic consequences of HD and ARM are continence related problems. Defecation appears to be a very complex process in which anatomical, physiological, and neurological factors are finely tuned in order to obtain such a simple thing as fecal continence. Due to congenital anomalies or surgical procedures this process is disrupted leading to a high frequency of continence problems or constipation in HD and ARM. Continence reported in HD is about 65% in most recent studies (Rescorla et al., 1992; Heij, De Vries, Bremer, Ekkelkamp, & Vos, 1995; Marty et al., 1995; Moore, Albertyn, & Cywes, 1996). In one study only 20% of patients obtained normal continence (Heij et al., 1995), a discrepancy which cannot be explained by the authors on the basis of patient selection or follow-up method. The figures for ARM are worse; normal continence, is reached by maximally 60% of patients in one study (Rintala, Mildh, & Lindahl, 1992), and of these only 15% had optimal continence (i.e. no signs whatsoever of smearing of feces in underwear or constipation). Rintala et al. (1992) were the only authors who compared continence of ARM patients with normal controls. In normal controls 100% had normal continence and of these 76% had optimal continence. Younger children appear to have the greatest problems as is shown in a study by Langemeijer and Molenaar (1991) who found that none of 50 children aged 4 to 7 years were continent, although 40% reached pseudo continence with daily enemas. In a study of 50 children with HD or ARM Bouman, Koot and Hazebroek (2000) found that almost one-third of children with ARM had moderate to serious fecal incontinence versus none of the children with HD. Diseth and Emblem (1996) reported that of 33 adolescents with ARM 77% had impaired control of continence with 40% having occasional staining and 37% having intermittent or constant soiling. The figures for adults are somewhat better as is shown in the study of Rintala et al. (1992) and Hassink, Rieu, Brugman, and Festen (1994). Although Hassink et al. (1994) reported that none of 56 adults reached complete continence, 84% of them had "socially acceptable" continence. An age effect is also shown by Ditesheim and Templeton (1987). Continence increased with increasing age, with 33% of children aged 2.5 to 9 years, 58% of adolescents aged 10 to 16 years, and 63% of adults aged 17 to 24 years having normal continence. Apart from gastrointestinal problems, urologic problems are reported in 24 to 29% of patients with ARM (Boemers, De Jong, Van Gool, & Bax, 1996; Misra, Mushtaq, Drake, Kiely, & Spitz, 1996). These problems concern incontinence, vesico-ureteric reflux, recurrent urinary tract infections, and eventually renal failure. However, concerns of parents about fecal incontinence appear to be much greater than about urinary incontinence and urologic problems (Boemers et al., 1996).

Psychological and social functioning

Psychological and social functioning of HD and ARM are the most extensively studied among congenital abdominal anomalies. As in IBD a difference must be made between studies assessing the prevalence of psychiatric disorders and studies assessing the amount of emotional or behavioral problems in children with HD or ARM. Using the Child Assessment Schedule (CAS) Ludman, Spitz, and Kiely (1994) found that 29% of 160 children with ARM aged 6 to 17 years had a mild to moderate psychiatric disorder most of which were internalizing disorders. Diseth and Emblem (1996) even found that 58% of 33 adolescents with ARM had a psychiatric disorder, also predominantly internalizing. In 19 adolescents with HD Diseth et al. (1997) did not find increased rates of psychiatric disorder.

Several studies have assessed the rates of behavioral and emotional problems using the Child Behavior CheckList (CBCL) and related questionnaires (Teacher's Report Form [TRF], Youth Self-Report [YSR]). The outcomes of these studies are contradictory. Diseth found no increased behavioral and emotional problems in adolescents with ARM (Diseth & Emblem, 1996) and with HD (Diseth et al., 1997). There is a contradiction in the fact that in the study of adolescents with ARM, Diseth and Emblem (1996) found 58% with psychiatric disorder, while CBCL and YSR total problems scores were in the normal range. The explanation by the authors that internalizing problems are often underreported seems insufficient and it raises questions about the methodology used in the study. Higher rates of emotional and behavioral problems were found in studies by Ludman et al. (1994) on 160 children and adolescents with ARM, by Ginn-Pease et al. (1991) on 34 children with ARM, and by Bouman et al. (2000) on 50 children with ARM and HD. Until now there are no indications that children with HD or ARM have lower self-esteem. In the studies by Ginn-Pease et al. (1991) and Bouman et al. (2000) mean scores on, respectively, the Piers-Harris Self-Concept Scale and the Self-Perception Profile for Children were within normal limits. There are, however, indications that age plays a role in the development of psychosocial problems in children with HD or ARM. Adolescents with ARM seem to be at greater risk for emotional and behavioral problems (Diseth & Emblem, 1996) or negative self-concept (Ginn-Pease et al., 1991).

Because incontinence is supposed to have the most negative influence on psychosocial functioning of patients with ARM and HD, most studies have assessed the relationship between incontinence and psychosocial outcome measures. Ginn-Pease et al. (1991) found increased rates of maladjustment for children who were incontinent compared to continent children. Other authors however did not find increased psychiatric disorders of behavioral and emotional problems for incontinent children compared to continent children (Ludman et al., 1994; Diseth & Emblem, 1996; Diseth et al., 1997; Bouman et al., 2000). However, Diseth found a negative influence of incontinence on overall psychosocial functioning using the Children's Global Assessment Scale (CGAS) (Diseth & Emblem, 1996; Diseth et al., 1997). No negative influence of incontinence on self-concept of children with ARM was found by Ginn-Pease et al. (1991) or Bouman et al. (1999b).

Social problems related to continence are reported for 12% to 39% of adults with ARM (Hassink et al., 1994; Rintala et al., 1992). Ditesheim and Templeton (1987) developed a QL measure focusing on the social limitations due to continence problems. Items included in the measure were school attendance, limitations in social relations, and restrictions in physical activities. Based on this measure the QL could be rated as good, fair, or poor. Seventy-two percent had good, 23% fair, and 5% poor QL. However, this conclusion is not relevant to QL in general because in this study QL was directly related to the effects of continence problems on social functioning.

Diseth and Emblem (1996) found that the duration of anal dilation in children with ARM in early childhood was negatively correlated to mental health and psychosocial functioning. No other studies have approached this problem, but it is an important finding because it indicates that frequent painful medical procedures in early childhood may have a long-standing negative influence on the psychological development of a child.

It can be concluded that HD and ARM are congenital anomalies which have long-term negative consequences for physical, psychological, and social functioning. Fecal incontinence is an embarrassing problem which affects a large proportion of children with HD and ARM. Many children with HD and ARM who have continence problems are functioning very well. However, in adolescence incontinence may have a more negative influence on QL. It appears that incontinence is not the sole determinant of QL in these children; other factors, such as having a congenital anomaly regardless of its consequences, or undergoing frequent painful medical procedures, may be of equal importance for the QL of these children. This is supported by the results of a large follow-up study of 140 children with several congenital abdominal disorders (Bouman, Koot, Verhulst, & Van Gils, 1999c). In this study the children with congenital abdominal anomalies did function worse than normative groups in several aspects (intelligence, school level, problem behavior) but very few specific aspects of the different anomalies influenced QL.

CONCLUSION

In conclusion it can be said that there are ample indications that it is necessary to continue QL research in children with congenital abdominal anomalies. The most adequate strategy seems to be to use generic QL measures which cover the physical, psychological, and social domains in a comprehensive way . Only for some anomalies will specific measures have to be added, such as measures for continence in HD and ARM. More efforts should be made to identify factors that determine QL. These efforts may help to implement adequate treatment and preventive measures.

References

Aaronson, N.K.A. (1991). Methodological issues in assessing the quality of life of cancer patients. *Cancer, 67,* 844–850.

Ahmed, A., & Spitz, L. (1986). The outcome of colonic replacement of the esophagus in children. *Progress in Pediatric Surgery, 19,* 37–54.

Anderson, K.A., Noblett, H., Belsey, R., & Randolph, J.G. (1992). Long-term follow-up of children with colon and gastric tube interposition for esophageal atresia. *Surgery, 111,* 131–136.

Apley, J. (1959). *The child with abdominal pains.* Oxford, United Kingdom: Blackwell Scientific Publications.

Apley, J. (1975). *The child with abdominal pains.* Oxford, United Kingdom: Blackwell Scientific Publications.

Apley, J., & Hale, B. (1973). Children with recurrent abdominal pain: How do they grow up? *British Medical Journal, 3,* 7–9.

Biller, J.A., Allen, J.L., Schuster, S.R., Treves, S.T., & Winter, H.S. (1987). Long-term evaluation of esophageal and pulmonary function in patients with repaired esophageal atresia and tracheoesophageal fistula. *Digestive Diseases and Sciences, 32,* 985–990.

Boemers, M.L., De Jong, T.P.V.M., van Gool, J.D., & Bax, K.M.A. (1996). Urologic problems in anorectal malformations. Part 2: Functional urologic sequelae. *Journal of Pediatric Surgery, 31,* 634–637.

Borge, A.I.H., Nordhagen, R., Moe, B., Botten, G., & Bakketeig, L.S. (1994). Prevalence and persistence of stomachache and headache among children. Follow-up of a cohort of Norwegian children from 4 to 10 years of age. *Acta Paediatrica, 83,* 433–437.

Bouman, N.H., Koot, H.M., Tibboel, D., & Hazebroek, F.W.J. (2000). Children with congenital diafragmatic hernia are at risk for lower levels of cognitive functioning and increased emotional and behavioral problems. *European Journal of Pediatric Surgery, 10,* 3–7.

Bouman, N.H., Koot, H.M., & Hazebroek, F.W.J. (1999a). Long-term physical, psychological, and social functioning of children with esophageal atresia. *Journal of Pediatric Surgery, 34,* 399–404.

Bouman, N.H., Koot, H.M., & Hazebroek, F.W.J. (1999b). Psychosocial functioning of children with Hirschsprung's disease and anorectal anomalies. *Submitted for publication.*

Bouman, N.H., Koot, H.M., Van Gils, A.P.J.M., & Verhulst, F.C. (1999c). Development of a health-related quality of life instrument for children: The Quality of Life Questionnaire for Children. *Psychology & Health, 14,* 829–846.

Büller, H.A. (1997). Problems in diagnosis of IBD in children. *The Netherlands Journal of Medicine, 50,* S8-S11.

Burke, P., Meyer, V., Kokoshis, S., Orenstein, D., Chandra, R., Nord, D.J., Sauer, J., & Cohen, E. (1989a). Depression and anxiety in pediatric inflammatory bowel disease and cystic fibrosis. *Journal of the American Academy of Child and Adolescent Psychiatry, 28,* 948–951.

Burke, P., Meyer, V., Kokoshis, S., Orenstein, D., Chandra, R., & Sauer, J. (1989b). Obsessive-compulsive symptoms in childhood inflammatory bowel disease and cystic fibrosis. *Journal of the American Academy of Child and Adolescent Psychiatry, 28,* 525–527.

Chatrath, R.R., El Shafie, M., & Jones, R.S. (1971). Fate of hypoplastic lungs after repair of congenital diaphragmatic hernia. *Archives of Diseases in Childhood, 46,* 633–635.

Chetcuti, P., Dickens, D.R.V., & Phelan, P.D. (1989). Spinal deformity in patients born with esophageal atresia and tracheo-esophageal fistula. *Archives of Diseases in Childhood, 64,* 1427–1430.

Chetcuti, P., Myers, N.A., Phelan, P.D., & Beasley, S.W. (1988). Adults who survived repair of congenital oesophageal atresia and tracheo-oesophageal fistula. *British Medical Journal, 297,* 344–346.

Chetcuti, P., Myers, N.A., Phelan, P.D., Beasley, S.W., & Dickens, D.R.V. (1989). Chest wall deformity in patients with repaired esophageal atresia. *Journal of Pediatric Surgery, 24,* 244–247.

Chetcuti, P., & Phelan, P.D. (1993). Gastrointestinal morbidity after repair of oesophageal atresia and tracheo-oesophageal fistula. *Archives of Diseases in Childhood, 68*, 163–167.

Chetcuti, P., Phelan, P.D., & Greenwood, R. (1992). Lung-function abnormalities in repaired oesophageal atresia and tracheo-oesophageal fistula. *Thorax, 47*, 1030–1034.

D'Agostino, J.A., Bernbaum, J.C., Gerdes, M., Schwartz, I.P., Coburn, C.E., Hirschis R.B., Baumgart, S., & Polin, R.A. (1995). Outcome for infants with congenital diaphragmatic hernia requiring extracorporeal membrane oxygenation: The first year. *Journal of Pediatric Surgery, 30*, 10–5.

Davenport, M., Rivlin, E., D'Souza, S.W., & Bianchi, A. (1992). Delayed surgery for congenital diaphragmatic hernia: Neurodevelopmental outcome in later childhood. *Archives of Diseases in Childhood, 67*, 1353–1356.

Daum, R. (1984). Spätergebnisse nach operativen Korrektur kongenitaler Bauchwanddefekte. [Late outcomes of surgical correction of abdominal wall defect.] *Monatschrift für Kinderheilkunde, 132*, 402–407.

Delepoulle, F., Martinot, A., Leclerc, F., Riou, Y., Remi-Jardin, M., Amegassi, F., Dubois, J.P., & Lequien, P. (1991). Devenir à longe terme des hernies diaphragmatiques congénitales. Etude de 17 enfants. [Long-term outcome of congenital diaphragmatic hernia. Study of 17 infants.]. *Archives Francaises de Pediatrie, 48*, 703–707.

Dera, M., Mies, U., & Martinus, J. (1980). Erste Ergebnisse der Studie zur psychosozialen Entwicklung von Kindern, die wegen bestimmter Fehlbildungen als Neugeborene operiert werden mussten. [First results of the study on psychosocial development of children who were operated as newborns for certain anomalies.] *Zeitschrift für Kinderchirurgie, 29*, 95–108.

Diseth, T.H., Bjornland, K., Novik, T.S., & Emblem, R. (1997). Bowel function, mental health, and psychosocial function in adolescents with Hirschsprung's disease. *Archives of Diseases in Childhood, 76*, 100–106.

Diseth, T.H., & Emblem, R. (1996). Somatic function, mental health, and psychosocial adjustment of adolescents with anorectal anomalies. *Journal of Pediatric Surgery, 31*, 638–643.

Ditesheim, J., & Templeton, J.M. (1987). Short-term vs long-term quality of life in children following repair of high imperforate anus. *Journal of Pediatric Surgery, 22*, 581–587.

Drossman, D.A. (1996). Inflammatory bowel disease. In B. Spilker (ed.), *Quality of life and pharmacoeconomics in clinical trials* (pp. 925–935). Philadelphia, PA: Lippincot-Raven Publishers.

Engström, I. (1991a). Family interaction and locus of control in children and adolescents with inflammatory bowel disease. *Journal of the American Academy of Child and Adolescent Psychiatry, 30*, 913–920.

Engström, I. (1991b). Parental distress and social interaction in families with children with inflammatory bowel disease. *Journal of the American Academy of Child and Adolescent Psychiatry, 30*, 904–912.

Engström, I. (1992). Mental health and psychological functioning in children and adolescents with inflammatory bowel disease: a comparison with children having other chronic illnesses and with healthy children. *Journal of Child Psychology and Psychiatry, 33*, 563–582.

Engström, I., & Lindquist, B.L. (1991). Inflammatory bowel disease in children and adolescents: a somatic and psychiatric investigation. *Acta Paediatrica Scandinavica, 80*, 640–647.

Falconer, A.R., Brown, R.A., Helms, P., Gordon, I., & Baron, J.A. (1990). Pulmonary sequelae in survivors of congenital diaphragmatic hernia. *Thorax, 45*, 126–129.

Faull, C., & Nicol, A.R. (1986). Abdominal pain in six-year-olds: An epidemiological study in a new town. *Journal of Child Psychology and Psychiatry, 27*, 251–260.

Finch, S.M., & Hess, J.H. (1962). Ulcerative colitis in children. *American Journal of Psychiatry, 118*, 819–826.

Finney, J.W., Lemanek, K.L., Cataldo, M.F., Katz, H.P., & Fuqua, R.W. (1989). Pediatric psychology in primary health care: Brief targeted therapy for recurrent abdominal pain. *Behavior Therapy, 20*, 283–291.

Freyschuss, U., Lännergren, K., & Frenckner, B. (1984). Lung function after repair of congenital diaphragmatic hernia. *Acta Paediatrica Scandinavica, 73*, 589–593.

Garber, J., Zeman, J., & Walker, L.S. (1990). Recurrent abdominal pain in children: Psychiatric diagnosis and parental psychopathology. *Journal of the American Academy of Child and Adolescent Psychiatry, 29*, 648–656.

Garret, J.W., & Drossman, D.A. (1990). Health status in inflammatory bowel disease. Biological and behavioral considerations. *Gastroenterology, 99,* 90–96.

Ginn-Pease, M.E., King, D.R., Tarnowski, K.J., Green, L., Young, G., & Linscheid, T.R. (1991). Psychosocial adjustment and physical growth in children with imperforate anus or abdominal wall defects. *Journal of Pediatric Surgery, 26,* 1129–1135.

Griffiths, A.M., Nicholas, D., Smith, C., Munk, M., Stephens, D., Durno, C., & Sherman, P.M. (1999). Development of a quality-of-life index for pediatric inflammatory bowel disease: Dealing with differences related to age and IBD type. *Journal of Pediatric Gastroenterology and Nutrition, 28,* S46–52.

Halsband, H., & Von Schwabe, C. (1989). Langzeitergebnisse und Lebensqualität bei Kindern mit Omphalocele und Gastroschizis. [Long-term outcomes and quality of life of children with omphalocele and gastroschizis.] *Langenbecks Archiven für Chirurgie,* 951–955.

Hassink, E.A.M., Rieu, P.N.M.A., Brugman, A.T.M., & Festen, C. (1994). Quality of life after operatively corrected high anorectal malformation: A long-term follow-up study of patients aged 18 years and older. *Journal of Pediatric Surgery, 29,* 773–776.

Heij, H.A., De Vries, X., Bremer, I., Ekkelkamp, S., & Vos, A. (1995). Long-term anorectal function after Duhamel operation for Hirschsprung's disease. *Journal of Pediatric Surgery, 30,* 430–432.

Helzer, J.E., Stillings, W.A., Chamas, S., Norland, C.C., & Alpers, D.H. (1982). A controlled study of the association between ulcerative colitis and psychiatric diagnoses. *Digestive Diseases and Sciences, 27,* 513–518.

Helzer, J.E., Chamas, S., Norland, C.C., Stillings, W.A., & Alpers D.H. (1984). A study of the association between Crohn's disease and psychiatric illness. *Gastroenterology, 86,* 324–330.

Herbst, J.J. (1992). Inflammatory bowel disease. In R.E. Behrman (ed.), *Nelson textbook of pediatrics* (pp. 966–970). Philadelphia, PA: W.B. Saunders Company.

Hyams, J.S. (1996). Crohn's disease in children. *Pediatric Clinics of North America, 43,* 255–277.

Hyams, J.S., Burke, G., Davis, P.M., Rzepski, B., & Andrulonis, P.A. (1996). Abdominal pain and irritable bowel syndrome in adolescents: A community based study. *Journal of Pediatrics, 129,* 220–226.

Hyams, J.S., Grand, R.J., Colodny, A.H., Schuster, S.R., & Eraklis, A. (1982). Course and prognosis after colectomy and ileostomy for inflammatory bowel disease in childhood and adolescence. *Journal of Pediatric Surgery, 17,* 400–405.

IJsselstijn, H., Tibboel, D., & Hop, W.C.J. (1997). Long-term pulmonary sequelae in children with congenital diaphragmatic hernia. *American Journal of Respiratory and Critical Care Medicine, 155,* 174–180.

Kerr, A.A. (1977). Lung function in children after repair of congenital diaphragmatic hernia. *Archives of Diseases in Childhood, 52,* 902–903.

Kieffer, J., Sapin, E., Berg, A., Beaudoin, S., Bargy, F., & Helardot, P.G. (1995). Gastroesophageal reflux after repair of congenital diaphragmatic hernia. *Journal of Pediatric Surgery, 30,* 1330–1333.

Kirschner, B.S. (1996). Ulcerative colitis in children. *Pediatric Clinics of North America, 43,* 235–254.

Langemeijer, R.A.T.M., & Molenaar, J. (1991) Continence after posterior sagittal anorectoplasty. *Journal of Pediatric Surgery, 26,* 587–590.

Langham, M.R., Kays, D.W., Ledbetter, D.J., Frentzen, D., Sanford, L.L., & Richards, D.S. (1996). Congenital diaphragmatic hernia. Epidemiology and outcome. *Clinics in Perinatology, 23,* 671–688.

Langholz, E., Munkholm, P., Krasilnikoff, P.A., & Binder, V. (1997). Inflammatory bowel disease with onset in childhood. Clinical features, morbidity, and mortality in a regional cohort. *Scandinavian Journal of Gastroenterology, 32,* 139–147.

Larsson, L.T., & Kullendorf, C.M. (1990). Late surgical problems in children born with abdominal wall defects. *Annales Chirurgiae et Gynaecologiae, 79,* 23–25.

Lask, B., Jenkins, J., Nabarro, L., & Booth, I. (1987). Psychosocial sequelae of stoma surgery for inflammatory bowel disease in childhood. *Gut, 28,* 1257–1260.

Lehner, M. (1984). Ösophagusatresie und Lebensqualität. *Zeitschrift für Kinderchirurgie, 45,* 209–211.

Lindahl, H., Rintala, R., & Sariola, H. (1993). Chronic esophagitis and gastric metaplasia are frequent late complications of esophageal atresia. *Journal of Pediatric Surgery, 28,* 1178–1180.

Lindham, S. (1984). Long-term results in children with omphalocele and gastroschizis. A follow-up study. *Zeitschrift für Kinderchirurgie, 39*, 164–167.

Ludman, L., Spitz, L., & Kiely, E.M. (1994). Social and emotional impact of faecal incontinence after surgery for anorectal abnormalities. *Archives of Diseases in Childhood, 71*, 194–200.

Lund, D.P., Mitchell, J., Kharasch, V., Quigley, S., Kuehn, M., & Wilson, J.M. (1994). Congenital diaphragmatic hernia: The hidden morbidity. *Journal of Pediatric Surgery, 29*, 258–264.

Marty, T.L., Seo, T., Matlak, M.E., Sullivan, J.J., Black, R.E., & Johnson, D.G. (1995). Gastrointestinal function after surgical correction of Hirschsprung's disease: Long-term follow-up in 135 patients. *Journal of Pediatric Surgery, 30*, 655–658.

Misra, D., Mushtaq, I., Drake, D.P., Kiely, E.M., & Spitz, L. (1996). Associated urologic anomalies in low imperforate anus are capable of causing significant morbidity: A 15-year experience. *Urology, 48*, 281–283.

Moore, S.W., Albertyn, R., & Cywes, S. (1996). Clinical outcome and long-term quality of life after surgical correction of Hirschsprung's disease. *Journal of Pediatric Surgery, 31*, 1496–1502.

Nobuhara, K.K., Lund, D.P., Mitchell, J., Kharasch, V., & Wilson, J.M. (1996). Long-term outlook for survivors of congenital diaphragmatic hernia. *Clinics in Perinatology, 23*, 873–887.

Prugh, D.G. (1951). The influence of emotional factors on the clinical course of ulcerative colitis in children. *Gastroenterology, 18*, 339–354.

Puntis, J.W.L., Ritson, D.G., Holden, C.E., & Buick, R.G. (1990). Growth and feeding problems after repair of oesophageal atresia. *Archives of Diseases in Childhood, 65*, 84–88.

Rabbett, H., Elbadri, R., Northover, H., Dady, I., Firth, D., Hillier, V.F., Miller, V., & Thomas, A.G. (1996). Quality of life in children with Crohn's disease. *Journal of Pediatric Gastroenterology and Nutrition, 23*, 528–533.

Raymer, D., Weininger, O., & Hamilton, J.R. (1984). Psychological problems in children with abdominal pain. *The Lancet, 1 (8374)*, 439–440.

Reid, I.S., & Hutcherson, R.J. (1976). Long-term follow-up of patients with congenital diaphragmatic hernia. *Journal of Pediatric Surgery, 11*, 939–942.

Rescorla, F.J., Morrison, A.M., Engles, D., West, K.W., & Grosfeld, J.L. (1992). Hirschsprung's disease. Evaluation of mortality and long-term function in 260 cases. *Archives of Surgery, 127*, 934–942.

Rintala, R., Mildh, L., & Lindahl, H. (1992). Fecal continence and quality of life in patients with an operated low anorectal malformation. *Journal of Pediatric Surgery, 27*, 902–905.

Robertson, D.F., Mobaireek, K., Davis, G.M., & Coates, A.L. (1995). Late pulmonary function following repair of tracheoesophageal fistula or esophageal atresia. *Pediatric Pulmonology, 20*, 21–26.

Robinson, J.O., Alvarez, J.H., & Dodge, J.A. (1990). Life events and family history in children with recurrent abdominal pain. *Journal of Psychosomatic Research, 34*, 171–181.

Saeki, M., Tsuchida, Y., Ogata, T., Nakano, M., & Akiyama, H. (1988). Long-term results of jejunal replacement of the esophagus. *Journal of Pediatric Surgery, 23*, 483–489.

Sanders, M.R., Shepherd, R.W., Cleghorn, G., & Woolford, H. (1994). The treatment of recurrent abdominal pain in children: A controlled comparison of cognitive behavioral family intervention and standard pediatric care. *Journal of Consulting and Clinical Psychology, 62*, 306–314.

Spieth, L.E., & Harris, C.V. (1996). Assessment of health-related quality of life in children and adolescents: An integrative review. *Journal of Pediatric Psychology, 21*, 175–193.

Steinhausen, H.C., & Kies, H. (1982). Comparative studies of ulcerative colitis and Crohn's disease in children and adolescents. *Journal of Child Psychology and Psychiatry, 23*, 33–42.

Stevenson, J., Simpson, J., & Bailey, V. (1988). Research note: Recurrent headaches and stomachaches in preschool children. *Journal of Child Psychology and Psychiatry, 29*, 897–900.

Stolar, C.J.H., Crisafi, M.A., & Driscoll, Y.T. (1995). Neurocognitive outcome for neonates treated with extracorporeal membrane oxygenation: Are infants with congenital diaphragmatic hernia different? *Journal of Pediatric Surgery, 30*, 366–72.

Swartz, K.R., Harrison, M.W., Campbell, J.R., & Campbell, T.J. (1986). Long-term follow-up of patients with gastroschizis. *The American Journal of Surgery, 151*, 546–549.

Tarnowski, K.J., King, D.R., Green, L., & Ginn-Pease, M.E. (1991). Congenital gastrointestinal anomalies: Psychosocial functioning of children with imperforate anus, gastroschizis, and omphalocele. *Journal of Consulting and Clinical Psychology, 59*, 587–590.

Touloukian, R.J., & Spackman, T.J. (1971). Gastrointestinal function and radiographic appearance following gastroschizis repair. *Journal of Pediatric Surgery, 6*, 427–434.

Tunell, W.P., Puffinbarger, N.K., Tuggle, D.W., Taylor D.V., & Mantor, P.C. (1995). Abdominal wall defects in infants. Survival and implications for adult life. *Annals of Surgery, 221*, 525–530.

Turnbull, G.K., & Vallis, T.M. (1995). Quality of life in inflammatory bowel disease: The interaction of disease activity with psychosocial function. *The American Journal of Gastroenterology, 90*, 1450–1454.

Ure, B.M., Slany, E., Eupasch, E.P., Gharib, M., Holschneider, A.M., & Troidl, H. (1994). Long-term functional results and quality of life after colon interposition for long-gap oesophageal atresia. *European Journal of Pediatric Surgery, 5*, 206–210.

Vanamo, K., Peltonen, J., Rintala, R., Lindahl, H., Jääskeläinen, J., & Louhimo, I. (1996). Chest wall and spinal deformities in adults with congenital diaphragmatic defects. *Journal of Pediatric Surgery, 31*, 851–854.

Vanamo, K., Rintala, R.J., Lindahl, H., & Louhimo, I. (1996). Long-term gastrointestinal morbidity in patients with congenital diaphragmatic defects. *Journal of Pediatric Surgery, 31*, 551–554.

Vanamo, K., Rintala, R., Sovijärvi, A., Jääskeläinen, J., Turpeinen. M., Lindahl, H., & Louhimo, I. (1996). Long-term pulmonary sequelae in survivors of congenital diaphragmatic defects. *Journal of Pediatric Surgery, 31*, 1096–1100.

Van Der Meer, S.B. (1993). Chronische recidiverende buikpijn bij schoolkinderen. [Chronic recurrent abdominal pain in school-aged children.] *Tijdschrift voor Kindergeneeskunde, 61*, 69–75.

Van Meurs, K.P., Robbins, S.T., Reed, V.L., Karr, S.S., Wagner, A.E., Glass, P., Anderson, K.D., & Short, B.L. (1993). Congenital diaphragmatic hernia: Long-term outcome in neonates treated with extracorporeal membrane oxygenation. *Journal of Pediatrics, 122*, 893–899.

Walker, L.S., & Greene, J.W. (1989). Children with recurrent abdominal pain and their parents: More somatic complaints, anxiety, and depression than other patient families. *Journal of Pediatric Psychology, 14*, 231–243.

Walker, L.S., Garber, J., Van Slyke, A., & Greene, J.W. (1995). Long-term health outcomes in patients with recurrent abdominal pain. *Journal of Pediatric Psychology, 20*, 233–245.

Wischermann, A., Holschneider, A.M., & Hubner, U. (1995). Long-term follow-up of children with diaphragmatic hernia. *European Journal of Pediatric Surgery, 5*, 13–18.

Wohl, M.B., Griscom, N.D., Strieder, D.J., Schuster, S.R., Treves, S., & Zwerdling, R.G. (1977). The lung following repair of congenital diaphragmatic hernia. *Journal of Pediatrics, 90*, 405–414.

Wood, B., Watkins, J.B., Boyle, J.T., Nogueira, J., Zimand, E., & Carroll, L. (1987). Psychological functioning in children with Crohn's disease and ulcerative colitis: Implications for models of psychological interaction. *Journal of the American Academy of Child and Adolescent Psychiatry, 26*, 774–781.

Chapter 9

ASTHMA

Davina J. French

Current estimates of the prevalence of asthma in childhood range from 11–12% in the UK (Hilton, 1994) and 9.5% in the USA (Nelson et al., 1997) to 16–17% in Australia (Bauman et al., 1992; Forero, Bauman, Young, & Larkin, 1992). Some studies suggest that the lower of these figures represent significant under-diagnosis; in one US study a further 8.5% of children suffered asthma symptoms without diagnosis (Joseph, Foxman, Leickly, Peterson, & Ownby, 1996). Diagnosis may occur at any age and, among young children, is more common in boys. The very existence of between one in five and one in ten children with asthma in every classroom suggests that — to the extent that asthma has any negative impact on the quality of life (QL) — this impact is likely to be widespread.

Medically asthma is described as variable, reversible airways obstruction (Warner et al., 1989). For the individual this is experienced as episodes of coughing and wheezing which vary in frequency and severity. Although intermittent there is likely to be a pattern to these episodes since many children's asthma will have a strong atopic or allergic component. The most common allergen or "trigger" in children is the house dust mite (*Dermatophagoides pteronyssinus*) (Price, 1994) with pollens, moulds and animal dander also among the more regular culprits. Frequently this hyper-responsiveness of the airways will also be triggered by environmental irritants such as cold air and cigarette smoke, and by exertion. For many children with mild asthma their experience will be almost entirely limited to shortness of breath during and after exercise. In contrast to some of the medical conditions outlined in this volume the severity of asthma symptoms varies widely both between individuals and within individuals over time. The same child may experience eight to ten months of the year without impairment then suffer moderately severe symptoms for a short pollen or mould season. More commonly experiences will vary on a day-to-day basis.

Placing these medical features of asthma into the typical daily life of a child suggests that a sufferer may experience any or all of the following:

- frequent waking at night, since house dust mite is especially prevalent in mattresses and bedding;
- inability to sustain physical activities such as physical education and playground games;
- a risk of worsening asthma symptoms where allergens cannot be controlled, for example on school excursions or visits to the homes of others;
- the loss of a household pet if it is found to be the source of an allergic response;
- for sufferers of more severe forms of the disease increased school absence and periods of hospitalization during lengthy symptomatic episodes.

These are largely direct impacts of the symptoms of asthma, which themselves have the potential to lead to further indirect impacts. For example frequent broken nights may lead to under-performance in the classroom while school absence and exclusion from playground games may impair self-concept and social development. In addition, the daily management of the illness falls mainly to the child and his or her family. Medications are administered principally via an inhaler device, the use of which may draw unwanted attention to the user. In well-controlled asthma the need for medication may be restricted to preventative doses in the morning and evening but, even so, a fast-acting bronchodilator must be carried at all times in case of encounters with unexpected triggers. The ability to use these delivery devices is generally limited to children aged five years and over. The under fives need techniques which are both more time-consuming and more prone to cause systemic side-effects (Warner et al., 1989). Some of the drugs required to control severe asthma have been associated with a range of cognitive, behavioral and emotional side effects especially likely to impact upon a child's progress at school (Bender, 1995).

The wide range of functional effects of asthma symptoms and its treatments suggests that for some children many areas of life may be impaired. Schipper, Clinch, and Powell (1990) propose four broad components of health-related QL or dimensions along which the impact of chronic illness may be felt: physical limitation; emotional distress; social and relationship difficulties and somatic sensation (the discomfort associated with the illness itself). For the paediatric asthma patient all of these are relevant; physical limitation may be experienced at school and at home and emotional and social development may also be placed at risk.

The prior discussion has outlined the features of asthma that may impair QL on any or all of its dimensions. Impact is also likely to occur across the entire age range, although the changing concerns of the developing child and adolescent are likely to lead this impact to vary in nature. Especially in the case of young children the impact on the QL of parents and care-givers is also likely to be considerable and should not be overlooked. Broken nights, curtailed outings and sudden hospitalizations are likely to affect the whole family, as are measures to reduce allergens in the home.

This chapter will review a broad literature on the impact of childhood asthma, and discuss any age or sex differences found in these effects. It will then move on to a specific focus on quality of life, and how this can be operationalised in the context of asthma. The measures available to assess QL in childhood asthma will be described and evaluated. Finally, the future of QL assessment in this population and the role of valid assessment procedures in the improvement of QL will be discussed.

THE IMPACT OF ASTHMA

The literature on QL in childhood asthma is fairly new and quite limited. However, the range of studies investigating the psychosocial and educational effects of asthma is much larger. These studies can contribute to our accumulating knowledge of the impacts of childhood asthma where it is clear that they are addressing relevant dimensions of QL. This chapter will therefore review a diverse range of studies whose outcomes can be viewed as components of QL even where it does not appear as a named variable.

SCHOOL ATTENDANCE

For most children over the age of five the most salient feature of their daily lives is likely to be school attendance and the activities undertaken there. Research findings support the earlier claim that these are likely to be significant areas of QL impairment for some children with asthma. Children with asthma have been noted in a number of studies to suffer markedly higher rates of school absence. Fowler, Davenport, and Garg (1992) report an average of 7.6 days lost per year in their group of 5 to 17 year olds with asthma, compared with 2.5 days in a group of well controls. Twenty-one percent of these asthmatics had missed 11 or more days in the past year, with only 3% of controls reporting this level of absence. Importantly this study was able to rule out the effects of maternal education and ethnicity, both influential variables in school attendance and achievement. Missing out on school may have a wide range of effects on a child's functioning and QL, including their achievement in the classroom and their social integration with their peer group.

LEARNING DIFFICULTIES

Fowler et al. (1992) also report that children with asthma, after accounting for demographic variables, are 1.7 times more likely to suffer a learning difficulty than their healthy peers. This figure remains higher than normal, an odds ratio of 1.4:1, even when school absence is accounted for, suggesting that several factors associated with having asthma may be influential. In contrast, a number of studies (e.g. Gutstadt et al., 1989; O'Neil, Barysh, & Setear, 1985) have found that having asthma *per se* does not appear to impair school achievement, although it may interact with other predictors, for example low socioeconomic status (Gutstadt et al., 1989). Specific neuro-cognitive impairments, particularly of memory and attention, are known to be associated with the use of orally administered corticosteroids (Bender, 1995). While these effects are thought to be temporary, and this treatment is only used in short courses for more severe cases, the possibility of vital links in the learning chain being missed cannot be ruled out.

ACTIVITY RESTRICTIONS

A child's days at school are filled with far more than learning to read and write, and it is in some of the less academic areas that asthma has its greatest impact. Bremberg and Kjellman (1985) found that 78% of their sample of children with asthma reported activity restriction during physical education lessons. French, Christie, and West (1994) found a significant difference in the level of the enjoyment of playtime games between asthmatic and non-asthmatic children. Townsend et al. (1991) report the results of interviews with children attending hospital asthma clinics — 85% reported limitation when running and 30% suffered restriction when playing with friends. Just over half of these children reported feeling different because of their asthma, although on average they were less bothered by this than other aspects of their illness. Several other studies also suggest that impairment of social role functioning is limited. For example studies by Kashani, Konig, Shepperd, Wilfley, and Morris (1988) and Nassau and Drotar (1995) both found that the social competency of children with asthma does not differ from healthy controls. Qualitative work with children and adolescents (French et al., 1994) has revealed that concern with the social impact of asthma does not emerge until the mid-teens and so may be obscured in the above studies which looked at younger children or wider age ranges.

EMOTIONAL EFFECTS

Quality of life includes the dimension of emotional impairment, which may take the form of depression, anxiety or undue worry for the future. In young children, whose ability to express these emotions is limited, it may also be observed as problem behavior as youngsters struggle to understand their feelings. A range of studies has shown behavioral and emotional impacts of asthma, however these are seldom widespread and cofactors are often implicated. Bussing, Halfon, Benjamin, and Wells (1995) report that children who have asthma plus another medical condition are significantly more likely than healthy controls to display a range of current behavior problems including anxiety and depression, hyperactivity and peer conflict. For children with asthma alone only levels of anxiety and depression were significantly elevated. Children with severe asthma were also very much more likely (30% compared with 5%) to have suffered an emotional or behavioral problem during their lifetime. In a further study Bussing, Burkett, and Kelleher (1996) found that 43% of a group of children with mainly mild to moderate asthma experienced clinical levels of anxiety, significantly more than a matched control group. In these children separation anxiety was particularly prevalent; the authors suggest that this may be the result of repeated visits to hospital. MacLean, Perrin, Gortmaker, and Pierre (1992) also report that children who have asthma are at greater risk of poor psychological adjustment, and that this is increased if the asthma is severe and is compounded by low socioeconomic status and the occurrence of negative life events.

While levels of clinically significant psychological impairment may only be elevated in particular cases the occurrence of sub-clinical levels of emotional impact is much greater. It is these less severe but more regular emotional events which aggregate to produce significant impairment in the emotional component of QL. Townsend et al. (1991) report that 49% of children feel frightened by an asthma attack, and are very bothered by it, and 62% feel frustrated. Butz and Alexander (1993) report that 65% of children feel panic associated with an attack of asthma. Eksi, Molzan, Savasir, and Guler (1995) interviewed the mothers of children with asthma who reported high levels of overly dependent and of oppositional behavior. Walsh and Ryan-Wegner (1992) found that illness was the most frequent life stressor reported by children with asthma, and although some stressors such as parental separation were ranked as more severe, illness was rated as more severe than moving house or changing schools. Clearly having asthma is a source of negative emotional experience for many children and has the potential, for some, to result in serious mental health problems.

EFFECTS ON PARENTS

The impact of asthma on a child's life is not likely to occur in isolation, the QL of parents may also be impaired. In Townsend et al.'s study half of the parents they interviewed felt angry or upset when the child had an asthma attack, 81% experienced worry over their child's illness, 70% suffered sleep interruption and 51% experienced interference with their own work. Shulz, Dye, Jolicoeur, Cafferty, and Watson (1994) report the results of a qualitative study in which parents raised a wide range of impacts of their child's asthma. These included career limitations, increased housework, restricted social life and increased tension at home. In discussing the QL effects of childhood asthma it would therefore be inappropriate to exclude measures of family as well as patient impact.

AGE AND GENDER EFFECTS

Asthma prevalence varies with both age and sex; a number of explanations have been offered for these variations but no consensus has been reached (Sweeting, 1995). Prevalence declines after the mid-teens as some children appear to "outgrow" their asthma, however Price (1994) reports that more than 30% of teenagers who become asymptomatic will experience a recurrence during adulthood. While some figures (e.g. Hilton, 1994) suggest that up to half of the children who are diagnosed with asthma will outgrow it, others (e.g. Forero et al., 1992) show prevalence declining only from 16% to 12% and only in boys.

In children aged up to 10 years an increased prevalence of asthma in boys has been shown in a number of studies in the UK (Hilton, 1994) and the USA (Gold et al., 1993; Nelson et al., 1997). The ratio of male to female sufferers in this age group is likely to be at least 1.5:1 and in individual studies has been found to be almost 3:1 (Nelson et al., 1997). During the teenage years prevalence increases in girls and decreases in boys with rates being equal by around 14–15 years of age (Gergen, Mullally, & Evans, 1988; Forero et al., 1992).

Asthma is not a progressive illness — that is it does not worsen with longer duration — although with increasing age wheeze takes over from cough as the primary symptom. The impact of asthma on QL is, however, far from stable since QL is about the patient's perceptions and is thus determined by an interaction of the illness itself with the concerns, abilities and activities of the individual. Age differences observed in both the objective and subjective impact of asthma are consistent with the typical developmental changes taking place during childhood and adolescence. For example deaths from childhood asthma are most likely to occur during adolescence (Warner et al., 1989) despite the fact that greater physical and cognitive maturity should enable the adolescent to self-manage more effectively. These deaths are largely avoidable and may be associated with the lower compliance levels seen in adolescents (Christiaanse, Lavigne, & Lerner, 1989). Smoking during the teenage years has been shown to increase respiratory symptoms (Gold et al., 1993). Despite this, youngsters with asthma are no less likely to smoke than their peers (Forero et al., 1992), and in some studies do so at higher rates than healthy controls (Forero, Bauman, Young, Booth, & Nutbeam, 1996).

Such behavior may be part of a syndrome of feelings and actions often experienced by teenagers including the need to gain independence from parents and to conform with peers (Lemanek, 1990). Taking regular medication and avoiding trigger factors can interfere with these important developmental tasks and may help to explain why some studies have found that teenagers with asthma report greater loneliness (Forero et al., 1996) and lower self-esteem (Seigel, Golden, Gough, Lashley, & Sacker, 1990) than healthy teenagers. Focus group work with teenagers has supported this line of argument, with youngsters in the 13 to 15 year age range raising issues such as the use of medication in public and the need to avoid cigarette smoke as major social concerns. Adolescents with asthma frequently cited the reactions of their peers as their greatest asthma-related concern (French et al., 1994).

There is also some evidence that the educational impact of asthma may be cumulative since although Gudstadt et al. (1989) were not able to link absence during the current semester with poor school performance, they did find that earlier onset and longer duration of asthma were predictive of lowered performance. This pattern has also been observed, and more extensively investigated, in youngsters with insulin-dependent diabetes mellitus (Kovacs, Goldston, & Iyengar, 1992). These authors concluded that setbacks in school achievement were likely to be the result of repeated school absences, which have also been noted in children with asthma (see above). The impact of asthma on school functioning may therefore be worse for teenagers than for younger children, particularly during the years that an examinable syllabus must be covered.

There is some suggestion that on average boys experience more severe illness than girls (McNichol & Williams, 1973) and are disproportionately more likely to need hospital treatment (Skobeloff, Spivey, St Clair, & Schoffstall, 1992). Studies have also shown that the observable components of school functioning — educational achievement and behavior — are more likely to be impaired in boys with asthma than in girls (Fowler et al., 1992; Bussing et al., 1995). Learning and behavior problems are however markedly more frequent among male children in the general population (Sweeting, 1995) and the increased rates in children with asthma may not reflect an illness specific component.

In summary, while age and sex differences are apparent in the impact of asthma on quality of life, they are limited to those that might be predicted from our general knowledge of the ways in which boys and girls, and older and younger children, differ. In particular we might expect the importance of different dimensions of QL to differ with the age of the child. This prediction however rests upon assumptions about how QL is to be defined and measured. It is to the more specific definition of quality of life in childhood asthma that this chapter will now turn.

QUALITY OF LIFE IN CHILDHOOD ASTHMA
DEFINITION

In order to define the scope of the following review of instruments that purport to measure QL in childhood asthma, it is necessary to examine the degree of overlap between the construct of asthma-specific QL and the range of physical and psychological impacts of asthma reviewed above. Spieth and Harris (1996) offer a general definition of QL as the subjective and objective impact of dysfunction associated with illness or injury, medical treatment or health policy (p. 176). Richards and Hemstreet (1994), in the specific field of asthma, distinguish between (objective) impairment and QL, which they define as how much the impairment (subjectively) matters. In a foundational work in this literature Schipper et al. (1990) propose that health-related QL represents the functional effects of an illness, and its subsequent therapy upon the patient, *as perceived by the patient* (p. 16, my emphasis). It is to this important aspect of QL that the reader's attention is drawn — QL should be a matter of patient perception, or patient experienced impact. Thus the literature reviewed above on the educational, functional and emotional impact of asthma is addressing QL to the extent that the child him or herself is concerned by the impact. This review will therefore be restricted to those instruments that assess the impact of the disease on the individual from the perspective of that individual. This is most aptly achieved using self-reports however in the case of childhood QL proxy reports, most often by parents, are not uncommon (Osman & Silverman, 1996). These proxy measures are included where it is clear that the items assess aspects of functional status that are likely to be perceived as salient by the child.

Since asthma has been demonstrated to impact upon a child in a number of ways — educational, social, emotional and physical — it is also argued here that QL in childhood asthma is likely to be multidimensional. This is consistent with the views of Vivier, Bernier, and Starfield (1994) who propose that an appropriate range of health outcomes for paediatric patients includes physical and emotional well-being, activity and achievement as well as longevity and disease status. Adult asthma QL measures (Hyland, Bellesis, Thompson, & Kenyon, 1996; Juniper, Guyatt, Ferrie, & Griffith, 1993; Wisniewski et al., 1997) also display multidimensionality, both conceptually and when factor analyzed. This review will therefore be restricted to measures that aim to assess more than disease status. At the very least those included all address functional limitation as well as symptoms. The most extensive of them, like the measures of asthma-specific QL in adults, include both emotional and functional components as well as symptom reports.

In summary a number of characteristics are argued to be important features of QL measures for childhood asthma. The following questions will therefore be asked of each measure.

- How many of the likely dimensions of impact — physical symptoms, emotions and daily activities at home and at school — does the instrument address?
- How was the content of the instrument derived, and is this consistent with a conceptualization of QL as patient-centred?
- Who reports, and does the measure assess aspects of QL for which a different informant may be more accurate?

- Does the instrument meet the general requirements of reliability and validity?
- Has it been shown to be useful in clinical or research settings?

Finally, this chapter will only review in detail those measures that are asthma-specific. These include three self-report measures for the children themselves, two proxy reports of childhood QL, and one self-report measure of the QL of those who care for children with asthma. A brief account will then be given of those generic measures that have a history of successful application with paediatric asthma patients. More detailed accounts of these measures may be found in other chapters of this volume.

MEASURES

Life Activities Questionnaire for Childhood Asthma

The Life Activities Questionnaire for Childhood Asthma (Creer et al., 1993), is intended for the assessment of functioning in a single QL domain — daily activities. The prior review suggests that this is a highly salient domain for children with asthma and it seems likely that some users will nominate these activities as the primary target of their intervention. Within the principle of selecting a measure that closely matches the intended outcomes it is therefore likely to be a useful questionnaire for some applications. The instrument contains 71 items under seven headings: physical activities, work activities, outdoor activities, emotional behaviors, home care, eating and drinking, and miscellaneous. These are rated by the child on a five point ordinal scale from "total restriction" to "no restriction". The items were derived from information gathered systematically from patients and so are likely to be a fair reflection of the activities that children actually undertake and experience restriction in. Each section also provides space for respondents to nominate their own activities although it is not clear how these are to be scored.

Initial reaction to a report of 71 items is that this would be too long for a paediatric self-report measure. The items are however in the form of a checklist of largely single words, e.g. walking, swimming, dusting, vacuuming, and so the reading requirement, beyond the instructions, is not great. The data reported by Creer et al. (1993) are from a postal survey and so the time needed for completion is not known. The sample age range was however 5 to 17 years and the authors report that parents were asked to assist where necessary. It seems likely that children below the age of about 8 years would need considerable assistance, particularly in the use of the response scale. The test-retest reliability over one month is an acceptable 0.76 for the total scale. Cronbach's *alpha* is reported as 0.97 for the total scale, although since *alpha* is strongly influenced by the number of items in a scale this value may not be comparable to those reported for shorter instruments or subscales. Validity estimates are not presented but inspection of the scores reported suggests that the instrument is hitting its target. For example the greatest average restriction is reported for those activities most strongly associated with the known clinical aspects of asthma, including working in strong odours or with chemicals, being around pets or cigarette smoke, running, dusting and vacuuming.

This instrument is targeted specifically at a single component of QL and the available evidence suggests that it is likely to be useful for this purpose. Caution is however likely to be necessary with young children, especially pre-readers, and with samples outside North America. The process of basing the items on patients' responses has led to good content validity for this population but the content is, necessarily, constrained by the lifestyles of the respondents. Items therefore include some climate specific activities such as raking leaves and shovelling snow, but not others such as going to the beach and watering the garden. Some terms are also highly specific to North American English, such as "Horsing around" and "Hayride". These problems are however present at some level in all measures and care is always needed when using instruments developed in other countries.

Index of Perceived Symptoms in Asthmatic Children

The Index of Perceived Symptoms in Asthmatic Children (Usherwood, Scrimgeour, & Barber 1990), assesses impact in the broad areas of symptoms and activity limitation. Factor analysis reveals three factors: Disability, which asks in general terms about interference with activities at home and at school, Nocturnal Symptoms and Daytime Symptoms. Responses are on a five point ordinal scale from "every day" to "not at all". The measure is completed by parents and the items were refined through pilot work with parents. All but one of the items do however ask directly about impact on the child. Whilst self-report may be preferred for these aspects of QL the careful piloting of the instrument has resulted in items which parents are, at least on the face of it, able to answer. For example they are asked "has your child's education suffered?" rather than "has your child been restricted at school?" and "has your child *complained of* being short of breath?" which might otherwise be difficult to observe. While the scope might be narrowed by this approach, the accuracy of the proxy reports is likely to be maximised.

Data are reported from a sample of 5 to 14 year olds. Good internal consistency was obtained but test-retest reliability is not reported. The authors do not discuss another important issue in the use of proxy reports — the agreement between two care-givers completing the instrument about the same child. Two observers are not exposed to the same aspects of the child's life, and so their reports are unlikely to be 100% concordant, nevertheless the reporting of such a figure is valuable. Such information allows the user to ascertain the potential importance of a problem raised by Bender (1996) of the instrument being completed by different informants in different phases of a study. In the absence of such information it would be wise to take steps to ensure that the same proxy completes the questionnaire on all occasions. The authors also suggest that the instrument may be useful as a means of communicating with individual patients about their illness; in this case the parent who accompanies the child is likely to be the appropriate respondent.

Items from the index have been used in a number of epidemiological studies (e.g. Peat, Gray, Mellis, Leeder, & Woolcock, 1994; Gray, Peat, Mellis, Harrington, & Woolcock, 1994) where their reproducibility has also been established.

Asthma Functional Severity Scale

The Asthma Functional Severity Scale (Rosier et al., 1994) is a six item, parent completed measure which provides a single score comprised of symptom and activity limitation components. The items were selected by "experienced judgement" (p. 1439) — that is, the primary input was from physicians rather than patients. This begs a question regarding whose opinions of the important functions impaired by asthma are reflected in the instrument. Factor analysis indicates that the scale is unidimensional and the relatively low *alpha* of 0.65 is not surprising for a scale of only six items. Reproducibility over time is not reported. Item response theory has been used to estimate calibrated scale scores and perhaps more usefully, four bands of functional severity based on the raw scores.

The statistical techniques employed rest on the assumption that there is a single latent trait of functional severity underlying item responses, one which is distinct from physiological severity (Rosier et al., 1994). Construct validity estimates are consistent with this distinction — the severity scale scores show a moderate correlation with a generic measure of functional severity, the FSII(R) (Stein & Jessop, 1990), but are weakly related to lung function. These findings may however also be attributable to common method variance since the FSII(R) is also parent-completed. There is also factor analytic evidence from a number of studies in children (Christie, French, Sowden, & West, 1993; Usherwood et al., 1990) and adults (Wisniewski et al., 1997) that items about symptoms and about activity limitation factor out separately when both are present in sufficient numbers. Whilst there are likely to be large scale epidemiological studies in which this scale is invaluable for its brevity, and its provision of a "standardised" score, it seems unlikely that it would be the measure of choice for treatment evaluations. Again the authors suggest that it may be useful in clinical consultations. Data are reported on children aged 8 to 16 years and the authors refer to the scale as suitable for "school-age children". The applicable age range is likely to be limited only by an item asking about "your child's sporting activities".

Paediatric Asthma Quality of Life Questionnaire

The Paediatric Asthma Quality of Life Questionnaire (PAQLQ) (Juniper et al., 1996b), bears a strong resemblance to its adult partner, the Asthma Quality of Life Questionnaire (AQLQ; Juniper et al., 1993) and has been developed using similar techniques. The instrument is self-report, but has so far been reported only when administered by a trained interviewer. This takes 10 to 15 minutes for the 23-item questionnaire. Satisfactory psychometric characteristics are reported across the entire age range of 7 to 17 years (Juniper, Guyatt, Feeny, Griffith, & Ferrie, 1997). The items assess a wide range of symptoms, emotions and activities, producing three subscale scores with these labels. Three of the activity items require the child to select the three activities that bother them most. The child is first asked to produce these spontaneously and then offered a list to select from. The authors indicate that it would be appropriate to alter this list to suit varying cultures and climates. In addition to these "individualised" items the remaining items are based on extensive consultation with patients. The subscales are however identified *a priori* rather than through factor analysis and evidence for their independence is not reported.

The PAQLQ has excellent psychometric properties as an instrument for treatment evaluation — intraclass correlation coefficients of reproducibility range from 0.84 to 0.95 over 1 month in stable patients and all subscales show strong correlations (0.40 to 0.71) with changes in global ratings of asthma impact. Juniper et al. (1996b) report both the minimal important difference and the sample size required to detect this with varying levels of power. The requirement for n per group in parallel group studies ranges from 36 to 61 patients. The technique of establishing minimal important differences on the basis of patient reports is a valuable one and reflects the experience of the authors in this field. The instrument is well suited to treatment evaluations but less useful for between-group comparisons since 3 of the 23 items are not common across respondents. Scores show strong correlations with generic QL and with appropriate clinical parameters. Both empirically and theoretically the content validity of the instrument is good and it should be expected, in studies where interviewer administration is feasible, to perform well. Juniper et al. (1997) report that there is also a self-completion version of the questionnaire and that the reading skills needed to complete it are currently under investigation. To date all psychometric data refer to the interviewer-administered version.

The adult form of this measure is now widely used in treatment evaluation and performs better than alternatives in comparative studies (Rutten-van Molken et al., 1995). The pediatric version is showing similar properties, for example in demonstrating the efficacy of a hospitalization program for difficult-to-control asthmatics (Gavin et al., 1997).

The Childhood Asthma Questionnaires

The Childhood Asthma Questionnaires (CAQs; Christie et al., 1993; French, Christie, & Sowden 1994) were developed in the United Kingdom for use in clinical trials. They consist of three developmentally appropriate forms — both content and format vary to suit children of different ages. Form A is for children aged 4 to 7 years and includes instructions for parents to help pre-readers, forms B for 8 to 11 year olds and C for 12 to 16 year olds are intended for independent completion. All use a graphic of smiley and sad faces to aid understanding. In this way self-reports are obtained from children of all ages on subscales that include emotions (termed Distress) and activities (termed Active Quality of Living). The frequency of physical symptoms (Severity) is also reported on forms B and C. Item content for the measures was derived through extensive focus group work with children and their parents; the subscale structure was also empirically derived through factor analysis. The questionnaires take 15 to 20 minutes to complete, with adult assistance needed for non-readers. Younger children may give their responses by coloring in the smiley faces, which can increase administration times.

Internal consistency and reproducibility are reported for the three forms separately — coefficients are generally in the acceptable range. Reproducibility ranges from 0.68 to 0.84 in forms B and C but falls to 0.6 in form A. There must still be some doubt over the reliability of reports obtained from the youngest children. Examples of validity estimates include consistent moderate correlations between Distress and Active Quality of Living and parent reports of impact on the family (French & Christie, 1996). The subscales have consistently been shown to be distinct from one another and do not all improve in response to interventions. In particular the Distress scale is reported to show relatively stable individual differences which are somewhat resistant to change in pharmaceutical trials (e.g. Langton Hewer, Hobbs, French, & Lenney, 1995). Current data suggest however that the Severity and Active Quality of Living subscales are sensitive to change in clinical trials. Longitudinal validity estimates are consistent with a sensitive instrument, for example change in Active Quality of Living scores on form C show a correlation of 0.37 with change in lung function over a six month period (Langton Hewer, French, Hobbs, & Lenney, submitted). Studies such as Langton Hewer et al. (1995, 1996) suggest sample size requirements in the range of n = 30 per group for parallel group designs. This requirement must be met separately for each of the questionnaire forms since their scores are not directly comparable.

The Childhood Asthma Questionnaires have been used in a number of clinical trials of asthma medications including those cited above. They have also been adapted for use in Australia (French, Carroll, & Christie, in press) and have been translated into French (Auquier, P., personal communication, April 1997) and Russian (Smolenov, I., personal communication, July 1997). The self-completed nature of these measures makes them especially suitable for multi-centre clinical trials where bias brought about by the administration of an instrument by different interviewers must be avoided.

Paediatric Asthma Caregiver's Quality of Life Questionnaire

The Paediatric Asthma Caregiver's Quality of Life Questionnaire (PACQLQ; Juniper et al., 1996a), is the only disease-specific instrument that assesses the QL of those caring for children with asthma. It contains 13 items which give 2 subscale scores, emotions and activities; caregivers do not, of course, have symptoms themselves. The measure is easy to self-complete and takes only five minutes. Its content is based on the extensive interviews with parents reported by Townsend et al. (1991). Items cover emotional issues such as parents' frustration, anger and worry over their child's condition and activity impacts such as changed plans and sleepless nights. One month reproducibility coefficients are all 0.80 or higher. The instrument shows moderate to high correlations with ratings of the child's health status and with a generic instrument, the Impact-on-Family Scale (Stein & Reissman, 1980).

Data reported by Juniper et al. (1996a) and by recent users of the instrument (Gavin et al., 1997; Sorkness, McGill, & Decker, 1997) suggest that the PACQLQ is valuable both for treatment evaluations and for more descriptive explorations in this neglected area. For controlled treatment trials the authors recommend a sample size of 16 to 26 patients per group, depending on power requirements. Psychometric data are reported for the parents of 7 to 17 year olds, however Sorkness et al. (1997) used the instrument successfully with the parents of 3 to 5 year olds and inspection of the item content is consistent with this use.

Generic Measures of Quality of Life Suitable for Children with Asthma

The Functional Status II (R) (Stein & Jessop, 1990) and the Impact-on-Family Scale (Stein & Reissman, 1980) have both been used as measures against which to validate asthma specific measures. As such they hold promise for use with paediatric asthma patients. The Impact-on-Family Scale in particular contains a number of items that closely parallel those of the PACQLQ (Juniper et al., 1996a) and are similar to the concerns of parents reported by Townsend et al. (1991). These include questions about work and lifestyle restrictions and emotional distress. The paediatric version of the Rand Health Status measure (Eisen, Ware, Donald, & Brook, 1979) is also related to asthma status in potentially useful ways (Osman & Silverman, 1996). Since most children who suffer from asthma are only mildly affected, and only in specific ways, it seems likely that most generic measures will be less sensitive than disease-specific measures for this population. The Impact-on-Family Scale appears to have considerable potential for use with this population, especially in the assessment of impact of asthma in preschool children. More detailed reviews of these and other generic measures may be found in Chapters 3 and 7 of this volume.

SUMMARY

A wide range of QL assessment instruments for children with asthma is now available. Multi-dimensional measures assessing social, emotional, physical and functional components (French et al., 1994; Juniper et al., 1996b) may be the instruments of choice for descriptive studies and those trialing broad ranging interventions. For studies which focus upon improvement in a particular component of QL more specific measures are also available (Creer et al., 1993; Rosier et al., 1994). Most recently assessments of the QL of parents of children with asthma have also become possible (Juniper et al., 1996a). If the disease-specific approach is preferred to a generic instrument then asthma must surely be one of the few truly well served conditions. There are however some remaining questions in the field, and gaps in coverage. These will be addressed in the following section.

FUTURE DIRECTIONS

Profitable directions for future investigation can be divided into three basic areas — development of further measures, exploration of the methodological aspects of QL assessment in this population, and the increased use of QL assessment to enhance patient care.

DEVELOPMENT OF MEASURES

Considering both the preceding review and the frequent (unsolved) queries to the author from researchers worldwide, the most obvious and pressing need for further QL measures lies with the preschool population. Asthma is almost as prevalent in preschool children as in older age groups (Taylor & Newacheck, 1992) yet the range of instruments reviewed provides no coverage for children younger than 4 years. Even when instruments are completed by parents the references to school achievements and activities limit the applicable age range. The assessment of QL in these young children is unusually difficult, and will necessarily involve proxy reports — the problem is not however insoluble. Many of the questions in existing instruments could reasonably be asked about younger children, for example, "How often has asthma stopped your child from doing all the things that a boy or girl should at his/her age?" Usherwood et al. (1991) and "How often did your child wake at night with cough or wheezing?" Rosier et al. (1994).

These could be accompanied by questions about behavioral signs of anger or frustration, and items about treatment-related behavior problems similar to those in the Asthma Problem Behaviour Checklist (Creer, Marion, & Creer, 1983). In addition the impact upon parents of caring for such a young child with asthma is likely to be appreciable, and the content of the PACQLQ (Juniper et al., 1996a) is largely appropriate. In fact the advanced state of measurement development in the field of childhood asthma means that little work would be required to develop these much-needed instruments. The necessity of using proxy reports does however raise an issue which has yet to be addressed — it is to this and other methodological issues that this discussion will now turn.

METHODOLOGICAL ISSUES

Many paediatric QL instruments, both generic and disease-specific, rely upon proxy reports, usually from parents. Little is known about the relationship between proxy reports of QL and the children's own perceptions, but evidence from studies of behavioral and emotional problems is suggestive. Cross-informant reports of behavioral and emotional problems show little agreement in large population studies (Achenbach, MacConaughy, & Howell, 1987) or in children with chronic illness (Varni, Katz, Colegrove, & Dolgin, 1995). In a sample of children with cystic fibrosis (Thompson, Gustafson, Hamlett, & Spock, 1992) levels of maternal adjustment were more predictive of mothers' reports of psychological problems than of child self-reports of similar problems, suggesting one source for the discrepancy.

In one of the few studies more closely related to the current question, Dadds, Stein, and Silver (1995) found that mother's proxy reports of functional status in a range of chronic illnesses were not related to her own psychological adjustment. The only study of QL reports in children with asthma is less supportive. Guyatt, Juniper, Griffith, Feeny, and Ferrie (1997) conclude that "parents of younger children do not have a good idea of what their asthmatic children are experiencing", while parents of older children can add "little if any additional information" to the child's own reports (p. 167). Clearly the emotional component of QL is especially vulnerable to disagreements between informants and we should expect especially large differences in reports. There may be smaller differences in reports of observable components such as functional disability. Further evidence is however needed to establish the circumstances under which proxy reports might add to, or substitute for, self-reports of QL in children with asthma.

A further issue worthy of investigation is the influence of children's cognitive and emotional development on their perceptions of QL and their ability to self-report. It has been noted earlier in this chapter that the focus of the impact of asthma varies with age, with young children having different concerns to teenagers. The capacity of children to self-report also differs across the age range and so they are likely to need different degrees of assistance to complete self-report measures. These developmental changes have been dealt with in different ways by different authors — the PAQLQ (Juniper et al., 1996b) contains some individualized items and may be administered by self-report or interview whilst the CAQs (Christie et al., 1993) appear in three developmentally appropriate forms. While the latter approach makes fewer compromises with the changing needs of the population, it has drawbacks for clinical use. Sample size requirements must be met individually for each age-appropriate form and longitudinal studies over more than 2 or 3 years are not practical since scores on the differing forms are not equivalent. The different forms with their changing use of graphics to assist with completion are, however, highly acceptable to children.

As in most QL applications there is no "best measure" since needs vary widely. In general terms, where the study involves a wide age range, unless the sample is very large, a single version questionnaire is likely to be first choice. Similarly studies of very long duration (more than two years) would benefit from the single form approach. For studies of a single age group though, the principles of specificity apply. The questions on separate age-appropriate are highly specific to the children's concerns and activities as well as to their disease and so are likely to enhance content validity.

APPLICATIONS FOR QUALITY OF LIFE ASSESSMENT

QL assessment is now an accepted component of clinical trials in adult and paediatric asthma. An appreciation of the importance of QL outcomes in paediatric asthma research is demonstrated by the publication of three recent review papers (Bender, 1996; Osman & Silverman, 1996; Juniper, 1997). Despite these recent advances in outcome measurement and in the pharmaceutical treatments available for asthma, substantial morbidity remains (Price, 1994). It is likely that contributors to this situation include both unwillingness and inability on the part of the patient to adhere to treatments that have proven efficacy in clinical trials. Important improvements in QL for children with asthma may therefore be brought about by patient education — to promote more effective self-management — and by attention to the burden of treatment placed upon the individual. Patients who feel more confident to manage their illness, or are able to do so with less effort, are likely to report reduced QL impairment even where there is no change in clinical outcomes.

The role of quality of life assessment in evaluating educational interventions and management changes is now being recognized. Early examples include Gavin et al. (1997) who showed improvements in perceived competence and QL following intensive multi-disciplinary intervention, and Langton Hewer et al. (1996) who propose that quality of life is the primary outcome of interest in trials where the most salient change for patients is frequency of medication use. In these and other applications attention to the patient's perceptions of the impact of the entire intervention, not just improvement in lung function, is likely to lead to treatments which improve functioning without imposing further burdens upon the patient. One of the most fruitful areas for identifying means of improving QL is therefore the investigation of the complex relationship between knowledge, self-management decisions and quality of life outcomes in this group of patients.

There is also little or no information on psychological and social correlates of HRQOL in asthma. Those few studies in other chronic conditions, for example Wikby and colleagues (1993a, 1993b) in adults with diabetes, suggest that factors such as life situation and life events play an important role. This is also true for psychological adjustment in children with asthma (MacLean, et al., 1992), but the distinction between psychosocial adjustment and quality of life has been made above and so the non-illness predictors of QL may differ in ways that can inform patient care.

CONCLUSIONS

In the field of pediatric asthma QL assessment is well advanced, with a range of measures available. Those conditions with less well advanced assessments can learn not only from the technical achievements, which demonstrate that paediatric disease-specific instruments can perform well in clinical settings, but from the rapid uptake of QL as an outcome measure. The measures reviewed above are becoming widely used and have readily found acceptance among both physicians and patients. Their inclusion in recent treatment evaluations has proved a rich source of information for those whose aim is to enhance patient care. QL assessment, especially by self-report, is gaining an established place in asthma studies — for example the number of presentations at the American Thoracic Society annual meeting rose by 500% between 1992 and 1997. Paediatric studies have remained a small but significant proportion of these and their growth can encourage those researchers and clinicians whose endeavour is in other chronic paediatric conditions.

References

Achenbach, T.M., McConaughy, S.H., & Howell, C.T. (1987). Child/adolescent behavioral and emotional problems: Implications of cross-informant correlations for situational specificity. *Psychological Bulletin, 101,* 213–232.

Bauman, A., Mitchell, C.A., Henry, R.L., Robertson, C.F., Abramson, M.J., Comino, E.J., Hensley, M.J., & Leeder, S.R. (1992). Asthma morbidity in Australia: an epidemiological study. *Medical Journal of Australia, 156,* 827–831.

Bender, B.G. (1995). Are asthmatic children educationally handicapped? *School Psychology Quarterly, 10,* 274–291.

Bender, B.G. (1996). Measurement of quality of life in pediatric asthma clinical trials. *Annals of Allergy, Asthma and Immunology, 77,* 438–447.

Bremberg, S.G., & Kjellman, N.I.M. (1985). Children with asthma: how do they get along at school? *Acta Paediatrica Scandinavica, 74,* 833–840.

Bussing, R., Burkett, R.C., & Kelleher, E.T. (1996). Prevalence of anxiety disorders in a clinic-based sample of pediatric asthma patients. *Psychosomatics, 37,* 108–115.

Bussing, R., Halfon, N., Benjamin, B., & Wells, K.B. (1995). Prevalence of behavior problems in US children with asthma. *Archives of Pediatrics and Adolescent Medicine, 149,* 565–572.

Butz, A.M., & Alexander, C. (1993). Anxiety in children with asthma. *Journal of Asthma, 30,* 199–209.

Christiaanse, M.E., Lavigne, J.V., & Lerner, C.V. (1989). Psychosocial aspects of compliance in children and adolescents with asthma. *Developmental and Behavioral Pediatrics, 10,* 75–80.

Christie, M.J., French, D.J., Sowden, A., & West, A. (1993). Development of child-centered disease-specific questionnaires for living with asthma. *Psychosomatic Medicine, 55,* 541–548.

Creer, T.L., Marion, R.J., & Creer, P.P. (1983). Asthma Problem Behavior Checklist: Parental perceptions of the behaviour of asthmatic children. *Journal of Asthma, 20,* 97–104.

Creer, T.L., Wigal, J.K., Kostes, H., Hatala, J.C., McConnaughy, K., & Winder, J.A. (1993). A Life Activities Questionnaire for childhood asthma. *Journal of Asthma, 30,* 467–473.

Dadds, M.R., Stein, R.E.K., & Silver, E.J. (1995). The role of maternal psychological adjustment in the measurement of children's functional status. *Journal of Pediatric Psychology, 20,* 527–544.

Eisen, M., Ware, J.E., Donald, C.A., & Brook, R.H. (1979). Measuring components of children's health status. *Medical Care, 17,* 902–921.

Eksi, A., Molzan, J., Savasir, I., & Guler, N. (1995). Psychological adjustment of children with mild and moderately severe asthma. *European Child and Adolescent Psychiatry, 4,* 77–84.

Forero, R., Bauman, A., Young, L., Booth, M., & Nutbeam, D. (1996). Asthma, health behaviors, social adjustment and psychosomatic symptoms in adolescence. *Journal of Asthma, 33,* 157–164.

Forero, R., Bauman, A., Young, L., & Larkin, P. (1992). Asthma prevalence and management in Australian adolescents: results from three community surveys. *Journal of Adolescent Health, 13,* 707–712.

Fowler, M.G., Davenport, M.G., & Garg, R. (1992). School functioning of US children with asthma. *Pediatrics, 90,* 939–944.

French, D.J., Carroll, A., & Christie, M.J. (1998). Health-related quality of life in Australian children with asthma: Lessons for the cross-cultural use of quality of life instruments. *Quality of Life Research, 7,* 409–419.

French, D.J., & Christie, M.J. (1996). Developing outcome measures for children: the example of "Quality of Life" assessment for paediatric asthma. In A. Hutchinson, E. McColl, & M. Christie (Eds.), *Health outcomes in primary and outpatient care.* Chur: Harwood Academic Publishers.

French, D.J., Christie, M.J., & Sowden, A.J. (1994). The reproducibility of the Childhood Asthma Questionnaires: measures of quality of life for children with asthma aged 4–16 years. *Quality of Life Research, 3,* 215–224.

French, D.J., Christie, M.J., & West, A. (1994). Quality of Life in Childhood Asthma: Development of the Childhood Asthma Questionnaires. In M.J. Christie & D.J. French (Eds.), *The assessment of quality of life in childhood asthma.* Chur: Harwood Academic Publishers.

Gavin, L.A., Brenner, M., Klinnert, M., Glenn, K., Price, M., & Bartleson, B. (1997). Outcome of day hospitalization for children and adolescents with severe asthma. *American Journal of Respiratory and Critical Care Medicine, 155,* A306.

Gergen, P.J., Mullally, D.I., & Evans III, R. (1988). National survey of prevalence of asthma among children in the United States, 1976 to 1980. *Pediatrics, 81,* 1–7.

Gold, D.R., Rotnitzky, A., Damokosh, D.I., Ware, J.H., Speizer, F.E., Ferris, B.G., & Dockery, D.W. (1993). Race and Gender Differences in Respiratory Illness Prevalence and their Relationship to Environmental Exposures in Children 7 to 14 Years of Age. *American Review of Respiratory Disease, 148,* 10–18.

Gray, E.J., Peat, J.K., Mellis, C.M., Harrington, J., & Woolcock, A.J. (1994). Asthma severity and morbidity in a population sample of Sydney school children: part I — prevalence and effect of air pollutants in coastal regions. *Australian and New Zealand Journal of Medicine, 24,* 168–175.

Gudstadt, L.B., Gillette, J.W., Mrazek, D.A., Fukuhara, J.T., LaBrecque, J.F., & Strunk, R.C. (1989). Determinants of school performance in children with chronic asthma. *American Journal of Diseases of Children, 143,* 471–475.

Guyatt, G.H., Juniper, E.F., Griffith, L.E., Feeny D.H., & Ferrie, P.J. (1997). Children and adult perceptions of childhood asthma. *Pediatrics, 99,* 165–168.

Hilton, S. (1994). Management of childhood asthma in general practice. In M.J Christie & D.J. French (Eds.), *The assessment of quality of life in childhood asthma.* Chur: Harwood Academic Publishers.

Hyland, M.E., Bellesis, M., Thompson, P.J., & Kenyon, C.A.P. (1996). The constructs of asthma quality of life: psychometric, experimental and correlational evidence. *Psychology and Health, 12,* 101–121.

Joseph, C.L., Foxman, B., Leickly, F.E., Peterson, E., & Ownby, D. (1996). Prevalence of possible undiagnosed asthma and associated morbidity among urban school children. *Journal of Pediatrics, 129,* 735–742.

Juniper, E.F. (1997). How important is quality of life in pediatric asthma? *Pediatric Pulmonology, 15,* 17–21.

Juniper, E.F., Guyatt, G.H., Feeny, D.H., Ferrie, P.J., Griffith, L.E., & Townsend, M. (1996a). Measuring quality of life in the parents of children with asthma. *Quality of Life Research, 5,* 27–34.

Juniper, E.F., Guyatt, G.H., Feeny, D.H., Ferrie, P.J., Griffith, L.E., & Townsend, M. (1996b). Measuring quality of life in children with asthma. *Quality of Life Research, 5,* 35–46.

Juniper, E.F., Guyatt, G.H., Feeny, D.H., Griffith, L.E., & Ferrie, P.J. (1997). Minimum skills required by children to complete health-related quality of life instruments for asthma: comparison of measurement properties. *European Respiratory Journal, 10,* 2285–2294.

Juniper, E.F., Guyatt, G.H., Ferrie, P.J., & Griffith, L.E. (1993). Measuring quality of life in asthma. *American Review of Respiratory Disease, 147,* 832–838.

Kashani, J.H., Konig, P., Shepperd, J.A., Wilfley, D., & Morris, D.A. (1988). Psychopathology and self-concept in asthmatic children. *Journal of Pediatric Psychology, 13,* 509–520.

Kovacs, M., Goldston, D., & Iyengar, S. (1992). Intellectual development and academic performance of children with insulin-dependent diabetes-mellitus: A longitudinal study. *Developmental Psychology, 28,* 676–684.

Langton Hewer S., French, D., Hobbs, J., & Lenney, W. (Submitted). Quality of life assessments in older children receiving Salmeterol for chronic severe asthma. *European Respiratory Journal.*

Langton Hewer, S., Hobbs, J., French, D., & Lenney, W. (1996). Improvement in quality of life assessment in children with chronic severe asthma on inhaled Salmeterol. Presented at the *Annual Conference of the European Respiratory Society,* Stockholm, September.

Langton Hewer, S., Hobbs, J., French, D., & Lenney, W. (1995). Pilgrim's progress: The effect of Salmeterol in older children with chronic severe asthma. *Respiratory Medicine, 89,* 435–440.

Lemanek, K. (1990). Adherence issues in the medical management of asthma, *Journal of Pediatric Psychology, 15,* 437–458.

MacLean, W.E., Perrin, J.M., Gortmaker, S., & Pierre, C.B. (1992). Psychological adjustment of children with asthma: effects of illness severity and recent stressful life events. *Journal of Pediatric Psychology, 17*, 159–171.

McNichol, K.N., & Williams, H.B. (1973). Spectrum of asthma in children. I. clinical and physiological components. *British Medical Journal, 4*, 7–11.

Nassau, J.H., & Drotar, D. (1995). Social competence in children with IDDM and asthma: child, teacher and parent reports of children's social adjustment, social performance and social skills. *Journal of Pediatric Psychology, 20*, 187–204.

Nelson, D.A., Johnson, C.C., Divine, G.W., Strauchman, C., Joseph, C.L., & Ownby, D.R. (1997). Ethnic differences in the prevalence of asthma in middle class children. *Annals of Allergy, Asthma and Immunology, 78*, 21–26.

O'Neil, S.L., Barysh, N., & Setear, S.J. (1985). Determining school programming needs of special population groups: a study of asthmatic children. *Journal of School Health, 55*, 237–239.

Osman, L., & Silverman, M. (1996). Measuring quality of life for young children with asthma and their families. *European Respiratory Journal, 21* (supplement), 35s–41s.

Peat, J.K., Gray, E.J., Mellis, C.M., Leeder, S.R., & Woolcock, A.J. (1994*). Differences in airway responsiveness between children and adults living in the same environment: an epidemiological study in two regions of New South Wales. *European Respiratory Journal, 7*, 1805–1813.

Price, J.F. (1994). Asthma — A growing problem. In M.J. Christie & D.J. French (Eds.), *The assessment of quality of life in childhood asthma*. Chur: Harwood Academic Publishers.

Richards, J.M., & Hemstreet, M.P. (1994). Measures of life quality, role performance, and functional status in asthma research. *American Journal of Respiratory and Critical Care Medicine, 149*, S31–S39.

Rosier, M.J., Bishop, J., Nolan, T., Robertson, C.F., Carlin, J.B., & Phelan, P.D. (1994). Measurement of functional severity of asthma in children. *American Journal of Respiratory and Critical Care Medicine, 149*, 1434–1441.

Rutten-van Molken, M., Custers, F., Doorslaer, E., et al. (1995). Comparison of performance of four instruments in evaluating effects of salmeterol on quality of life. *European Respiratory Journal, 8*, 888–898.

Schipper, H., Clinch, J., & Powell, V. (1990). Definitions and conceptual issues. In B. Spilker (Ed.), *Quality of life assessments in clinical trials*. New York: Raven Press.

Schulz, R.M., Dye, J., Jolicoeur, L., Cafferty, T., & Watson, J. (1994). Quality-of-life factors for parents of children with asthma. *Journal of Asthma, 31*, 209–219.

Seigel, W.M., Golden, N.H., Gough, J.W., Lashley, M.S., & Sacker, I.M. (1990). Depression, self-esteem and life events in adolescents with chronic diseases. *Journal of Adolescent Health Care, 11*, 501–504.

Skobeloff, E.M., Spivey, W.H., St. Clair, S.S., & Schoffstall, J.M. (1992). The influence of age and sex on asthma admissions. *JAMA, 268*, 3437–3440.

Sorkness, C.A., McGill, K.A., & Decker, C.A. (1997). Quality of life of caregivers of head start children with asthma. *American Journal of Respiratory and Critical Care Medicine, 155*, A721.

Spieth, L.E., & Harris, C.V. (1996). Assessment of health-related quality of life in children and adolescents: an integrative review. *Journal of Pediatric Psychology, 21*, 175–193.

Stein, R.E.K., & Jessop, D.J. (1990). Functional Status II(R): A measure of child health status. *Medical Care, 28*, 1041–1055.

Stein, R.E.K., & Reissman, C.K. (1980). The development of an impact-on-family scale: preliminary findings. *Medical Care, 18*, 465–472.

Sweeting, H. (1995). Reversals of fortune? Sex differences in health in childhood and adolescence. *Social Science and Medicine, 40*, 77–90.

Taylor, W.R., & Newacheck, PW (1992). Impact of childhood asthma on health. *Pediatrics, 90*, 657–662.

Thompson, R.J., Gustafson, K.E., Hamlett, K.W., & Spock, A. (1992). Psychological adjustment of children with cystic fibrosis: the role of child cognitive processes and maternal adjustment. *Journal of Pediatric Psychology, 17*, 741–755.

Townsend, M., Feeny, D.H., Guyatt, G.H., Furlong, W.J., Seip A.E., & Dolovich, J. (1991). Evaluation of the burden of illness for pediatric asthmatic patients and their parents. *Annals of Allergy, 67,* 403–408.

Usherwood, T.P., Scrimgeour, A., & Barber, J.H. (1990). Questionnaire to measure perceived symptoms and disability in asthma. *Archives of Disease in Childhood, 65,* 779–781.

Varni, J.W., Katz, E.R., Colegrove, R., & Dolgin, M. (1995). Adjustment of children with newly diagnosed cancer: cross-informant variance. *Journal of Psychosocial Oncology, 13,* 23–38.

Vivier, P.M., Bernier, J.A., & Starfield, B. (1994). Current approaches to measuring health outcomes in pediatric research. *Current Opinion in Pediatrics, 6,* 530–537.

Walsh, M., & Ryan-Wenger, N.M. (1992). Sources of stress in children with asthma. *Journal of School Health, 62,* 459–463.

Warner, J.O., Gotz, M., Landau, L.I., Levinson, H., Milner, A.D., Pedersen, S., & Silverman, M. (1989). Management of asthma: A consensus statement. *Archives of Disease in Childhood, 64,* 1065–1079.

Wikby, A., Hornquist, J.-O., Stenstrom, U., & Andersson, P.-O. (1993a). Background factors, long-term complications, quality of life and metabolic control in insulin dependent diabetes. *Quality of Life Research, 2,* 281–286.

Wikby, A., Stenstrom, U., Hornquist, J.-O., & Andersson, P.-O. (1993b). Coping behavior and degree of discrepancy between retrospective and prospective self-ratings of change in quality of life in Type 1 diabetes mellitus. *Diabetic Medicine, 10,* 851–854.

Wisniewski, M., Emmett, A., Petrocella, V., Kalberg, C., Cox, F., Rickard, K., & Bowers, B. (1997). Principal component analysis of the Asthma Quality of Life Questionnaire (AQLQ) to examine the addition of information to clinical and symptom measures in patients with asthma. *American Journal of Respiratory and Critical Care Medicine, 155,* A721.

Chapter 10

CANCER

Christine Eiser

Childhood cancer is a rare disease, affecting some 13 in every 100,000 children (data from the US National Cancer Institute; Miller, Young, & Novakovi, 1995). Before the 1950s, the disease was inevitably and rapidly fatal. Since that time, new treatments involving a combination of chemotherapy, radiotherapy and, less frequently, surgery have been developed and have resulted in significant improvements in survival. In the UK, overall survival increased from 26% for children treated between 1962–70 to 65% for those treated between 1986–1988 (Robertson, Hawkins, & Kingston, 1994). For some cancers (for example, retinoblastoma, Hodgkin's disease) survival rates more in the order of 90% have been reported (Stiller, 1994). Consequently, treatment of childhood cancer is frequently hailed as one of the great successes of modern medicine.

As survival has increased, the question of quality of life, rather than quantity or length of survival has become a critical issue. Treatment is aggressive, lengthy and very painful. Children can experience multiple hospitalisations, physical side-effects as a consequence of treatment and many restrictions on their everyday activities. The hope is that after a period of intense treatment (usually 6 months to 2 years depending on the specific cancer) children will be well and cancer-free. Disappointingly, such an outcome cannot be guaranteed, and many children experience long-term complications as a result of the treatment, or may not survive at all.

This chapter will consider the ways in which cancer may possibly affect QL in a) the family and b) the child, making special note of how the impact may differ depending on the child's developmental level. Having established the potential value of QL measures, it is important to define QL and consider the main theoretical orientations. Measures that are currently available will be described, together with details of their development and psychometric properties. The chapter will conclude by considering the potential value of QL measures, particularly in evaluating the outcomes of clinical trials, and assessing the efficacy of psychosocial interventions.

IMPLICATIONS OF CANCER FOR QUALITY OF LIFE
EFFECTS ON THE FAMILY

Parents' relationships

Childhood cancer can have far-reaching implications for the whole family (Kupst, 1992), and one of the first things that pediatricians warn parents is that the diagnosis will affect everyone. While the focus of attention, at least immediately after the diagnosis, is the sick child, parents themselves face many challenges; to their parenting skills, to their relationship together, and to their work commitments. At the same time, they are likely to feel exhausted; both by the physical demands of caring for a sick child, and by the emotional demands created by the awareness that the child has a life-threatening condition. Parents, perhaps more than their children, realise that there is a possibility of recurrence and can become hypervigilant about the child's health.

Although it is reasonable to assume that family QL will be jeopardized during treatment, it is to be hoped that more normal relationships can be achieved after treatment. At least for some mothers, there is now some evidence that compromised QL, in the form of continued anxiety and loneliness, can continue well beyond the active treatment phase (van Dongen-Melman et al., 1995). Given the extended follow ups and need for care and treatment beyond the initial treatment phase, it is not surprising that many parents report continuing anxiety about their child.

Healthy siblings

Having a chronically ill brother or sister is one of the most stressful events that can happen to a child. As parents are necessarily preoccupied by the needs of the sick child, siblings can feel left out and ignored. For parents, what to do about their healthy children is a source of much anxiety. Younger siblings are often left with friends and relations and older siblings may be expected to take on considerable responsibility for running the house and caring for other children. Inevitably, the needs of healthy siblings can be overlooked. Parents may withhold information so as not to upset siblings, but this can have the effect of creating even more anxiety. Most work suggests that siblings of a child with cancer are at risk of behavioral and emotional difficulties (Carpenter & Sahler, 1991), though there are occasional reports that the experience can have positive outcomes. Horwitz and Kazak (1990) reported that preschool siblings whose brother or sister had cancer were more helpful and considerate compared with age-matched controls who had no experience of how illness can affect others.

EFFECTS ON THE CHILD

During active treatment

Treatment for cancer potentially affects all aspects of the child's QL. During the active part of treatment, almost all children experience physical limitations; they may be tired and lacking in energy. They experience unpleasant side-effects and symptoms. These include nausea, mouth ulcers, alopecia (the loss of hair from all over the body) and skin complaints. Children experience changes in food preferences; disturbances in taste and a combination of mouth ulcers and sickness can sometimes have a long-lasting impact on food choices and eating habits. Chemotherapy can have a significant effect on mood and behavior. Parents often report that their children experience sleep disturbance, listlessness and aggression (Drigan et al., 1992), though there have been surprisingly few systematic reports about the frequency or intensity of these mood changes.

It is easy to see how parents might be tempted to overprotect sick children. As a result, they may restrict their children's activities, and this in turn becomes a source of conflict (Cappelli et al., 1989). Conflict can also be created because of communication difficulties. In particular, the very early literature suggested that many children and adolescents were aware of the seriousness of their disease but deliberately did not discuss their fears in order not to distress their parents further (Binger, 1969). In their study of a Dutch population, van Veldhuizen and Last (1991) reported that one-quarter of children interviewed did not want to ask their parents questions about the illness as they feared this would upset them.

Although every attempt is made to encourage children back to school as soon as possible, it is inevitable that their schooling is interrupted. This can affect their academic progress as well as interfere with participation in normal school activities.

On completion of treatment

However, on the assumption that physical side-effects are short-lived and necessary for long-term survival, most children and parents are able to cope effectively. Most parents do expect that, following completion of therapy, the child will be free of symptoms. In this respect, many are very disappointed. Not only can children experience a wide variety of late-effects, but also parents are increasingly confronted with information that the child may be subject to new and as yet unknown risks in the future. Current work suggests that survivors may experience growth impairment and infertility, respiratory or cardiac damage, as well as educational and behavioral problems (Hawkins & Stevens, 1996). As physicians become more knowledgeable about the nature of damage which may be associated with radiotherapy and chemotherapy, it has been thought necessary and ethically appropriate to warn parents about possible late-effects. In some cases, the purpose of this is simply to inform. In other cases, the purpose is to ensure that parents (and the children as they grow older) are aware of risks that may be run, and avoid activities that might exaggerate that risk. Information is also given in the hope that it will encourage children to attend follow-up clinics, thereby allowing early identification and treatment of late-effects should they occur, as well as facilitating accurate record-keeping with regard to specific problems associated with different therapies.

Both during and after completion of treatment, it is clear that QL is potentially jeopardised. Yet many children and their families seem to cope with setbacks with remarkable fortitude. Increasingly, questions are being asked about how far treatment can be justified; how far is it right to administer increasingly aggressive treatment with the goal of possible long-term survival, particularly where such survival itself is compromised? In addition, can parents and clinicians make such decisions for children? Parents may feel that all treatment is justified for the chance of survival, while children may be less certain, especially where they are the ones who must enter adult life handicapped by infertility, compromised mobility or intellectual potential.

THE IMPORTANCE OF DEVELOPMENTAL LEVEL

Although these potentially adverse effects have been well-documented (Eiser, 1995), it has less often been recognised that the specific implications may well vary with the developmental level of the child. More generally, QL considerations as a function of developmental stage have been recognised with respect to diabetes (Anderson, 1990) and physical illness (Perrin & Gerrity, 1984) but can also be applied to childhood cancer. The following schema draws largely on the theoretical perspectives of Erikson (1959).

Infants

According to Erikson (1959), it is important for the young child to acquire a sense of trust in adults. Small children may be adversely affected by periods of separation from their parents. Although many hospitals offer accommodation for parents, it is inevitable that children experience some enforced separations, either because parents must spend some time at home with their other children, or because hospital policies do not encourage parents to be present during medical procedures. At a time when children should be developing a basic trust in adults, they are likely to experience multiple physical assaults, through injections and other painful procedures. Parents may feel particularly helpless because it is not possible to explain what is happening to the child, or prepare them in advance for painful procedures.

Children

For school age children, a diagnosis of cancer is again likely to result in many experiences of separation from parents. Children may feel different from others, partly through sickness or tiredness, partly because they are less able to keep up with peers and normal activities (Tebbi, 1985; Spirito, DeLawyer, & Stark, 1991). Ross and Ross (1984) reported that children with leukemia are often teased on return to school, and this can be because of hair loss or visible changes in weight gain. Some children report that this teasing is at least as bad as the physical pain from the disease or diagnostic procedures.

Children with cancer have been reported to be lonely or isolated and have difficulties with peer relationships (Noll et al., 1991). Difficult peer relationships can have negative consequences for integration in school. Children "must be prepared to handle teasing, questions, and comments from peers, in addition to allaying their own concerns about feeling different and unattractive" (La Greca, 1990). Although hospital policy is generally to encourage children to return to school as soon as possible after diagnosis, many experience some difficulties. Absences (Eiser, 1980; Charlton et al., 1991) and in extreme cases, school phobia, have been reported (Lansky et al., 1975). School absence also has implications for cognitive development and attainment of normal academic success. Teachers report that they are uncertain about how to handle sick children, especially in setting limits to behavior (Eiser & Town, 1987). Teachers' lack of knowledge about childhood cancer and their own fears about the disease can further compromise the child's successful integration in school, as teachers' response to their own uncertainty is to make allowances and communicate lowered expectations.

Adolescents

The key developmental tasks of adolescence are attainment of independence from the nuclear family and adoption of appropriate work and career choices. Cancer, like any other serious illness, very much compromises the individual's ability to achieve these goals. Adolescents may be forced into a position of dependence on parents while also being less able to participate in a normal social life. Treatment can be specially disruptive for education during adolescence, and many are forced to interrupt their studies or delay taking major examinations.

Adolescents, often more than younger children, are concerned about changes in their physical appearance as a result of cancer. The problem is particularly acute for newly diagnosed patients who must endure very visible changes in their appearance. Loss of hair has frequently been cited as a major cause of concern in young people (van Veldhuizen & Last, 1991; Varni & Setoguchi, 1991). Even after completion of therapy, there can be permanent changes in appearance. At the extreme, patients with a bone tumor may have been treated by an amputation which poses a major challenge to the attainment of a normal body image. Some survivors experience difficulties in regaining normal body-weight, and are unable to lose the weight gained during chemotherapy. For others, linear growth may be compromised as a result of chemotherapy and treatment with growth hormone replacement therapy may be necessary.

RATIONALE FOR QUALITY OF LIFE MEASUREMENT

The development of QL scales in pediatric oncology has been justified on several grounds. Most commonly, measures are developed in order to distinguish between different therapies; the question is whether one treatment results in less consequences for QL compared with another, assuming of course, the same implications for survival. A measure which was sensitive enough to detect differences between treatments in terms of the implications for QL would be very valuable. Such a measure would need to be brief and easy to administer to large populations of children, probably by a non-trained administrator, usually while the child was attending a routine clinic appointment. Such a scale would also need to be very sensitive to small changes in QL and at the same time, not subject to learning effects due to repeated administrations.

Secondly, others have suggested that QL measures have most potential in evaluating intervention programmes. Scales for this purpose may also need to be brief since it might be necessary to sample a broad spectrum of behaviors and attitudes that might be affected by an intervention.

Thirdly, QL scales may be needed to make treatment decisions in the context of limited financial resources. Should very expensive treatment be offered when the chances of success are remote? Should such treatment be administered where the child's survival is likely to be of very short duration, or where irreversible and major handicap is likely to result? Such an approach is extremely controversial, since the implication could be that treatment would be withheld in situations where QL was perceived to be below a minimum defined standard. Issues surrounding the definition of such a standard would clearly be subject to much debate.

Fourthly, there is an issue of when it is useful to administer QL scales. Clinicians often accept that some compromise to QL is inevitable during treatment (Bradlyn et al., 1996). However, it is to be hoped that in the longer term, QL among long-term survivors will not differ from that experienced by the rest of the population. As awareness of the range and incidence of late-effects among survivors has increased, the question of QL among survivors has become pertinent. This has resulted in a focus in recent scales toward assessment of QL among survivors. Such scales may not need to be as brief in that there is less urgency for the scales to be completed during hurried clinic visits. There may however, be a need for a different emphasis in content; it may be necessary to include additional domains specifically of relevance to survivors (e.g. fertility and sexual functioning).

CURRENT CONCEPTUALIZATIONS OF QUALITY OF LIFE

Definitions of QL have varied greatly (Calman, 1987), but, especially with regard to work with children, can be categorized as follows:

The Multidimensional approach emphasises the comprehensive nature of QL. For example, Bradlyn et al. (1996, p. 1333–4) propose:

"Quality of life in pediatric oncology is multidimensional. It includes, but is not limited to, the social, physical, and emotional functioning of the child and adolescent, and when indicated, his/her family. Measurement of QL must be from the perspective of the child, adolescent, and family, and it must be sensitive to the changes that occur throughout development".

The Cost-effectiveness approach is based on decision theory. A number of decision models are in use, and share many features. Common to many is the idea of expressing the benefits of treatment in terms of well-years.

The Goal orientated approach uses pragmatic task analysis to focus on perceived differences between an individual's hopes and expectations and their present experience (Calman, 1987; Ruta et al., 1994). According to this approach, good QL is achieved where there is a closer match between an individual's actual, or real self, and their ideal or future self.

Common to most definitions is the assumption that QL is the result of an interaction between the individual's physical health, psychological health, level of independence and social relationships. Most QL measures include an *ad hoc* selection of items, or domains. This selection is invariably driven by intuitive beliefs about the meaning of QL and not based on any theoretical framework which takes into account the meaning of QL for children and their families. Mulhern et al. (1989) has suggested that a minimal requirement is that QL scales should include measures of physical and social functioning, and self-esteem. Although it is possible to identify the following approaches to measurement of QL, in practice, scale developers have often not specified which specific approach they adopt, or have drawn on more than one methodology.

METHODOLOGICAL APPROACHES TO DEFINITION AND MEASUREMENT OF QUALITY OF LIFE

The psychometric approach

The psychometric approach to scale construction is widely used in the social sciences and involves a number of stages (Oppenheim, 1992). First, items must be selected to cover the whole range of attitudes in order to reflect both an underlying "latent variable," and variation, or error associated with the item or statement being considered. It is therefore important to include lots of items or "multiple indicators" in order to partial out this variance. Second, factor analyses are conducted to determine a construct common to all. In the context of health care, the most useful original sources are patients' interviews, and more recently focus groups. This preliminary stage is often overlooked and can be poorly reported in journals since it relies on the use of "soft" or interview data. Clearly, the source of the original items is crucial. Consideration needs to be given to the particular concerns of special groups, such as children. Although there may be some overlap between children and adults in terms of their perceptions of the impact of a disease on QL, children also have a unique perspective and one that may best be represented through careful preparatory work. Measures which rely on clinicians or nurses to provide the items are likely to be less adequate as the basis for measures of patient evaluated QL. Some modifications to the method have been reported in order to make assessment reflect individual QL more satisfactorily (Joyce, 1994).

This is the most common approach in pediatric oncology and has been used in measures developed by Goodwin, Boggs, and Graham-Pole (1994), Eiser et al. (1995) and Varni et al. (1998a,b). The appropriateness of the method is dependent on satisfactory selection of the original items and it is essential that these are elicited directly from the patient group involved. It is likely to be most useful in research generally, or in assessing interventions.

The cost-effectiveness approach

The cost-effectiveness model is derived from economic decision theory and is based on subjective preferences of treatment effects. Respondents are asked to imagine a specified health condition and to express their relative preference for that condition as a choice between quantity and quality of life (between a shorter life with less dysfunction and a longer life with more dysfunction). Responses are quantified in terms Quality Adjusted Life Years (QALYs). This approach is described in detail in the earlier chapter by Kaplan (Chapter 4).

The goal-orientated approach

An emerging hypothesis in adult work is that good QL is a consequence of a match between perceived current functioning and expectations for the future. Poorer QL occurs where individuals perceive a gap between these two perceptions of self. There are implications for interventions in that these should address unrealistic expectations and bring future expectations in line with current functioning, making patients more realistic or practical. This approach leads to an assessment of QL whereby patients rate their current and expected future functioning in a number of different domains on conventional Likert scales. Difference scores are then computed.

Whether or not such a theoretical framework is appropriate for use with children rests critically on whether or not children are able to make judgments about their future functioning. However, some work suggests that, with simple instructions, the idea of a future self is within the grasp of 3–4 year olds (Eder, 1990).

This model, developed in the adult sphere appears to have some potential as a basis for measuring QL. It has advantages in having clear implications for rehabilitation. One disadvantage is that, as currently conceptualized, the model takes no account of clinical status, i.e. in some cases (of serious or life-threatening illness) a large gap between current and perceived future functioning may be realistic.

MEASURES OF QUALITY OF LIFE
PARENT-COMPLETED MEASURES

The Play Performance Scale for Children (PPSC)

The Play Performance Scale for Children (PPSC; Lansky et al., 1985) is the original, most simple and most frequently cited indicator of QL used for children with cancer. It is a relatively simple "downward extension" of the Performance Scale described by Karnofsky et al. (1948) for work with adult cancer patients. Parents are asked to record play activity in terms of 10 graded statements ("fully active, normal" scored as 100 through to "unresponsive", scored as 0). It is quick to administer and easy to score. It was originally considered suitable for a relatively wide age-range (1–16 years) though has recently been thought to lack sensitivity, particularly for older children and those functioning at near normal levels.

Mulhern et al. (1989) compared the efficacy of the PPSC over a simple visual analogue scale. Both were completed by parents and physicians of 120 cancer patients. Comparisons were made between children who were hospitalised, treated as out-patients or had completed therapy. There was some evidence that the PPSC discriminated between the groups better than the visual analogue scale. Scores on the Play Performance Scale were lower for hospitalised patients compared with out-patients or those who had completed therapy, suggesting a degree of validity. However, there were no differences between the two non-hospitalised groups, indicating less sensitivity for those functioning near normal levels.

This scale has been used widely in research and remains popular. At a clinical level, it is quick and easy to administer and can be used by those with no special training. More critically, it is not a sensitive instrument, and there is no facility for children to make ratings for themselves. The PPSC is frequently treated as a kind of "gold standard" against which new measures are compared, although the wisdom of this is hard to accept, given its clear limitations.

TABLE 10.1 LEVEL OF IMPAIRMENT RATINGS FOR THE SOCIAL ACTIVITY DOMAIN OF THE QUALITY OF WELL-BEING SCALE (BRADLYN ET AL., 1993).

1. NO LIMITATIONS FOR HEALTH REASONS.
2. LIMITED IN OTHER ROLE ACTIVITY, HEALTH RELATED.
3. LIMITED IN PRIMARY ROLE ACTIVITY, HEALTH RELATED.
4. PERFORMED NO MAJOR ROLE ACTIVITY, HEALTH RELATED BUT DID PERFORM SELF-CARE.
5. PERFORMED NO MAJOR ROLE ACTIVITY, HEALTH RELATED, AND DID NOT PERFORM OR HAD MORE HELP THAN USUAL IN PERFORMANCE OR ONE OR MORE SELF-CARE ACTIVITIES, HEALTH RELATED.

The Quality of Well-Being Scale

The Quality of Well-Being Scale (Bradlyn et al., 1993), is a slightly modified version of the Quality of Well-Being Scale for adults (Kaplan & Anderson, 1990). In this model, health status is assessed in three areas; physical functioning, social/role functioning and mobility. In addition, patients are shown a list of 27 symptoms and asked to identify any that have affected them within the previous 6 days. A structured 15 minute interview format is used. Estimates of the level of impairment in each area are based on interview responses (see Table 10.1).

Validation was reported in relation to ratings made on the PPSC and information from medical records about treatment toxicity. Physicians rated treatment toxicity on a global score (1 = mild to 5 = severe), based on information about bone marrow suppression, nausea and vomiting, acute and long term risk of hematopoietic functioning and nutritional status.

Limited data is currently available. The scale was completed by parents of 30 children, aged between 4 and 18 years, and appeared to distinguish between children on the basis of medical data as would be expected. Criticisms of this scale are that it involves a more complex and time-consuming method of data-collection and needs trained personel for administration. Again, there is no parallel form for children to make their own ratings. The 3 dimensions which are assessed (physical functioning, social/role functioning and mobility) perhaps do not reflect as comprehensive a view of QL as is implicit within most definitions.

Multi-attribute health status classification system

The multi-attribute health status classification system (Feeny et al., 1995) based on the Health Utility Index (Torrance et al., 1982), has been used primarily for work in neonatal intensive care and oncology. In this model, four attributes or components of health were identified

TABLE 10.2   ITEMS FROM THE COGNITION DOMAIN (FEENY ET AL., 1995)

1. ABLE TO REMEMBER MOST THINGS, THINK CLEARLY AND SOLVE DAY-TO-DAY PROBLEMS.
2. ABLE TO REMEMBER MOST THINGS, BUT HAVE A LITTLE DIFFICULTY WHEN TRYING TO THINK AND SOLVE DAY-TO-DAY PROBLEMS.
3. SOMEWHAT FORGETFUL, BUT ABLE TO THINK CLEARLY AND SOLVE DAY-TO-DAY PROBLEMS.
4. SOMEWHAT FORGETFUL, AND HAVE A LITTLE DIFFICULTY WHEN TRYING TO THINK OR SOLVE DAY-TO-DAY PROBLEMS.
5. VERY FORGETFUL, AND HAVE GREAT DIFFICULTY WHEN TRYING TO THINK OR SOLVE DAY-TO-DAY PROBLEMS.
6. UNABLE TO REMEMBER ANYTHING AT ALL, AND UNABLE TO THINK OR SOLVE DAY-TO-DAY PROBLEMS.

and each attribute consisted of between four and eight levels of function. Proponents of this schema argue that one of the merits lies in the potential to determine almost a thousand health states, by combining the scores on each level from each attribute.

In the initial development of the multi-attribute health status classification, parents of children in the general population were asked to identify important components of health for their children. From these data, six domains were identified: sensation, emotion, cognition, mobility, self-care and pain. A seventh domain: fertility was added, as this was felt to be important to parents of children treated for cancer, though not an issue for parents of healthy children. For each attribute, three to five levels of functioning were identified (see Table 10.2, for an example). The child's health status score is a computation of functioning on the different levels for each domain.

The link between these health status measurements and QL is assessed using a technique called the standard gamble. Respondents are asked to consider a specific health state. Then they must choose between remaining in this health state or take a gamble, the gamble being between sudden death and enjoying perfect health. These preferences are then varied until the respondent is unable to choose between the two. This is called the utility score; the better the state of health the higher the utility score.

There are some problems with the schema itself. The attributes are not completely independent. For example, if you score badly on the mobility attribute it is almost inevitable that you will also score badly in terms of self-care. In part recognition of some of these problems, later versions dropped the self-care attribute. The system does not easily allow for better than average functioning. Thus, in terms of cognition for example, ratings are made from severe morbidity to normality.

Thus, the system fails to recognise children who function better than average.

This system has been adopted with some enthusiasm by a number of workers and is especially popular among paediatricians. It is most commonly used to compare alternative treatments. The main advantages include brevity and ease of administration. It is possible for a clinician to complete the instrument within a few minutes. From this point of view, it seems ideal for work in a busy clinic. The measure has been used successfully by Billson and Walker (1994) to elicit data directly from children. It may prove useful as a very brief screening instrument in the comparison of different therapies, but may need to be supplemented with additional measures to yield a comprehensive picture of QL.

The Pediatric Oncology Quality of Life Scale

The original items for the Pediatric Oncology Quality of Life Scale (Goodwin, Boggs, & Graham-Pole, 1994) were generated by health professionals, parents of cancer patients and patients themselves. Parents were asked to generate written statements about how their child's life was affected by cancer. Adolescents were asked to report the impact themselves. Younger children were simply asked to describe the "good" and "bad" things about having cancer. From the original item pool, 44 items were selected as representative of the most commonly reported themes.

A questionnaire was then constructed using these 44 items and respondents were asked to rate each one on a series of 7 point scales (never to very frequently). This measure was completed by 210 parents. On the basis of factor analysis and further refinement of the scale, the authors finally developed a 21 item scale. Validity was established in relation to the Play Performance Scale for Children (Lansky et al., 1985), the Child Behavior Checklist (Achenbach & Edelbrock, 1983) and the Reynolds Adolescent Depression Scale (Reynolds, 1987).

The final scale measures three components of QL; physical functioning and restriction from normal activity, emotional distress, and response to active medical treatment. Although there were no age differences in total scores, there were significant age differences on two of the three subscales. Older children were more restricted in terms of physical functioning and normal activity than younger children. On the subscale measuring emotional distress, children aged 8–12 years showed more distress compared with younger or older children. There were no age effects on the subscale measuring response to treatment.

The authors report good internal reliability for the total score and for the 3 separate subscales. The measure also appears to have adequate validity, at least in terms of discriminating between children depending on time since diagnosis. In addition, scores on the subscales correlated with the validity measures as expected. For example, scores on the physical functioning subscale correlated with the PPSC but not with the Child Behavior Checklist or depression measure.

This measure was designed for use by parents of children from preschool through to adolescence. Age differences on subscale scores suggest that the impact of cancer on QL may be age-dependent, at least as far as parents are concerned. There are indications that adolescents are more affected in terms of physical functioning compared with younger children, while children between the ages of 8–12 years are most affected in terms of emotional functioning.

The authors argue that parents are a reliable and accurate source of information about their children and that parent-completed measures have some advantages over child-completed measures. This is clearly a point of view, and many would see the limitation of this measure to centre on lack of a child version. The arbitrariness of the domains which are used in QL work is highlighted by comparing the domains used in this measure (physical functioning and restriction from normal activity, emotional distress, and response to active medical treatment) with those (physical functioning, social/role functioning, mobility) reported by Bradlyn et al. (1993). Although both include 3 subscales, there is clear overlap only for the subscale measuring physical functioning.

MEASURES FOR CHILDREN AND PARENTS

The Pediatric Cancer Quality of Life Inventory (PCQL and PCQL-32)

The Pediatric Cancer Quality of Life Inventory (PCQL; Varni et al., 1998) includes 84 items organised around five domains: physical functioning (8 items), disease-related and treatment related symptoms (28 items), psychological functioning (13), social functioning (23) and cognitive functioning (12). Ratings are made on a series of 4-point Likert scales (where 0 = never a problem to 3 = always a problem) and respondents are asked to think back over a 1 month period. The PCQL includes a child form for 8–12 year olds and an adolescent form for 13–18 year olds. There are identical forms for parents, which differ only in terms of the use of "developmentally appropriate language" and whether they are written in the first or third person. Initial psychometric data were based on responses from 291 children, aged 8–18 years.

For both children and adolescents, concordance with parent ratings were mostly in the medium effect size range (suggesting parents do have a different perception from their children/adolescents, but there is still a correlation between the values). Lower concordance was found for subjective ratings (emotional distress) compared with functional status.

A potential problem relates to the length of the scale (which includes 84 items). In anticipation of this, the same group (Varni et al., 1998b) subsequently reported a short form (PCQL-32). The number of items in each domain was reduced (disease and treatment related symptoms = 9 items, physical functioning = 5 items, psychological functioning = 6 items, social functioning = 5 items, cognitive functioning = 7 items). Ratings were made on 4 point scales as before.

The authors report satisfactory internal consistency, clinical and construct validity and suggest that the brief form is potentially suitable for research involving evaluation of randomized clinical trials. It should be noted that the item means were mostly under 1.0. Although the standard deviations were larger, suggesting a degree of variability in response, the low item means suggest that to a large extent patients did not rate the impact of cancer on their lives to be very significant. It is not clear if this is because patients included in the study were well and not severely affected or if the items used were not entirely appropriate.

The Perceived Illness Experience Scale — the PIE

The Perceived Illness Experience Scale (PIE; Eiser, Havermans, Craft, & Kernahan, 1995), represents an attempt to develop a measure of QL which captures the specific interests and concerns of the child with cancer. Following the approach recommended by Oppenheim (1992), a series of indepth interviews were first conducted with children and adolescents to determine their own perceptions of the impact of cancer.

The interviews were analysed using a content analysis guided by a review of the literature. Nine major themes were identified, including *physical activity, appearance, peer relationships, integration in school, emotion and manipulation, parental behavior, disclosure, preoccupation with illness and impact of treatment*. Each theme was assessed by four items and ratings were made on 5 point Likert scales. The items were rated by 41 children (mean age = 14.6 years) and 35 of their parents. In addition, they also completed a set of related measures in order to obtain preliminary validation data. These included measures of physical functioning and physical and psychological symptoms (Watson, Law, & Maguire, 1992; Walker & Greene, 1991).

The Flesch (1948) scoring system was used to determine the ease of readability of the scale. This scoring is based on the average number of words per sentence and the average number of syllables per 100 words. Reading ease scores range from "very easy" (90–100) (equivalent to 4 years of schooling) to "very difficult" 0–30 (equivalent to 15 years of schooling). Analysis suggested that readability of the scale was within a range from "fairly easy" to "standard" (Flesch reading ease = 60–70).

Evidence for the validity of the PIE was inferred from significant correlations between the number of reported physical symptoms and the total score on PIE. Scores on the physical functioning measures also correlated with the activity subscale and the family subscale suggesting that children with more limited physical functioning experienced more difficulties with parents imposing restrictions on their activities. In addition there were positive correlations between the total score on PIE and number of psychological symptoms reported. Disappointingly, the scale failed to distinguish between those who were still on maintenance therapy and those who had completed treatment. The only exception was the school subscale where those who had completed treatment reported less impact than those on treatment.

Ratings made by mothers correlated well with those made by children. Significant correlations were found on all but two subscales (disclosure and treatment). In both cases, mothers reported less impact on QL compared with their children. In order to assess test-retest reliability, mothers were asked to complete the measures again after a 2 month interval. Test-retest scores were in fact good for the total score (r = 0.92) and satisfactory for all subscales (range = 0.51–0.85).

This scale was developed to reflect the child's view of the illness and as a consequence some issues, such as worrying about relapse or minding if people ask questions about the illness, are unique to this measure. However, many would not consider it a comprehensive measure of QL and certainly it would need to be supplemented by a measure of physical functioning if a comprehensive view of QL was needed.

Subsequently modifications to the PIE scale have been made. It was felt that the two items to measure activity were insufficient and two additional items were added. In addition, a subscale to measure attitudes to food was added, since many children, including those who had been off-treatment for some time, suggested that their diets remained restricted because of changes in taste and food habits resulting from chemotherapy.

Further work with this revised scale provides additional evidence for the reliability and validity of the scale (Eiser, Kopel, Cool, & Grimer, 1999). Internal reliability for the separate subscales and total scale were confirmed. There were significant correlations between mothers' and children's ratings, suggesting that the instrument can be used as a good proxy measure. High correlations between the PIE and other established scales (the SF36, Ware et al., 1994; and Functional Evaluation of Reconstructive Procedures, Enneking et al. 1993) were taken as evidence of construct validity.

MEASUREMENT CRITIQUE

Early measures were simple downward extensions of adult QL measures (e.g. Lansky et al., 1985; Bradlyn et al., 1993). More recently, the approach has been more child-centered, with researchers going to some pains to collect preliminary data from children in order to ensure that their views are represented (e.g., Eiser et al., 1995).

The issue of establishing validity is problematic, since to date, there is no widely accepted gold standard. Most new measures report validity in relation to the PPSC (Lansky et al., 1985). Yet this scale is also widely criticised, particularly in that it lacks sensitivity for work with children functioning at near normal levels. Choice of the PPSC as the key instrument against which to determine the validity of a new instrument does little more than establish a correlation between the two measures. Since it is not clear that the PPSC is a comprehensive measure of QL for children, it follows that establishing a correlation between the PPSC and any other measure does not satisfactorily establish the validity of the new instrument.

There are also difficulties in establishing the psychometric properties of new scales in that conventional statistical procedures (e.g. factor analysis) require relatively large samples of respondents. Given the low incidence of cancer in children, it is only possible to collect adequate sample sizes through collaboration. Small sample sizes mean that only one currently available QL measure (Goodwin, Boggs, & Graham-Pole, 1994) has been subject to factor analysis (and this is based on parent- rather than child-completed data). In other cases, the different themes or domains have been defined intuitively and are not supported by statistical techniques.

Proxy ratings

Although parents have a unique perspective on their child's health and well-being, provision must be made for the child to rate their own QL wherever possible. There are indications from other work that parents may not always be able to answer for their child, and indeed, are more able to judge certain behaviors (e.g., acting out or aggressive reactions) compared with internalizing problems (e.g., anxiety). Parental ratings of the child's QL are also affected by the parent's own health status. Although there are some inconsistencies in the findings, it seems that mothers who are themselves depressed rate their child more negatively compared with mothers who are not depressed.

It is important that QL measures reflect a child's concerns and are not simply scaled down versions of adult measures. It is likely that parents may be more concerned about the long-term consequences of treatment than children, or may be anxious about the consequences of the illness for the child's future health or work potential. Children's QL is more likely to be affected by the immediate consequences of the disease and they are less concerned with future issues. QL measures need to focus on the specific concerns of childhood.

Response mode

For older children and adolescents, it may be possible for ratings to be made using Likert scales as in adult measures, though simpler multiple choice or yes/no formats may be more appropriate for younger children. Juniper et al. (1997) attempted to determine the age and skills required for children to complete different QL measures. Children from 7 years of age were able to use Likert style rating scales. The skills required to complete the "standard gamble" are more complex, and were found to be too difficult for children below 11–12 years of age. Other work (Eder, 1990) suggests that children from 5 years are able to make the kind of real self/ideal self-judgments necessary in the goal-orientated approach. Nevertheless, there is surprisingly little work concerned with children's understanding of rating scales and different response modes, and scale developers need to pay more attention to this.

Reading level

In general, more attention needs to be paid to the content of the items that make up the QL scale, and the way in which the items are expressed. Estimates of reading age need to be an integral part of assessments of the efficacy of any new measure for children, although to date information about reading age has been provided for only one scale (Eiser et al., 1995).

FUTURE DIRECTIONS
APPLICATIONS OF QUALITY OF LIFE MEASURES

Although considerable progress has been made in the development of QL scales, it has yet to be established that they have a role in routine clinical practice, or in research. In this section, I would like to consider how far QL scales have been used for the purposes for which they were developed. It was hoped that QL scales would be used particularly in evaluating clinical trials, as an adjunct to survival data; and in evaluating the efficacy of interventions. It is perhaps premature, but it is important to make some preliminary assessment of the performance of QL scales in practice.

CLINICAL TRIALS WORK

Despite the fact that many have argued that one of the principal purposes of a QL scale may be for use in clinical trials, only 3% of 70 Phase III trials in pediatric oncology included a measure of QL, compared with 75% which included a measure of treatment toxicity (Bradlyn, Harris, & Spieth, 1995). In part, this can be attributed to a reticence on the part of clinical trial organisers to include QL measures, a reflection of a view that scale development is in its infancy and that no available scale is sufficiently robust to justify inclusion. In discussing why QL measures have not been more routinely included in evaluations of clinical trials, Bradlyn, Harris, and Spieth (1995) suggest there is a need to educate researchers and clinicians about the merits and limitations of available measures. Clinicians are often skeptical about the value of "soft" data, and many demand that scales have more robust psychometric properties than is currently possible.

In part, also, pediatricians may believe that QL is necessarily compromised during treatment and therefore be reluctant to include a measure which might result in unwelcome findings. QL measures have real potential in this field. Chemotherapy may be delivered in high doses for a few days and followed by a rest period, or patients may receive a lower dose over a longer period of time. Information about the relative merits of these approaches (assuming no difference in survival rates) would be very relevant when developing new clinical trials.

INTERVENTIONS

Reducing procedural distress

One of the potential applications of QL measures has always been to assess the efficacy of psychosocial interventions. Some practical changes in the administration of therapy have resulted in improvements in QL for children undergoing treatment. There has been an improvement in the control of nausea with new anti-emetic therapy. Central venous catheters minimise the need for venepuncture and it is now possible to perform many unpleasant procedures when the child is under sedation or general anesthesia. Despite these practical changes, treatment remains distressing and for this reason, psychological interventions to help the child manage pain control have been advocated. The question is becoming increasingly important as to whether or not interventions really improve the child's QL and can be justified in terms of cost effectiveness.

Children undergo regular and extremely painful procedures during the course of treatment. Some experience conditioned anxiety and nausea; others can become extremely difficult and noisy patients, contributing to levels of staff distress as well as upsetting other patients. Attempts to reduce behavioral distress are therefore important, not only for the patient but also through influencing the QL in the clinic more generally.

Several studies indicate that procedural distress can be effectively targetted by training parents (Blount et al., 1989; Powers et al., 1993), though these studies have not tended to include a formal measure of QL. More recently, Kazak et al. (1996a) used a structured QL measure to assess the efficacy of an intervention to reduce treatment related distress. Children were newly diagnosed patients with leukemia undergoing routine procedures. In this study, two interventions were compared. The first involved a pharmacological intervention (n = 45); the second a combined psychological and pharmacological intervention (n = 47). The intervention was delivered at 1, 2 and 6 months following diagnosis. Results were compared with a control group of 70 children who had received the same treatment with no supportive intervention. Outcome measures included the Perception of Procedures Questionnaire (Kazak et al., 1995), Parent-Stress Index (Abidin, 1990) and the Pediatric Oncology Quality of Life Scale (Goodwin, Boggs, & Graham-Pole, 1994). Parents and staff separately rated child distress on 7 point Likert scales.

First, of particular relevance for this review was the finding that both mothers and fathers reported improved QL for their child over the 6 months of the study. This suggests that the POQL Scale (Goodwin, Boggs, & Graham-Pole, 1994) is sufficiently sensitive to pick up changes over this period. As anticipated, mothers in the combined pharmacological/psychological intervention reported less child distress than those in the pharmacological intervention only. These conclusions were also supported by nurses' ratings of child distress. However, there were no differences on the other measures of Parent-Stress or quality of life (though data based on the Perception of Procedures Questionnaire approached significance). The results persisted at 6 months. Mothers in the combined intervention group reported lower child distress than mothers in the pharmacological intervention or control group.

The more negative finding as far as QL research is concerned is that this scale was not sensitive enough to record QL changes associated with an intervention to reduce procedural distress; a purpose for which QL measures are hopefully appropriate. It remains to be seen whether or not other QL measures fare better, or whether the problem was inherent in the design of the intervention itself. This study also highlights the real difficulties associated with intervention work; simply by introducing the intervention, staff became more knowledgeable and sympathetic to the idea of psychological interventions (Kazak et al., 1996b). Such shifts in staff attitudes are likely to dilute the effectiveness of any intervention, and make the attainment of intervention efficacy especially difficult.

Educational and social skills

Most interventions have, however, focused on the school experience. In part, this reflects a long-standing concern about the effects of treatment (notably CNS irradiation) on children's learning capacity (Eiser 1991), and in part, it reflects a more recent concern that children treated for cancer have poorly developed social skills, and may be lonely or isolated compared with healthy peers (Noll et al., 1991). There are now relatively large numbers of research findings which point consistently to educational and social risks at least for some survivors. Given the accumulated findings, it seems appropriate that attention should now be paid to developing interventions to reduce these problems. Intervention research is, of course, notoriously difficult, and consequently very few studies can be identified. To date, evaluation of most interventions have relied on general outcome indicators, but this is an area where QL measures may make a contribution.

Some 40% of children and adolescents with chronic conditions experience school related problems at some time. Children with cancer can experience very long absences (Eiser, 1980) and this will inevitably create difficulties with academic work as well as jeopardise social relationships. In recognising that the return to school following extended absence can be very difficult, many centres employ specialist nurses or social workers to liaise with the school and prepare the staff and pupils for the child's return. Most usually, this involves a class discussion of the issue, led by the specialist nurse. A more formal programme has been described by Katz and colleagues (Katz, Varni, Rubenstein, Blew, & Hubert, 1992). This programme involves four components: (a) preliminary intervention, assessing the child's school behaviour and parental involvement with an aim to arrange appropriate remedial help through the diagnostic period; (b) conferences with school personnel to help them plan for the child's return, (c) classroom presentations, in the child's presence to provide peers with age-appropriate information; and (d) follow-up contact after the child's return to provide any further help. Follow-up evaluations of this programme resulted in positive reports from teachers, parents and children, though it is not clear that there were long-term implications for achievement.

Other programmes have been directed more specifically at helping the child with cancer acquire the social skills to cope with school life. It is inevitable that the child with cancer may have to answer questions about what has happened to their hair, why they go to hospital so often, why they do not have to do PE. Varni et al. (1993) developed a social skills training programme to provide the child with the necessary skills to deal with these questions. The programme consisted of 3 modules, each of 1 hour duration. A social-cognitive problem solving module taught children to identify problems, consider their cause, and explore alternative ways of resolution. The assertiveness training module taught children how to express their thoughts and concerns to others. The "handling teasing and name calling" module taught children how to cope with verbal and physical teasing associated with changes in physical appearance. Children also took part in two follow-up sessions at 3 and 6 weeks following their return to school.

Parents reported fewer behavior problems and greater school competence for children who went through the problem-solving skills training compared with a group who received standard return to school instruction at 9 months follow-up. These results are encouraging. Use of QL as an outcome measure would enable a more comprehensive assessment of the efficacy of an intervention than relying on general measures of behavior problems. QL measures, especially those which can be completed by children would be useful.

Clearly, return to school can be a difficult time for children with cancer, but there are indications that this can be eased by sensitive intervention. Whether or not these interventions during the early stages of the disease have an impact on later functioning remains to be established.

Family relationships

The diagnosis of childhood cancer poses a considerable threat to normal parent–child relationships, and the adverse family experiences have been well-documented. Parents talk about the difficulties in involving healthy siblings and helping them to understand the reasons for disrupted family routines and parental absences. Programmes to help parents maintain normal family relationships, especially immediately following the diagnosis, would seem to be particularly important. Surprizingly then, there have been few reports of programmes to improve family-related QL and little attempt to evaluate them formally.

Meyer and Vadasy (1994) have reported a programme to improve general QL among siblings of a child with cancer. The programme involves a series of games and workshops, discussions and peer support activities. Although no formal evaluation has been conducted, the programme has been well-received and siblings have responded positively.

The potential for intervention at the family level is great, and much can be learned from interventions developed to help children with other chronic diseases and their families (Kaslow et al., 1997). The inclusion of QL measures in evaluations of family-based interventions should provide an important test of the value of the concept as well as provide insight into the further development of QL instruments.

NEW DEVELOPMENTS

A focus on QL seems to have advantages over emphases in earlier work on child maladjustment, depression or anxiety. Measures of QL have the merit of allowing the child to describe the good things about life, rather than focus on the problems, disadvantages and difficulties. QL work has also developed in parallel with demands to perceive the impact of disease from the child's perspective, rather than that of the clinician or parent. Both these emphases are laudable. QL scales have potential value in work with chronically sick children. However, these children inevitably experience difficulties and we must not fall into the trap of creating a QL industry. Numerous studies aimed at describing differences between sick groups, or between sick and healthy children on QL scales are unlikely to yield useful data for clinical practice. Where there are no differences, post hoc explanations need to be considered, that the scales lack sensitivity, or that somehow (process unknown) sick children have the same QL as healthy children, despite the often major disadvantages experienced. Where there are differences, what then? Some may be alleviated through appropriate interventions, but not all.

Most QL measures have been developed as general purpose instruments and focus on the QL of the child, as perceived by the parent or older child. In evaluating any scale, the purpose for which the instrument must be used needs to be considered. A brief, easy to administer scale may be ideal for work comparing different clinical trials, but will never provide a comprehensive view of the child's functioning or deepest concerns. There are circumstances in which it would be helpful to be able to make additional assessments, in order, for example to assess the total impact of treatment on the QL of the whole family. The challenges to the development of such an instrument are formidable. Although it is accepted that QL measures need to reflect the child's perspective, current instruments are only suitable for completion by older children or adolescents. More innovative measures suitable for younger children are essential.

Even a cancer specific scale may lack sensitivity for work with children with a brain tumor, bone tumor or some of the more rare cancers. In many cases, additional questions may need to be asked if a complete view of the child's QL is to be obtained. There are certainly difficulties in developing a scale which is both sensitive and appropriate for children with good prognosis cancers, such as Hodgkin's disease, and those with more life-threatening conditions such as is often the case with brain tumors.

For the moment, progress in treating child cancer seems to have peaked, with few major breakthroughs being achieved in recent years. At the same time, new treatments (such as bone-marrow transplants) impose huge burdens on children and families. In these circumstances, it is natural that attention should turn away from survival itself and toward the quality of survival. Treatment for cancer challenges the attainment of quality of life in numerous ways; not only through the practical demands of treatment, but also emotionally, since it is difficult to plan beyond the very short-term.

The need for quality of life measures, then, has been well-established. This need will not, however, be met by individuals or small groups of workers developing instruments in isolation. Development of a satisfactory instrument requires systematic and collaborative work involving different professionals and a number of centres of cancer care. The work needs to be multi-disciplinary involving pediatricians, nursing staff, psychometricians and health economists. Medical and nursing staff are necessary to ensure that the instrument taps the issues which are central to QL in children with cancer; they also need to be involved so that any instrument that is developed is acceptable for work in a pediatric oncology clinic. This need for clinical acceptability needs to be balanced with a professional approach to scale development. There is an established and well-developed literature concerned with scale development and the criteria for a satisfactory measure; it is essential that QL measures for children conform to these high standards of scale development.

Finally, the drive for highly validated, brief measures of QL should not be achieved at the expense of patient satisfaction. By this, I mean that children and their families give up time to participate in research, and they have their own views about the aims and value of such work. Many will feel let down when their involvement is limited to completion of a series of Likert scales. In many cases, good QL data will only be achieved by supplementing brief measures with more detailed inter-views, which give patients the opportunity to expand on their own experiences.

ACKNOWLEDGEMENT

The author is funded by the Cancer Research Campaign, London (CP1019/0101).

References

Abidin, R. (1990). *The Parenting Stress Index — Short form*. Charlottesville, VA: Pediatric Psychology Press.

Achenbach, T.M., & Edelbrock, C.S. (1983). *Manual for the Child Behavior Checklist and Revised Behavior Profile*. University of Vermont Department of Psychiatry, Burlington, VT.

Anderson, B.J. (1990). Diabetes and adaptations in family systems. In C.S. Holmes (Ed.), *Neuropsychological and behavioral aspects of diabetes* (pp. 85–101). New York: Springer-Verlag,.

Billson, A., & Walker, D.A. (1994). Assessment of health status in survivors of cancer. *Archives of Disease in Childhood, 70*, 200–204.

Binger, C.M. (1969). Childhood leukemia: Emotional impact on child and family. *New England Journal of Medicine, 280*, 414–418.

Blount, R., Corbin, S., Sturges, J., Wolfe, V., Prater, J., & James, L. (1989). The relationship between adult's coping behavior and child coping and distress during BMA/LP procedures. *Behavior Therapy, 20*, 585–601,

Bradlyn, A.S., Harris, C.V., & Spieth, L.E. (1995). Quality of life assessment in pediatric oncology: A retrospective review of phase III reports. *Social Science and Medicine, 10*, 1463–1465.

Bradlyn, A.S., Harris, C.V., Warner, J.E., Ritchey, A.K., & Zaboy, K. (1993). An investigation of the validity of well-being scale with pediatric oncology patients. *Health Psychology, 12*, 246–250.

Bradlyn, A.S., Ritchey, A.K., Harris, C.V., Moore, I.M., O'Brien, R.T., Parsons, S.K., Patterson, K., & Pollock, B.H. (1996). Quality of life research in pediatric oncology. Research methods and barriers. *Cancer, 78*, 1333–1339.

Calman, K.C. (1987). Definitions and measurement of quality of life. In N.K. Aaronson & J. Beckman (Eds.), *The quality of life of cancer patients* (pp. 1–9). New York: Raven Press.

Cappelli, M., McGrawth, P.J, MacDonald, N.E, Katsamis, J., & Lascalles, M. (1989). Parental care and overprotection of children with cystic fibrosis. *British Journal of Medical Psychology, 62*, 281–289.

Carpenter, P.J., & Sahler, O.J.Z. (1991). Sibling perception and adaptation to childhood cancer: Conceptual and methodological considerations. In J.H. Johnson & S.B. Johnson (Eds.), *Advances in child health psychology*. Gainesville, FL: University of Florida Press.

Charlton, A., Larcombe, I.J, Meller, S.T., Morris-Jones, P.H., Mott, M.G., Pottan, M.W., Trnmer, M.D., & Walker, I.J.P. (1991). Absence from school related to cancer and other chronic conditions. *Archives of Disease in Childhood, 66*, 1217–1222.

Chesler, M.A. (1995).The child with cancer and the family. Paper presented at the First International meeting in Psychosocial Oncology for Social Workers, University of York, UK.

Christie, M., & French, D. (1994). *Assessment of quality of life in childhood asthma*. Chur: Harwood Academic Publishers.

Dahlquist, L.M, Gil, K.M., Armstrong, D., Ginsberg, A., & Jones, B. (1985). Behavioral management of children's distress during chemotherapy. *Journal of Behavioral Experimental Psychiatry, 16*, 325–329.

Drigan, R., Spirito, A., & Gelber, R.D. (1992). Behavioral effects of corticosteroids in children with acute lymphoblastic leukemia. *Medical and Pediatric Oncology, 20*, 13–21.

Eder, R.A. (1990). Uncovering young children's psychological selves: Individual and developmental differences. *Child Development, 61*, 849–863.

Eiser, C. (1980). How leukaemia affects a child's schooling. *British Journal of Social and Clinical Psychology, 19*, 365–368.

Eiser, C. (1991). Cognitive deficits in children treated for leukaemia. *Archives of Disease in Childhood, 66*, 164–168.

Eiser, C. (1995). *Growing up with a chronic disease*. London: Jessica Kingsley Publishers.

Eiser, C., Cool, P., Grimer, R.J., Carter, S.R., Cotter, I.M., Ellis, A.J., & Kopel, S. (1997). Quality of life in children treated for a malignant primary bone tumour around the knee. *Sarcoma, 1*, 39–46.

Eiser, C., & Havermans, T. (1994). Treatment for childhood cancer and implications for long-term social adjustment: A review. *Archives of Disease in Childhood, 70,* 66–70.

Eiser, C., Havermans, T., Craft, A., & Kernahan, J. (1995). Development of a measure to assess the Perceived Illness experience after treatment for cancer. *Archives of Disease in Childhood, 72,* 302–7.

Eiser, C., Kopel, S., Cool, P., Grimer, R. (1999). The Perceived Illness Experience Scale (PIE): Reliability and validity revisited. *Child Care Health and Development, 25,* 179–190.

Eiser, C., & Town, C. (1987). Teachers' concerns about chronically sick children. Implications for pediatricians. *Developmental Medicine and Child Neurology, 29,* 56–63.

Erikson, E.H. (1959). Identity and the life-cycle. *Psychological Issues, 1,* 18–164.

Feeny, D., Furlong, W., & Barr, R.D. (1992). A comprehensive multi-attribute system for classifying health status of survivors of childhood cancer. *British Journal of Cancer, 10,* 923.

Feeny, D., Furlong, W., Boyle, M., & Torrance, G.W. (1995). Multi-attribute health status classification systems: Health Utilities Index. *PharmacoEconomics, 7,* 490–502.

Flesch, R.F. (1948). A new readability yardstick. *Journal of Applied Psychology, 32,* 221–233.

Goodwin, D.A.J., Boggs, S.R., & Graham-Pole, J. (1994). Development and validation of the Pediatric Oncology Quality of Life scale. *Psychological Assessment, 6,* 321–8.

Harris, J.C., Carel, C.A., Rosenberg, L.A, Joshi, P., & Leventhal, B.G. (1986). Intermittent high dose corticosteroid treatment in childhood cancer: Behavioural and emotional consequences. *Journal of American Academy of Child Psychiatry, 25,* 120–124.

Hawkins, M.M., & Stevens, M.C.G. (1996). The long term survivor. *British Medical Bulletin, 52,* 898–923.

Horwitz, W.A., & Kazak, A.E. (1990). Family adaptation to the child with cancer: Sibling and family system variables. *Journal of Clinical Child Psychology, 19,* 221–228.

Joyce, C.R.B. (1994). Requirements for the assessment of individual quality of life. In H. McGee & C. Bradley (Eds), *Quality of life following renal failure* (pp. 43–54). Chur: Harwood Academic Publishers.

Juniper, E.F., Guyatt, D.H., Feeny, D.H., Ferrie, P.J., Griffith, L.E., & Townsend, M. (1996). Measuring quality of life in the parents of children with asthma. *Quality of Life Research, 5,* 27–34.

Juniper, E.F., Guyatt, D.H., Feeny, D.H., Griffith, L.E., & Ferrie, P.J. (1997). Minimum skills required by children to complete health-related quality of life instruments for asthma: Comparison of measurement properties. *European Respiratory Journal, 10,* 2285–2294.

Kaplan, R.M., & Anderson, J.P. (1990). A General Health Policy model: An integrated approach. In B. Spilker (Ed.), *Quality of life assessment in clinical trials* (pp. 131–199). New York: Raven Press.

Karnofsky, D.A., & Buchenal, J.H. (1949). The clinical evaluation of chemotherapeutic agents in cancer. In C.M. Macleod (Ed.), *Evaluation of chemotherapeutic agents* (pp. 191–205). New York: Columbia University Press.

Kaslow, N.J., Collins, M.H., Loundy, M.R., Brown, F., Hollins, L.D., & Eckman, J. (1997). Empirically validated family interventions for pediatric psychology: Sickle cell disease as an exemplar. *Journal of Pediatric Psychology, 22,* 213–228.

Kazak, A., Blackall, G., Boyer, B., Brophy, B., Buzaglo, J., & Himelstein, B. (1996b). Implementing a pediatric leukemia intervention for procedural pain: The impact on staff. *Families, Systems and Health, 14,* 43–56.

Kazak, A., Penati, B., Boyer, B.A., Himelstein, B., Brophy, B., Waibel, M.K., Blackall, G.F., Daller, R., & Johnson, K. (1996a). A randomized controlled prospective outcome study of a psychological and pharmacological intervention protocol for procedural distress in pediatric leukemia. *Journal of Pediatric Psychology, 21,* 615–632.

Kazak, A., Penati, B., Waibel, M.K., & Blackall, G. (1995). The Perception of Procedures Questionnaire (PPQ): Psychometric properties of a brief parent report measure of procedural distress. *Journal of Pediatric Psychology, 21,* 195–207.

Kupst, M.J. (1992). Long-term family coping with acute lymphoblastic leukemia in childhood. In A.M. LaGreca, L.J. Siegel, J.L. Wallander, & C.E. Walker (Eds.), *Stress and coping in child health* (pp. 242–261). New York: Guilford Press.

La Greca, A.M. (1990). Social consequences of pediatric conditions: Fertile area for future investigation and intervention. *Journal of Pediatric Psychology, 15,* 285–307.

Lansky, L.L., List, M.A., Lansky, S.B., Cohen, M.E., & Sinks, L.F. (1985). Toward the development of a play performance scale for children. *Medical and Pediatric Oncology, 24*, 1837–1841.

Lansky, S.B., Lowman, J.T., Vats, T. & Guylay, J.E. (1975). School phobia in children with malignant neoplasms. *American Journal of Disease in Children, 129*, 42–46.

Meyer, D.J., & Vadasy, P.F. (1994). *Sibshops. Workshops for siblings of children with special needs.* Maryland: Paul Brookes.

Miller, R.W., Young, J.L., & Novakovic, B. (1995). Childhood cancer. *Cancer, 75*, 395–405.

Mulhern, R.K., Horowitz, M.E., Ochs, J., Friedman, A.G., Armstrong, F.D., Copeland, D., & Kun, L.E. (1989). Assessment of quality of life among pediatric patients with cancer. *Journal of Consulting and Clinical Psychology, 1*, 130–138.

Noll, R.B, LeRoy, S., Bukowski, W.M., Rogosch, F.A., & Kulkarni, R. (1991). Peer relationships and adjustment in children with cancer. *Journal of Pediatric Psychology, 16*, 307–326.

Noll, R.B., Bukowski, W.M., Davies, W.H., Kontz, K., & Kulkarni, R. (1993). Adjustment in the peer system of adolescents with cancer: A two-year study. *Journal of Pediatric Psychology, 18*, 351–364.

Oppenheim, A.N. (1992). *Questionnaire design, interviewing and attitude measurement.* London: Pinter Publishers.

Perrin, E.C., & Gerrity, B.S. (1984). Development of children with a chronic illness. *Pediatric Clinics of North America, 31*, 1–17.

Powers, S., Blount, R., Bachanas, P., Cotter, M., & Swan, S. (1993). Helping preschool leukemia patients and parents cope with injections. *Journal of Pediatric Psychology, 18*, 681–695.

Reynolds, W.M. (1987). *Reynolds Adolescent Depression Scale: Professional manual.* Odessa, FL. Psychological Assessment Resources.

Robertson, C.M., Kingston, M.M., & Hawkins, J.E. (1994). Late deaths and survival after childhood cancer: implications for cure. *British Medical Journal, 309*, 162–166.

Ross, D.M., & Ross, S.A. (1984). Childhood pain: the school-aged child's viewpoint. *Pain, 20*, 179–191.

Ruta, D.A., Garratt, A.M., & Leng, M. (1994). A new approach to the measurement of quality of life: The patient generated index. *Medical Care, 32*, 1109–1126.

Spirito, A., DeLawyer, D.D., & Stark, L.J. (1991). Peer relations and social adjustment of chronically ill children and adolescents. *Clinical Psychology Review, 11*, 539–564.

Stiller, C.A. (1994). Population based survival rates for childhood cancer in Britain, 1980–1991. *British Medical Journal, 309*, 1612–1616.

Tebbi, C. (1985). The role of social support systems in adolescent cancer amputees. *Cancer, 56*, 965–971.

Torrance, G.W., Boyle, M.H., & Horwood, S.P. (1982). Application of multi-attribute utility theory to measure social preference for health states. *Operations Research, 30*, 1043–1069.

van Dongen-Melman, J.E.W.M., Pruyn, J.F.A., de Groot, A., Koot, H.M., Hahlen, K., & Verhulst, F.C. (1995). Late psychosocial consequences for parents of children who survived cancer. *Journal of Pediatric Psychology, 20*, 567–586.

Varni, J.W., Katz, E.R., Colegrove, R., & Dolgin, M. (1993). The impact of social skills training on the adjustment of children with newly diagnosed cancer. *Journal of Pediatric Psychology, 18*, 751–768.

Varni, J.W., Katz, E.R., Seid, M., Quiggins, D.J.L., & Friedman-Bender, A. (1998a). The Pediatric Cancer Quality of life Inventory-32 (PCQL-32). Reliability and validity. *Cancer, 82*, 1184–.

Varni, J.W., Katz, E.R., Seid, M., Quiggins, D.J.L., Friedman-Bender. A., & Castro, C.M. (1998b). The Pediatric Cancer Quality of life Inventory: I. Instrument development, descriptive statistics, and cross-informant variance. *Journal of Behavioral Medicine, 21*, 179.

Varni, J.W., & Setoguchi, Y. (1991). Correlates of perceived physical appearance in children with congenital/acquired limb deficiencies. *Journal of Developmental and Behavioral Pediatrics, 12*, 171–175.

Walker, L., & Greene, J.W. (1991). The functional disability inventory: measuring a neglected dimension of health status. *Journal of Pediatric Psychology, 16*, 39–58.

Ware, J.E., Gandek, B., & the IQOLA Project Group. The SF-36 Health Survey: Development and use in mental health research and the IQOLA Project. *International Journal of Mental Health, 23*, 49–73.

Watson, M., Law, M., Maguire, G.P., Robertson, B., Greer, S., Bliss, J.M., & Ibbotson, T. (1992). Further development of a quality of life measure for cancer patients: The Rotterdam Symptom Checklist (revised). *Psycho-oncology, 1*, 35–44.

Chapter 11

CARDIOVASCULAR DISEASE

Alan M. Delamater
Lee Ann Pearse

Many children with cardiovascular disease who would have previously died as a result of their illness are now surviving due to recent advances in medical and surgical treatments. Along with improved survival rates, however, there has been increased concern regarding the long-term psychosocial and cognitive effects of cardiovascular disease and its treatment. While few studies have directly addressed the question of quality of life (QL), in recent years a number of studies have considered the effects which the disease and treatment process have on the psychosocial and cognitive functioning of children with various types of cardiovascular disease and treatments. When QL is mentioned in the medical literature, it may simply refer to "need for reoperation" (e.g., Elkins, Knott-Craig, McCue, & Lane, 1997).

This chapter will first provide an overview of medical issues regarding the major types of pediatric cardiovascular disease and their management. The impact of cardiovascular disease on children's psychosocial functioning and cognitive development will then be reviewed. The majority of research in this area has been conducted on children with congenital heart disease, who comprise the largest single group of children with cardiac problems. Studies addressing QL after heart transplantation will be highlighted. The chapter will conclude with a discussion of implications for clinical intervention and future research regarding QL.

MEDICAL ISSUES: DESCRIPTION, EPIDEMIOLOGY, AND TREATMENT

Cardiovascular disease in children can be divided into four main categories, including structural congenital heart disease (CHD), inflammatory cardiovascular disease, myocardial disease, and arrhythmias.

STRUCTURAL CONGENITAL HEART DISEASE

Structural CHD is defined as structural or functional heart disease that is present at birth. In the United States, approximately 10/1000 live births, or 1% of all children born each year, are diagnosed with CHD (Fyler, 1992). The severity of CHD can range from very benign defects that children will outgrow without any problems to those that have little to no surgical options and a shortened life span. Children may have very little to no symptoms to marked congestive heart failure, requiring medical and/or surgical intervention. In more severe cases with cyanosis, children may have significant limitations in their physical activity. Since there are multiple defects known, only several of the more common types of acyanotic and cyanotic defects will be discussed below.

Acyanotic Congenital Heart Disease

In acyanotic CHD the blood is shunted away from the body and to the lungs as a result of holes in the walls of the heart chambers. Ventricular septal defect is the most common type of CHD, excluding bicuspid aortic valves, comprising anywhere from 16–29% of cases (Gumbiner & Takao, 1990). In ventricular septal defect, there is a defect in the wall separating the right and left ventricles. It may occur as an isolated anomaly or in association with more complex disease. Patients with small defects are asymptomatic and many of these defects will close spontaneously; in these cases, there are no restrictions to children's physical activities. Moderate size defects may require medications early on to alleviate symptoms of heart failure, allowing for the opportunity of spontaneous closure of the defect as the child gets older. Surgical intervention is required for children who develop severe pulmonary hypertension or in cases of defects that result in intractable heart failure despite medications. With better echocardiogram capabilities available today, many children will not need to undergo cardiac catheterization prior to surgery.

Activity recommendations for those with a moderate degree of shunting through the defect usually involve moderate levels of exercise whereas those with large shunts will need to utilize low levels of exercise (Franklin, Allen, & Fontana, 1995). Postoperatively, the amount of exercise allowed for a patient will be determined by the amount of residual, if any, shunting as well as any additional problems, such as pulmonary hypertension, ventricular dysfunction, or any rhythm disturbances. A cardiac catheterization may be needed before specific recommendations regarding physical activity can be made (Graham, Bricker, James, & Strong, 1994).

Isolated atrial septal defects (ASD) comprise about 7–10% of CHD (Vick & Titus, 1990). This defect involves the wall separating the right and left atria. Atrial septal defects can also be part of more complex heart disease in the same manner as ventricular septal defect. Children with atrial septal defects generally do well during childhood, with very few symptoms attributed to their heart defect. As they get older, there is more shunting across the defect, which may lead to problems in the second or third decade of life such as rhythm disturbances and pulmonary hypertension. Many patients may live well into middle age or older before developing symptoms. Some atrial septal defects will close spontaneously but for those that do not, there are currently two treatment options: ASD closure in the catheterization lab or surgical closure. Postoperative recommendations depend on associated findings, such as pulmonary hypertension and rhythm disturbances (Graham, Bricker, James, & Strong, 1994). Patients that undergo closure via catheterization are treated similarly to postoperative patients, although they may have less problems with dysrhythmias due to the lack of suture lines. From a physical activity standpoint many will not have limitations imposed. Those that develop atrial dysrhythmias need to be evaluated before making an exercise plan (Franklin, Allen, & Fontana, 1995).

Other types of acyanotic CHD include those that cause obstruction to blood flow, either to blood leaving the heart or for blood moving through the blood vessels. Aortic stenosis (AS), accounting for 3–6% of CHD (Friedman, 1995), involves thickening of the aortic valve. In 85–90% of these cases, the diagnosis is made in children after their 2nd birthday and many will be either asymptomatic or have minimal symptoms. The severity of the obstruction dictates when one will need to come to some type of relief of the narrowing, whether in the catheterization lab or at surgery. Since one of the most frightening complications of aortic stenosis is sudden death, which generally occurs during or immediately after exercise, limitations are often placed on the activity level of the patient. Normal levels of physical activity are allowed when trivial or mild stenosis exists, as long as the EKG and/or the long term ambulatory monitoring is normal. Children with moderate aortic stenosis must undergo an exercise test prior to undergoing activities so a safe recommendation can be made. Generally these children are restricted to light activities that include recreational swimming, golf, and bicycling. Those with severe aortic stenosis are allowed to participate only at low levels of dynamic exercise, which would not include football or basketball. Because many of these children can be asymptomatic despite these gradients, and look and act normally, they and their peers may not understand why physical activity restrictions are being placed on them.

Cyanotic Congenital Heart Disease

Some children are born with heart defects that cause them to have less than normal oxygenation, called cyanotic heart defects. Most of these are noted shortly after birth and require rather immediate medical or surgical therapy. Most children with cyanotic CHD have abnormal exercise tolerance prior to surgery, which usually persists afterwards as well. This problem afterward may be a result of deconditioning. Other problems may exist postoperatively, such as rhythm disturbances, which will limit children's exercising capability. Overall, however, most patients grow up after surgical correction to have a relatively normal life, which includes some female patients going on to have children themselves (Fyler, 1992).

The most common cyanotic lesion is tetralogy of Fallot (TOF), accounting for 8–11% of CHD (Zuberbuhler, 1995). This problem includes a ventricular septal defect as well as some degree of obstruction to pulmonary blood flow. Depending on the amount of obstruction, the patient may not develop obvious cyanosis until after infancy. A murmur will be present, however, which in and of itself would lead to some type of evaluation. At least one and usually two surgeries are necessary to correct the defects associated with tetralogy of Fallot.

Transposition of the great arteries (TGA) is the most common cyanotic lesion presenting shortly after birth, and accounts for 5% of CHD (Fyler, 1992). This defect is made up of the aorta arising from the right ventricle and the pulmonary artery from the left ventricle. Surgical intervention is necessary within the first couple of weeks in simple transposition of the great arteries. The usual treatment now is the arterial switch operation. It is still too early to determine how these patients do in the long term, although there is optimism since the left ventricle is left as the systemic ventricle, rather than with the atrial switch where the blood is diverted at the atrial level and the right ventricle acts as the systemic ventricle. Those who have undergone atrial switch procedure can develop dysrhythmias as time goes on as well as develop right ventricular dysfunction which will limit their exercise tolerance.

Marfan's syndrome

Other children are born with syndromes that have structural cardiovascular disease as a component. Patients with Marfan's syndrome have an abnormal chemical makeup of their aorta, which makes it susceptible to rupture (Gersony, 1987). These patients are also tall for their age, and may feel peer pressure to play basketball. Because of the risk to the aorta, however, there is good consensus that these patients should not participate is sports where there is a chance of contact and thus an acceleration/deceleration type of injury. Also, beta blockers are often prescribed prophylactically in Marfan's, limiting their exercise capability.

Inflammatory cardiovascular disease

Another category of heart problems is inflammatory cardiovascular disease. These are acquired rather than congenital disorders, and include such problems as myocarditis, rheumatic heart disease, Kawasaki disease, and cardiovascular defects associated with connective tissue disease (Gersony, 1987; Newburger, 1992).

Certain viruses and bacteria may cause inflammation of the heart and lead to a disease called myocarditis. The actual incidence of this problem is unknown since some people who develop this are asymptomatic and the inflammation resolves spontaneously. However, others may develop severe congestive heart failure. Some children will die during the acute phase of the illness and a fraction will develop dilated cardiomyopathy, which may necessitate cardiac transplantation at some point.

Rheumatic fever is a problem that still exists in the US but not to the degree that it used to. However, it is a major public health problem elsewhere in the world, especially in third world countries, and is a leading cause of cardiac morbidity and mortality in children world-wide (Fyler, 1992). This disease can damage the valves of the heart, especially the mitral and aortic valves. If there is significant valve disease that does not respond to medical therapy, interventional catheterization or surgery may be necessary. Early in the course of the disease there is restriction on the amount of activity that a child is allowed to participate in, which may mean a prolonged period of bedrest or quiet activity. Prevention of recurrence in those who have rheumatic fever requires prophylaxis with antibiotics, usually given by monthly penicillin injections that are quite painful. The length of time for prophylaxis depends on several factors such as the age that the child develops rheumatic fever as well as environmental concerns, such as overcrowding.

Myocardial disease

Myocardial disease can present at any age. It can show up as thin, poorly contracting muscle, known as dilated cardiomyopathy, or thickened, hyperdynamic muscle known as hypertrophic cardiomyo-pathy (Gersony, 1987). These diseases may be inherited or may be secondary to medications taken to treat other diseases such as leukemia. The cause may not be found in a large number of patients. Clinically there may be few symptoms and the diagnosis suspected only when a chest x-ray is obtained for another reason and a large heart is seen. A new murmur or mitral insufficiency may be found then and the diagnosis made on echocardiographic evaluation.

As the disease progresses, children will experience a decrease in exercise tolerance and may start having heart rhythm disturbances. Those with the most severe cases of dilated cardiomyopathy may require a transplant in order for them to live. However, due to the shortage of available organs for transplant, many will die on the waiting list. Children with hypertrophic cardiomyopathy may be at risk for sudden death, which may be their first symptom of a heart problem. A family history of sudden death or cardiomyopathy may help lead to the diagnosis before symptoms develop.

Arrhythmias

Cardiac rhythm disturbances can develop during the prenatal period, infancy, or appear later in childhood or adulthood, and cause a variety of symptoms such as chest pain, dizziness, or syncope. Arrhythmias in childhood can result from CHD (both acyanotic and cyanotic subtypes), acquired heart diseases, or acquired systemic disorders (Walsh & Saul, 1992). Primarily as a result of improved diagnostic methods with electrocardiogram, children with arrhythmias have been identified more frequently in recent years. However, there is often difficulty confirming what sounds like an arrhythmia clinically but is not documented on tests such as Holter monitoring or event recorders. This can be frustrating for both patients and their families and the medical team, leading to multiple tests which are unrevealing although the patient still feels an abnormal sensation in their chest.

Some rhythm disturbances are common in children (e.g., premature atrial and ventricular beats) but are not associated with significant health risks in most cases. Severe untreated arrhythmia, however, may lead to sudden death. The primary risks associated with an arrhythmia are severe tachycardia (fast heart rate) or bradycardia (slow heart rate), leading to decreased cardiac output. The most common serious arrhythmias are bypass tracts such as Wolff-Parkinson-White (preexcitation) syndrome (a type of supraventricular tachyarrhythmia) and congenital heartblock (a type of bradyarrhythmia) (Gersony, 1987).

Depending on the cause of the rhythm disturbance, a patient may be treated medically with pharmacologic agents, or may need to undergo a procedure in the catheterization lab to evaluate the location of the abnormality resulting in the rhythm problem and then possibly treat it by performing an ablation. Rhythms that are too slow may result in the need for an implanted pacemaker. For some extreme cases unresponsive to these methods, heart transplantation may be needed. Problems with medical treatment of pediatric arrhythmias include dosage of medications, variable responses, side effects, and regimen adherence. Relatively little developmental, psychological, or behavioral research has been conducted with these patients.

Diagnosis and medical management

With today's technology, many children with CHD can be detected in utero by fetal echocardiograms. A recent study by Yagel et al. (1997) correctly detected in utero 85% of the cardiac anomalies noted at birth. Early detection in utero allows a family to get information on the type of defect from the medical team and together explore the options available to them. In some cases the choice may be for termination of the pregnancy. In other cases the mother will choose to continue the pregnancy and the team will help determine the best place for the infant to be born.

For those defects not determined in utero, CHD may come to the attention of a medical team after a murmur is first noted or a child is cyanotic or if the child is not growing as well or keeping up with his or her peers. The child may have other anomalies that prompt a physician to look for any possible associated heart disease. The initial evaluation includes a complete physical exam and usually a chest x-ray and an EKG. A working diagnosis is usually made at this point, taking into account the findings from the exam and the tests as well as the information obtained from a detailed history. Confirmation of the diagnosis is then usually done with an echocardiogram. Before the echocardiogram became as sophisticated as it is today, a cardiac catheterization was often needed to confirm the diagnosis. Today there are still some cases where complete information is not obtained with the echocardiogram, necessitating a cardiac catheterization. However, the latter is now used more for interventional purposes. When one is suspicious of a rhythm disturbance, monitoring can be done with

24-hour electrocardiograms (Holter monitors) or with devices that are utilized over a longer period of time for those episodes that occur sporadically (event monitors).

Other than the cardiac catheterization, the previous tests are all noninvasive and do not hurt. Many younger children do not like the chest x-ray, EKG, or echocardiogram, however, because they must hold still for a period of time. It may be necessary to sedate the younger children for an echocardiogram since that test can last 30 minutes or more when complex anatomy is found. These tests can be performed as outpatients, including most of the diagnostic cardiac catheterizations. The interventional cardiac catheterizations, which includes such procedures as closing a patent ductus arteriosus or dilating a stenotic valve may require an overnight stay in the hospital.

There is a wide variety of heart disease that can affect children, some quite benign and others very severe. It can present during infancy or not be known until adolescence. As a result of differences in location and severity of lesions, children and adolescents may experience various symptoms including fatigue, dyspnea (shortness of breath), poor exercise tolerance, growth failure, cough, cyanosis and chest pain. With mild versions of the disease no treatment is typically needed other than regular medical follow-up. Patients with mild to moderate disease could be expected to function normally, but those with severe disease will likely have decreased exercise tolerance and restricted physical activity. Because of their increased susceptibility to fatigue, headaches, and dizziness, cyanotic patients are advised to avoid high altitudes, abrupt changes in temperature, and situations in which dehydration could occur. Females with severe cyanotic CHD are at increased risk for problems related to pregnancy, but with corrective surgery, those with mild or moderate disease can have normal pregnancies.

There is no treatment for some cardiovascular conditions of childhood, ranging from the very mild (that do not require treatment) to the very severe (for which there is no real surgical option). The most severe defects are now surgically corrected during infancy. However, even though mortality rates are low, the surgery itself may result in adverse changes in functioning, including mental retardation, language and learning disorders, and movement and seizure disorders (Fallon, Aparicio, Elliott, & Kirkham, 1995; Ferry, 1987). Neurological problems following cardiac surgery have reported prevalence rates ranging from 2 to 25%. Imaging studies and autopsies of infants who have died have documented acquired brain lesions following open heart surgery, including evidence of diffuse hypoxic/ischemic injury, areas of focal infarction, and microscopic abnormalities in gray and white matter (Miller, Mamourian, Tesman, Baylen, & Myers, 1994; Muraoka et al., 1981).

Several new trends have developed in recent years in the surgical treatment of CHD: primary surgical repair during the noenatal period; use of low-flow cardiopulmonary bypass; use of extra-corporeal membrane oxygenation (ECMO); and interventional catheterization. In a clinical series of 304 neonates who underwent primary surgical repair, a total mortality rate of 11.8% was observed (Castaneda et al., 1989). Low-flow cardiopulmonary bypass rather than hypothermic circulatory arrest as a support technique during cardiac surgery has been shown to be associated with lower post-operative central nervous system perturbations and fewer neuropsychological deficits (Newburger et al., 1993; Oates, Simpson, Turnbull, & Cartmill, 1995). Extra-corporeal membrane oxygenation has been successfully used in life-threatening situations for cardiac support and as a bridge to transplantation when children decompensate after open-heart surgery or suffer acute decompensation due to chronic cardiomyopathy or viral myocarditis (del Nido, 1996; Klein et al., 1990). The neurodevelopmental effects of these procedures are discussed in a later section of this chapter.

As an alternative to open-heart surgery, interventional catheterization has been increasingly used for repair of certain types of CHD (Lock, Keane, Mandell, & Perry, 1992). For example, interventional catheterization has been used to treat patent ductus arteriosus and atrial septal defects. Angioplasty has also been shown to be efficacious for recurrent coarctation of the aorta and valvuloplasty has been successfully used for pulmonic and aortic stenosis.

Children with very severe CHD, acquired cardiac disease, or intractable arrhythmias may need heart transplantation. When other treatment options are exhausted and where neither open-heart repairs nor interventional catheterization is feasible, heart transplantation has become an accepted treatment approach (Addonizio, 1996; Baum & Bernstein, 1993). This operation was first performed successfully in children over 20 years ago. More than 1200 pediatric heart transplantations have been conducted through 1994, with 1-year survival of approximately 77% and 5-year survival of 70% (Addonizio, 1996; Hosenpud, Novick, Breen, Keck, & Daily, 1995). Survival rates and QL have improved dramatically in recent years as more transplants have been performed and techniques refined. However, approximately 20% of children may have neurologic complications following heart transplantation (Baum et al., 1993; Martin et al., 1992). The impact of transplantation on psychosocial and cognitive functioning is considered later in this chapter.

Medical treatment for acquired heart disease includes prophylactic drug regimens, and sometimes cardiac surgery is required to repair the structural damage to the heart. Although mortality is low with early diagnosis and treatment, acquired heart disease is still a significant cause of morbidity and mortality in children. Preventive interventions are therefore very important in the medical management of acquired heart disease. One of the major problems seen in clinical practice is nonadherence with prophylactic drug regimens. Despite the fact that these diseases pose a considerable health risk for children, few empirical studies with this patient population are available. More research addressing cognitive, psychosocial, and behavioral factors of children with acquired heart diseases is needed.

Follow-up at regular intervals is an important part of treatment. Patients may be seen anywhere from once a week to once a year, depending on the severity of the lesion. Pediatric cardiologists see many older children and adolescents whose defects were corrected in early childhood. Routine tests for evaluation and monitoring include chest radiographs, electrocardiograms, echocardiography, exercise testing, radionuclide studies, and cardiac catheterization. Because invasive procedures such as catheterization may be stressful for young patients, clinical practice for most patients routinely involves heavy sedation. After corrective surgery, some patients and parents may have unrealistic perceptions concerning physical activity restrictions or fear recurrence of heart-related problems, creating distress. Residual problems may exist, requiring further interventions including surgery. Further information on the medical aspects of CHD can be found in Gersony (1987) and Fyler (1992).

PSYCHOSOCIAL FUNCTIONING

A number of studies have examined the psychosocial functioning of children with CHD. While most of these studies have not directly addressed the question of QL, they nevertheless provide relevant information regarding behavioral and emotional functioning, from which QL can be inferred. Although early studies suggested a negative impact on behavior and emotions (e.g., Aurer, Senturia, Shopper, & Biddy, 1971; Green & Levitt, 1962) and family functioning (e.g., Apley, Barbour, & Westmacott, 1967), recent studies have identified some specific problems observed during early childhood, but fairly adaptive functioning later in childhood.

Some studies have focused on factors related to eating because children with CHD may have impaired growth (Baum, Beck, Kodama, & Brown, 1980) and have been described as having difficulty with feeding (Gudermuth, 1975). Results from one observational study suggested that the behavior of CHD infants may make feeding difficult, increasing their risk of growth problems (Lobo, 1992).

Marino and Lipshitz (1991) studied temperament in a sample of infants and toddlers with CHD. Infants with CHD were rated by their parents as more withdrawn, more intense in emotional reactions, and had lower thresholds for stimulation. Toddlers were rated as less active, rhythmic, and intense, and more negative in mood. However, there was no association between temperament and severity of CHD (as determined by oxygen saturation levels and physician ratings).

In another study related to temperament and parent–child interaction, Bradford (1990) examined factors related to young children's distress during diagnostic procedures. Observational ratings of distress during chest radiographs were made using reliable methods and parents were interviewed to identify possible psychosocial factors related to child distress. Forty-seven percent of the sample did not exhibit significant distress during the procedure. High child distress was associated with low stranger sociability and negative parenting style (i.e., use of force and reinforcement of dependency).

Kramer et al. (1989) studied personality in children with CHD compared with healthy controls. Although no differences were observed in younger children, among older children (9–14 years) there was some evidence suggesting increased feelings of anxiety, impulsiveness, and inferiority among those CHD patients with physical limitations as compared with healthy controls.

Alpern, Uzark, and Dick (1989) measured trait anxiety, self-competence, and locus of control in a study of CHD patients requiring pacemakers, 33% of whom had cyanotic CHD. The mean age of the study sample was 13 years. The control groups included CHD patients without pacemakers (50% with cyanotic CHD) and healthy children. Children with pacemakers reported a more external locus of control, but there were no group differences in anxiety and self-competence.

Content analysis of interviews with the children indicated those with pacemakers had fears of pacemaker failure and social rejection. While the non-pacemaker group and healthy controls viewed children with pacemakers as having significant emotional and social differences, children with pacemakers perceived themselves as no different than their peers. These findings indicate relatively healthy psychological adaptation in CHD children with pacemakers, possibly through the effective utilization of denial. However, the findings suggest such children may be at risk for social isolation and rejection, and difficulties with autonomy.

DeMaso et al. (1990) examined global psychological functioning in children with cyanotic CHD. Based on clinical interviews with parents, a behavioral symptom checklist, and observations during a testing protocol, ratings of global psychological functioning were made on a 5-point scale (from no impairment to severe impairment). Excellent inter-rater reliability was reported. Both groups of children with cyanotic CHD (transposition of the great arteries and tatralogy of Fallot) were rated as being lower in psychological functioning than the control group of healthy children who had spontaneous recovery of their heart problem. There was no difference between the cyanotic subgroups. Using multiple regression analysis, psychological functioning was predicted by degree of CNS impairment and IQ.

These authors then evaluated the effects of maternal perceptions and disease severity on the psychosocial adjustment of 4–10 year-old children with CHD (DeMaso et al., 1991). Predictor variables included measures of parenting stress, parental locus of control, and a measure of disease severity (based on number of hospitalizations, invasive procedures, outpatient visits, and a cardiologist's rating). The criterion measure was the total behavior problems score from the Child Behavior Checklist (CBCL). The mean T-score for total behavior problems for the group was 52.2, indicating good overall functioning. Similarly, the mean scores for parenting stress and locus of control were close to the means from the norms for these measures. Medical severity explained only 3% of the variance, while maternal perceptions accounted for the majority of variance (33%) in child adjustment.

Behavioral and emotional functioning (the CBCL and the Vineland Adaptive Behavior Scales) were measured by Morris et al. (1993) in a study of children surviving cardiac arrest. There was little evidence suggesting significant behavioral problems on the CBCL, although a significant proportion of the sample scored less than a standard deviation below the mean for norms on the Vineland subscales.

Spurkland, Bjornstad, Lindberg, and Seem (1993) examined behavioral functioning in adolescents with "complex" (i.e., cyanotic) CHD, in comparison with a group who had repaired atrial septal defects and were in good health. Measures included the CBCL, standardized clinical interviews for diagnosis of psychiatric disorders, and parent interviews to assess family dysfunction. The standardized bicycle ergometer stress test was used to measure physical capacity. Results showed patients with complex CHD had significantly lower physical capacity and more psychiatric diagnoses (42% vs. 27% of controls), with overanxious disorder and dysthymic disorder being the the most common diagnoses. Greater psychopathology was associated with more severe physical impairment. Only one-third of youths with complex CHD were functioning normally, with one-third having minor to moderate problems, and another third having serious dysfunction. Major psychiatric disorder was observed in just 4% of youths in the acyanotic group, with 54% functioning normally and 42% having minor to moderate problems. Behavior ratings by mothers revealed clinically significant problems in 19% of the complex group compared with only 4% in the acyanotic group. Similar levels (about 50%) of chronic family problems were apparent in both groups.

Casey, Sykes, Craig, Power, and Mulholland (1996) examined the behavioral adjustment of children with surgically-treated complex CHD compared to a control group of children with innocent heart murmurs. Behavior ratings by teachers indicated that children with CHD were more withdrawn than the control children. Parent ratings indicated that children with CHD had more social problems, engaged in fewer activities, and were more withdrawn. Family strain and exercise tolerance were significant predictors of teacher-rated school performance. Although measures of intellectual functioning were not available, teacher reports indicated that significantly more students with CHD were performing academically in the borderline or clinical range.

LONG-TERM PSYCHOSOCIAL ADJUSTMENT

Few studies are available on the longer-term psychosocial adjustment of children with CHD. Garson, Williams, and Redford (1974) evaluated personality factors (with the Cattell 16 PF Personality Inventory) in a study of patients with tetralogy of Fallot whose mean age was 19 years. Compared to test norms (based on college students), the study sample was more neurotic, with greater dependency, overprotection, weaker superego, more impulsivity, and less ambition. However, these findings are limited by the reliance on self-report and lack of an appropriate control group.

Baer, Freedman, and Garson (1984) examined psychological functioning with the Cattell 16 PF in a sample of young adults who had surgical correction for tetralogy of Fallot during childhood. The study sample represented 50% of available patients. Patients were divided into two groups based on younger (mean age of 6.5 years) or older (mean age of 12.5 years) age at surgery. Patients also completed an instrument measuring family conditions around the time of surgery and the Children's Report of Parental Behavior Inventory (yielding scores for acceptance, autonomy, and control). Results suggested that patients who had surgery later in childhood described their current personality as more timid and reserved, less venturesome, and more apprehensive than those who had surgery earlier in childhood, and recalled their parents as being more involved but less controlling and strict than those operated on at an earlier age.

Utens et al. (1994) investigated the long-term psychosocial outcome of young adults who had had surgical correction for CHD in childhood. On a self-report measure of emotional functioning, the young adults obtained better scores than the control group. No significant differences were found with regard to overall social functioning and occupational attainment, however, the young adults with CHD were more likely to be living with their parents.

In a study of 77 nonselected patients seen nearly 15 years after surgical repair of TOF, Meijboom, Szatmari, Deckers, Utens, Roelandt, Bos, and Hess (1995) evaluated health-related QL in association with medical status. The majority (82%) of patients rated their health as "excellent" or "good," and most (79%) had almost normal exercise capacity. However, there was no relationship between personal health assessments and medical symptoms and cardiac sequelae, which were substantial in the study sample.

In another study of long-term psychosocial functioning, 168 (of 463 potentially available) patients with various types of CHD were evaluated 25 years after their original examination (Brandhagen, Feldt, & Williams, 1991). Self-reported levels of psychological symptoms (using the SCL-90) revealed higher symptoms (particularly anxiety and depression) than expected based on norms. Psychological distress, however, was unrelated with the severity of the original cardiac defect.

PSYCHOSOCIAL ADJUSTMENT AND QUALITY OF LIFE AFTER HEART TRANSPLANTATION

One of the first studies of QL after pediatric heart transplantation was reported by Lawrence and Fricker (1987). Seven patients in the age range of 6 to 15 years were studied. As specific measures of children's QL were not available, the authors utilized a variety of measures to assess factors considered important to children's well being, including psychosocial adjustment, school behavior, and exercise tolerance. Measures of psychosocial adjustment included self-reports of self-image, projective drawings, personality and behavior ratings by parents, and interviews with parents. Pre-transplant data was not available, nor were data from a comparison group of children. However, this report was noteworthy in revealing how these survivors were competent in self-care, able to attend school regularly, and able to to engage in age-appropriate activities with friends, indicating improved QL. These authors' report of 10 patients similarly revealed dramatically improved functioning in many areas after transplantation despite the side effects of immunosuppression (Fricker, Griffith, Hardesty, Trento, Gold, Schmeltz, et al., 1987).

One important measure of QL is indicated by formal exercise testing. A recent study by Nixon, Fricker, Noyes, Webber, Orenstein, and Armitage (1995) showed that, despite being active and doing well, children had reduced exercise tolerance following heart transplantation. This finding confirmed an earlier study in which only 6 of 25 children had normal exercise performance after heart transplantation (Hsu, Garofano, Douglas, Michler, Quaegebeur, Gersony, & Addonizio, 1993).

Uzark, Sauer, Lawrence, Miller, Addonizio, and Crowley (1992) examined psychosocial adjustment two years after transplant in a group of 49 children who had a mean age of 10 years at the time of study. A control group was not obtained, but comparisons on standardized measures made to the normative samples. Parent behavior ratings (using the Child Behavior Checklist) indicated these children had significantly lower levels of social competence and more behavior problems than the normative population. In particular, depression was noted to be the most common psychological problem among these patients. Psychosocial problems of children were associated with greater family stress and fewer family resources for coping effectively with stress. Similarly, in a study of 65 children given heart or heart-lung transplants, compared with children receiving other cardiac surgery or healthy children, Wray,

Pot-Mees, Zeitlin, Radley-Smith, and Yacoub (1994) found increased behavioral problems at home in the transplanted children.

In one of the largest studies to date of long-term survivors of pediatric heart transplantation, Sigfusson and colleagues (Sigfusson, Fricker, Bernstein, Addonizio, Baum, et al., 1997) concluded that long-term survival with good QL can be achieved. In this study, 68 children who survived more than five years from transplantation were studed with a median follow-up of 6.8 years. QL was inferred by New York Heart Association classification status: before transplantation scores were either class 3 or 4 (indicating significant difficulties with breathing even with slight physical exertion), while all survivors were in class 1 at follow-up. Moreover, 45 of these long-term survivors were in full-time education, with 15 attending or graduated from college. Thirteen were working and only two were unemployed. However, these authors also reported that most patients had impaired peak exercise performance, and many faced problems related to chronic immunosuppression. Despite these difficulties, however, the authors concluded that good QL was achieved by attainment of age-appropriate activities. While this study is noteworthy in reporting improved QL, it is also significant in documenting significant health problems for many survivors, including complications of immunosuppression (such as hypertension), postrans-plantation coronary artery disease, and impaired exercise tolerance.

The post-transplantation regimen is very demanding and stressful, including daily doses of immunosuppressive medications that may have considerable side effects, as well as extensive medical follow-up including right ventricular endomyocardial biopsy. Regimen adherence problems may be especially significant, yet few studies have addressed this issue. One study of pediatric patients indicated 20% had significant nonadherence, increasing the chances of graft rejection (Douglas, Hsu, & Addonizio, 1993), while a study of adolescent patients also revealed adherence problems (Pahl, Zales, Fricker, et al., 1994). Sigfusson et al. (1997) reported that two deaths in their series of patients were directly related to nonadherence with immunosuppressive medication. In a study of adult patients, a higher incidence of hospital readmission and higher total medical costs was found in those who did not adhere well to the regimen (Paris, Muchmore, Pribil, Zuhdi, & Cooper, 1994).

Psychosocial adjustment of 24 adult survivors of heart transplantion was studied by Mai, McKenzie, and Kostuk (1990). The age range of patients was 15 to 56, with a mean age of 38 years. Evaluations were conducted prior to transplantation and 12 months later. Fourteen patients had a psychiatric diagnosis before transplantation, but at follow-up only 5 received psychiatric diagnoses. Post-operative regimen adherence was predicted by pre-operative psychiatric status. QL was considered to be significantly improved for the group at follow-up.

COGNITIVE FUNCTIONING
GENERAL AND DISEASE-RELATED ISSUES

There are a number of factors that influence neurodevelopment and cognitive functioning in children with cardiovascular disease. Infancy and early childhood are periods when many chronic diseases can have negative effects on brain development and cognitive functions because the brain develops rapidly during the first several years of life. Glial proliferation and myelination in the central nervous system take place most rapidly during the first year of life (Epstein, 1978, 1979). Interference with the process of brain development may have permanent adverse effects on cognitive functioning. In young children with cardiovascular disease, malnutrition may be present, and growth deficits are common.

There are also factors that may impact neurodevelopment that are specifically the result of the pathophysiology of cardiovasuclar disease. For example, there are a number of processes that can interrupt the flow of oxygenated blood to the brain, acutely or chronically, in children with CHD. In cyanotic CHD, reduced oxygenation of the blood can interfere with brain development and produce brain injury. The risk of cerebrovascular injury is increased for some children with CHD. In severe cases, low cardiac output and cardiac arrhythmias may also result in decreased blood flow to the brain, possibly compromising cognitive functioning. Children with severe heart disease may have cardiac arrests. Although they may be successfully resuscitated, these acute anoxic events could also have a negative impact on cognitive function. Finally, in some cases, CHD occurs in association with other defects forming a syndrome with related cognitive deficits such as Down's syndrome.

The effects of medical interventions constitute a second set of factors influencing cognitive functioning in children with CHD. Neurological sequelae of cardiac surgery are not uncommon. With better survival has come greater attention to the effects of different procedures, aiming to minimize neurological damage. Possible mechanisms include inadequate cerebral perfusion, hypoxia, microembolization (air and/or particulate matter), biochemical disturbances leading to neuronal damage, and hyperperfusion (Fallon, et al., 1995; Ferry, 1987; Miller et al., 1994).

Low-flow cardiopulmonary bypass and deep hypothermic circulatory arrest are two widely used support techniques, both of which can affect cerebral metabolism and hemodynamics leading to cerebral ischemia/reperfusion injury in some children (du Plessis et al., 1994). The maximum time of circulatory arrest with hypothermia to protect the brain without neurological sequelae is controversial. However, clinical experience suggests that the "safe period" is approximately 45 to 60 minutes. Low-flow cardiopulmonary bypass has been advocated as an alternative to complete circulatory arrest because it produces less neurological sequelae. However, due to microembolisms and hypoperfusion, this support technique also can produce adverse neurological events.

The use of extra-corporeal membrane oxygenation (ECMO) for cardiac support also carries risks for neurological damage (Mendoza et al., 1991). In many cases, ECMO involves permanent ligation of the right common carotid artery and right internal jugular vein; however, if ECMO is required in the immediate time period following cardiotomy, cannulation is performed through the sternotomy. Blood flow rate and velocity is affected by this procedure, and brain imaging during ECMO or immediately following decannulation has shown evidence of hemorrhage or lesions (Lott et al., 1990).

Heart transplantation also confers significant risk of neurologic complications, with neurological sequelae reported in at least 20% of heart transplant patients (Baum et al., 1993; Martin et al., 1992). In addition to the risks associated with open heart surgery and cardiopulmonary bypass discussed above, use of drugs such as cyclosporine and steroids can have adverse neurodevelopmental consequences (Stewart, Kenard, Waller, & Fixler, 1994).

Psychosocial variables common to children with significant chronic disease may also impact neurodevelopment and cognitive functioning. These include restrictions in physical activities, parental overprotection, reduced opportunities for peer socialization, and frequent and/or prolonged hospitalizations resulting in relative social isolation and absence from school.

In the following sections, studies that have investigated the impact of CHD on neurodevelopment and cognitive functioning will be reviewed, as these effects can have significant consequences for QL. First, studies that have examined cognitive outcomes for children with CHD as a whole will be discussed, with consideration of cyanotic and acyanotic disease. The neurodevelopmental impacts of different surgical and support techniques, including low-flow cardiopulmonary bypass, ECMO, and heart transplantation, will then be reviewed.

EFFECTS OF CONGENITAL HEART DISEASE ON COGNITIVE FUNCTIONING

A number of studies have compared cognitive functioning in children with cyanotic heart disease to children with acyanotic heart disease. The results of most studies have shown significantly lower cognitive functioning in the cyanotic group. In an early study, Linde, Rasof, and Dunn (1967), compared preschool aged-children with cyanotic CHD, acyanotic CHD, and two control groups of normal siblings and children from a well child clinic. The CHD children were assessed for intelligence prior to corrective cardiac surgery. Results showed significantly lower IQ for cyanotic compared with acyanotic children, and both CHD groups scored lower than the control groups. However, the mean IQ for the cyanotic group was in the normal range (mean of 96 vs. 104 for acyanotic). Furthermore, in the younger patients, physical disability measures and IQ scores were significantly related. In a 5-year follow-up of these children, Linde, Rasof, and Dunn (1970) found significant increases in IQ scores only for cyanotic children who had received corrective surgery.

Silbert, Wolff, Mayer, Rosenthal, and Nadas (1969) examined children with cyanotic CHD, children with acyanotic CHD with congestive heart failure, and children with acyanotic mild CHD. Children were tested between the ages of 4 and 8 years with standardized measures of intelligence, perceptual-motor, and gross motor coordination tests. Children with cyanotic disease had significantly lower IQ scores and did worse on the perceptual-motor and gross motor tasks. However, performance of the cyanotic group was in the normal range of intelligence.

More recent studies have also found lower cognitive functioning in children with cyanotic CHD. For example, Aram, Ekelman, Ben-Schachar, and Levinsohn (1985) studied children with CHD ranging in age from 3 months to 15 years. Using standardized intelligence, cyanotic children were compared with acyanotic and significantly lower IQ scores were observed for the cyanotic children (mean of 104 versus 113).

Kramer, Awiszus, Sterzel, van Halteren, and Classen (1989) compared intellectual functioning in children with CHD to control children who had benign heart murmurs. The CHD group was divided into those with and without significant symptoms with regard to physical capacity. The findings indicated that symptomatic children had significantly lower IQ scores than healthy controls. Although there were no significant differences between the symptomatic and asymptomatic CHD groups, the latter group had slightly higher scores. However, the study sample was heterogeneous with regard to cyanosis, type of defect, and history of surgery.

DeMaso, Beardslee, Silbert, and Fyler (1990) evaluated children with tetrology of Fallot (TOF), children with transposition of the great arteries (TGA), and a group of children originally diagnosed with acyanotic CHD but who had spontaneous recovery without medical intervention. All children in the study sample were diagnosed prior to one year of age and were tested between ages 5 and 6 years. The findings revealed children in both cyanotic groups had significantly lower IQ scores than the controls. Fourteen percent of children with TGA and 22% of those with TOF had IQ scores less than 79, compared with only 3% of the acyanotic children. Moreover, 40% of TGA and 45% of TOF children had clinically significant central nervous system impairment.

These studies indicate that as a group, children with cyanotic heart disease are more vulnerable with respect to overall cognitive development than children with acyanotic disease. However, several studies suggest that children with acyanotic heart disease also perform more poorly than normal controls. Linde, Rasof, and Dunn (1967) found that acyanotic children, tested prior to corrective surgery, had lower scores than control children. Yang, Liu, and Townes (1994) compared the test performance of Chinese children with acyanotic heart disease to a control group and reported that the scores of the acyanotic group were lower on tests of intelligence.

There is evidence supporting the idea that surgery conducted at earlier ages is associated with improved cognitive functioning of children with CHD. For example, in a study of young cyanotic children who had corrective surgery for TGA prior to testing, Newburger, Silbert, Buckley, and Fyler (1984) found IQ to be in the average range (mean of 102). While there was no difference compared with acyanotic children who had also received corrective surgery, for the cyanotic children there was a significant inverse correlation between age at repair (reflecting duration of hypoxia) and IQ; for the acyanotic group, however, there was no relationship between age at repair and IQ.

O'Dougherty, Wright, Garmezy, Loewenson, and Torres (1983) evaluated a number of neurodevelopmental outcomes in a sample of children with TGA, using standardized measures of intelligence, perceptual-motor functioning, and academic achievement. The children had open-heart surgical repair during early childhood (mean age of 2 years) and were tested at a mean age of 9.1 years. Although the mean IQ of the group was in the normal range, the distribution was bimodal, with more children than expected having borderline or lower intelligence (13%) or superior or very superior intelligence (16%). An inverse correlation was observed between age at surgery and IQ, perceptual-motor function, and academic achievement. Forty-two percent of the sample required special education programming at school. Age at surgical correction, growth failure, congestive heart failure, CNS infection, cerebrovascular stroke, lower socioeconomic status, and family stress were associated with poorer outcomes. These findings suggest that chronic hypoxia has adverse effects on neuro-development and cognitive functioning.

Wright and Nolan (1994) evaluated the impact of cyanotic CHD on children's school performance. They compared the academic and intellectual performance of children with TGA or TOF whose lesions had been corrected before age 2.5 to children with cardiac murmurs that did not require treatment. Children who had evidence of major nervous system trauma as a result of the cardiac lesion or its treatment were excluded from the study. Children with cyanotic CHD performed significantly worse on measures of intelligence academic achievement. However, the mean IQ score fell within the Average range while mean performance on academic measures was within the Low Average range. In addition, teacher ratings revealed significant differences between the groups with respect to arithmetic performance, with children in the cyanotic group more likely to be rated as below grade level in arithmetic. There was no statistically significant association between cognitive or academic functioning and any of the medical or surgical parameters including age at operation.

A number of studies have investigated specific neuropsychological deficits associated with CHD. Findings from several indicate that perceptual-motor skills are adversely affected by CHD (Rasof, et al., Wolff, Mayer, Rosenthal, & Nadas, 1969; Linde, Silbert, & Dunn, 1969; Newburger, 1984). As cyanosis, presumably due to hypoxia, has been linked with greater intellectual deficits, processes presumed to be more sensitive to hypoxia have been investigated. Although the actual effects of chronic hypoxia on the developing nervous system are unknown, inferences have been made based on findings from studies of adults with chronic obstructive airways disease (Prigatano & Levin, 1988) infants with perinatal hypoxia (Spreen, Risser, & Edgell, 1995). Based on these assumptions, researchers have examined attention and vigilance, and information processing capacity.

Several studies have shown deficits in attentional processes in children with cyanotic CHD. O'Dougherty, Wright, Loewenson, and Torres (1985) compared cyanotic children to a sample of control children matched for age, race, and socioeconomic status but with no history of sensory, neurologic, or learning problems. The cyanotic CHD group scored significantly lower on the WISC-R Freedom from Distractibility factor than would be expected based on the standardization sample; in addition, 23% of the CHD sample versus only 4% of the WISC-R standardization sample had a 30-point discrepancy between Verbal and Performance IQ. Although 80% of the CHD sample had IQ scores in the Average range or above, only 36% of the sample had academic achievement measures at or above grade level. There was also evidence that CHD children had more attentional problems on the continuous performance test (CPT) than normal control children.

Similarly, O'Dougherty, Nuechterlein, and Drew (1984) compared children with CHD to children with a DSM-III (R) diagnosis of attention deficit disorder (ADD) on a test of sustained attention (using the CPT). The two groups performed comparably with regard to overall vigilance, but the children with ADD displayed difficulty with inhibitory control whereas the CHD children had greater difficulty sustaining attention over time.

O'Dougherty, Berntson, Boysen, Wright, and Teske (1988) examined cardiac responses to non-signal stimuli and to signal stimuli in a vigilance task in children with CHD (cyanotic and acyanotic), children with ADD, and normal children. Overall task performance was lower in subjects with CHD and in the ADD group, but there were no differences between cyanotic and acyanotic children. Cardiac measures revealed that normal children displayed significantly larger heart rate deceleration to the target stimuli than did either of the clinical groups. Moreover, both clinical groups showed an exaggerated heart rate deceleration to vibrotactile stimuli. The magnitude of the cardiac response to somatosensory stimuli was predictive of task performance, with larger responses associated with higher error rates and lower perceptual sensitivity. For the normal control group, age was significantly related to false alarm rate, but this pattern was attenuated in the CHD and ADD groups, suggesting that normal age-related changes in attentional capacity may be disrupted for children with CHD and ADD. In addition, parent ratings for the children with CHD and ADD revealed significant problems with attention and hyperactivity.

However, Wright and Nolan (1994) found no relationship between medical or surgical parameters and measures of attentional and processing difficulties, suggesting that the nature of the cognitive and academic difficulties was not explained entirely by chronic hypoxia.

Two studies have examined the effects of surviving a cardiac arrest on the cognitive functioning of children with CHD. Morris, Krawiecki, Wright, and Walter (1993) examined neuropsychological performance of children, the majority of whom had CHD, who survived cardiac arrest with in-hospital resuscitation. The test battery was administered at some unspecified time after resuscitation. Results were compared to the normative mean of the various tests used in the study, rather than to a control group. Findings indicated that more children than expected scored less than one standard deviation below the normative means for the various tests used in the study. It was not known whether the observed deficits were due to cyanotic CHD or to cardiac arrest. However, a longer duration of cardiac arrest was associated with worse performance. Although this study is limited by the small and heterogenous sample, the findings suggest that children surviving cardiac arrest may be at increased risk for cognitive difficulties.

More recently, Bloom, Wright, Morris, Campbell, and Krawiecki (1997) compared children with CHD who had sustained a cardiac arrest in the hospital to a medically similar group of children with CHD to examine the additive impact of cardiac arrest on the functioning of children with CHD. The children in the cardiac arrest group had significantly lower scores on measures of general cognitive, motor, and adaptive behavior functioning, as well as greater disease severity. Forty-four percent of the cardiac arrest group performed at least one standard deviation below the mean on the general cognitive index, compared to only 6% of the children who had not sustained a cardiac arrest. Although the occurrence of a cardiac arrest alone did not add significantly to the prediction of outcome measures, the interaction of cumulative medical risk and the presence of a cardiac arrest was significant.

EFFECTS OF NEWER MEDICAL INTERVENTIONS

As noted earlier, there have been several new developments in the past decade regarding medical and surgical interventions for cardiac disease in children. Surgical repair for CHD is now routinely conducted during the neonatal period, as studies have demonstrated the advantages of early repair (Castaneda et al., 1989). With better survival rates, and with surgery being performed earlier during infancy (thereby reducing the impact of chronic hypoxia), increased attention has focused on neurological effects of various surgical and support techniques. In this section, studies evaluating neurodevelopment and cognitive functioning in relation to intraoperative variables (hypothermic circulatory arrest versus low-flow cardiopulmonary bypass), ECMO, and heart transplantation are discussed.

Hypothermic circulatory arrest and low-flow cardiopulmonary bypass

The effect of cardiovascular surgical support variables was studied by Bellinger et al. (1991) in a sample of children who received corrective cardiac surgery in early infancy. The children had standardized developmental evaluations after surgery when they were between 7 and 53 months of age to examine whether cardiopulmonary bypass perfusion variables were associated with later cognitive functioning. The sample was homogenous with respect to diagnosis and treatment: all had TGA repaired by the arterial switch operation using deep hypothermic circulatory arrest. The mean duration of deep hypothermic circulatory arrest was 64 ± 10 minutes (mean $\pm$ SD). Overall cognitive development score was in the normal range (mean of 101.2 ± 11.1). Duration of deep hypothermic circulatory arrest was not associated with cognitive performance. However, for core cooling periods of less than 20 minutes duration, shorter cooling periods were associated with significantly lower scores. These findings suggest that patients undergoing relatively long periods of deep hypothermic circulatory arrest may require some minimum time of cardiopulmonary bypass cooling to avoid central nervous system injury. A study by Newburger, Jonas, Wernovsky, Wypij, Hickey, et al. (1993) similarly documented reduced neurological sequelae and better outcome with the use of low-flow cardiopulmonary bypass.

Bellinger et al. (1995) conducted a randomized clinical trial of 171 children with TGA repaired by an arterial switch operation that used either predominantly total circulatory arrest or continuous low-flow cardiopulmonary bypass. Developmental and neurologic evaluations and magnetic resonance imaging (MRI) were performed at one year of age. Approximately one-fourth of the infants had a ventricular-septal defect; these children were older at the time of surgery so statistical analyses adjusted for the presence or absence of a ventricular septal defect. Subsequent analyses revealed that the presence of this defect was an independent risk factor for lower scores on developmental testing.

Results indicated that infants receiving circulatory arrest, compared with those receiving low-flow bypass, had a lower mean score on the Psychomotor Development Index of the Bayley Scales of Infant Development (a 6.5-point deficit) and a higher proportion had scores <80 (27 percent vs. 12 percent). These scores were inversely related to the duration of circulatory arrest. Neurologic abnormalities were more common among the children assigned to circulatory arrest; furthermore, the risk of neurologic abnormalities increased with the duration of circulatory arrest. The method of support was not associated with the prevalence of abnormalities on MRI scans of the brain, scores on the Mental Development Index of the Bayley Scale, or scores on a test of visual-recognition memory. However, perioperative electroencephalographic seizure activity was associated with lower scores on the Psychomotor Development Index and an increased likelihood of abnormalities on MRI scans of the brain.

In a follow-up study of these children, Bellinger, Rappaport, Wypij, Wernovsky, Newburger, et al. (1997) compared the developmental status based on parent-completed questionnaires. Responses to parental questionnaires completed when the children were 2.5 years old indicated that the children in the circulatory arrest group, especially those with a ventricular septal defect, manifested poorer expressive language.

Oates, Simpson, Turnbull, and Cartmill (1995) compared 114 children (51 with TOF, 30 with TGA, and 33 with ventricular septal defect) who had their defects repaired with the use of deep hypothermia and circulatory arrest to 54 children who had atrial septal defects repaired with the use of cardiopulmonary bypass. Intellectual and neuropsychological function was measured at an average of 9 to 10 years after the operation. Children with preoperative intellectual handicaps or postoperative neurologic complications were excluded. The only significant difference in the neuropsychological measures was that the bypass group had reaction times 2 to 3 seconds shorter on average than those of the hypothermic circulatory arrest group.

Although there were no significant differences in intelligence scores between the groups, a relationship between IQ scores and arrest time was found. Regression analysis of IQ against duration of arrest showed a significant decrease in IQ with increasing arrest time indicating a decrease of 3 to 4 points for each extra 10 minutes of arrest time.

Extracorporeal Membrane Oxygenation

Extracorporeal Membrane Oxygenation (ECMO) is a relatively new surgical procedure involving cardiopulmonary bypass of blood via cannulation of the right common carotid artery and right internal jugular vein (Klein, 1988). This life-saving technique is used for children whose risk of survival is less than 20% without ECMO (Short, Miller, & Anderson, 1987). For neonatal respiratory failure that is unresponsive to other interventions, ECMO is now considered a standard therapy. This procedure has also been applied to older (infants to preschool-age) children whose cardiopulmonary status deteriorates rapidly following surgery for repair of CHD (Klein, Shaheen, Whittlesey, Pinsky, & Arciniegas, 1990). In addition, increasing numbers of children are being placed on ECMO for acute decompensation of chronic cardiomyopathy or for a viral myocarditis (del Nido, 1996).

As ECMO has been used more over the past 15 years, research has examined the developmental functioning of these infants. Results have generally shown that, in terms of growth and intellectual functioning up to three years of age, children treated during the neonatal period with ECMO develop at or just below age-expected levels (Andrews, Nixon, Ciley, Roloff, & Barlett, 1986; Taylor, Glass, Fitz, & Miller, 1987). Longer-term follow-up studies into middle childhood have similarly indicated that most children appear to have normal growth and development using global measures, but neurologic complications have occurred in nearly 20% of cases (Hofkosh et al., 1991; Schumacher, Palmer, Roloff, LaClaire, & Barlett, 1991).

Less is known, however, about children who have received ECMO after cardiac surgery. Tindall, Rothermel, Delamater, Pinsky, and Klein (in press) examined neurodevelopment in 4–6 year-old children who had ECMO after cardiac surgery several years previous to the study, compared with cardiac controls (without ECMO) and normal control children. ECMO patients had deficits in left hand motor skill, as well as lower visual memory and visual-spatial constructive skills, compared with both cardiac and normal controls.

Heart transplantation

Little systematic data is available concerning cognitive development of children after heart transplantation. Clinical descriptive reports suggest that children do not have major abnormalities and that rehabilitation and QL is very good as children return to school and engage in age-appropriate activities (e.g., Backer et al., 1992; Starnes et al., 1989). QL in these medical reports is inferred by normal growth, attainment of developmental milestones, and low hospital readmission rate (e.g., Backer, Zales, Harrison, Idriss, Benson, & Mavroudis, 1991).

Trimm (1991) administered Bayley Scales of Infant Development five times over 30 months to 29 infants who received heart transplants before four months of age. Only two children had Mental Development Index scores less than 84 over the follow-up period, but 12 patients had scores less than 84 on the Psychomotor Development Index. In a more recent report of neurodevelopmental outcomes of children receiving transplants during infancy, Baum et al. (1993) found a mean Bayley Mental Developmental Index of 87 and Psychomotor Developmental Index of 90, with 67 percent of the sample having scores in the normal range.

Wray and Yacoub (1991) compared children who received heart transplants to children who had corrective open-heart surgery and healthy control children. The transplant group had lower developmental scores than the healthy controls, but mean scores were within normal limits. For children older than five years of age, however, the transplant group was significantly lower than both groups on developmental and academic achievement scores. Those with a history of cyanotic CHD, regardless of transplant or open-heart surgery, did worse.

Wray, Pot-Mees, Zeitlin, Radley-Smith, and Yacoub (1994) compared 65 children who had been given heart (n = 41) or heart-lung transplants (n = 24) to 52 children who had had other types of cardiac surgery and to 45 healthy children. The children in the transplant group ranged in age from 6 months to 16 years and the assessments were conducted 3 to 25 months following transplantation. The children with other types of cardiac surgery had various cyanotic and acyanotic conditions. A similar proportion of the transplant and cardiac surgery groups had been chronically ill since birth.

Results indicated that children given transplants had significantly lower scores on several developmental measures, particularly in children under 4.5 years of age. In this younger age group, the transplant and cardiac groups did not differ significantly from each other, but both groups performed significantly below the normal controls in all developmental areas. Performance on all tests, however, was within the normal range. Among children in the school-aged range, the transplant group had significantly lower IQ than the two comparison groups, and also performed significantly worse than the healthy group on tests of short-term memory, nonverbal reasoning, and speed of information processing. Their performance on the short-term memory subtests also was significantly lower than the cardiac group.

SUMMARY AND IMPLICATIONS

Few studies are available on QL in children with cardiovascular disease. When the construct of QL has been considered in the medical literature in this area, it has been concerned with the need for re-hospitalization or re-operation, formal tests of exercise capacity, physical growth, and/or return to age-appropriate physical activities and school (e.g., Backer et al., 1991; Elkins, et al., 1997; Nixon, et al., 1995; Sigfusson et al., 1997). Other than descriptive clinical reports (e.g., Lawrence & Fricker, 1987), the psychological literature in this area is remarkably limited in applying current assessment approaches, accounting for disease and functional status as well as psychological and social functioning (Spieth & Harris, 1996), to the study of QL in children and adolescents with cardiovascular disease.

However, a substantial amount of study has been directed toward the psychosocial and cognitive effects of cardiovascular disease, and most of this has focused on congenital heart disease. Other types of cardiovascular disease, such as acquired heart disease and arrhythmias, have received considerably less attention in the psychological research literature. More work in this area is needed, especially with adherence to prophylactic drug regimens, as this is a significant clinical issue related to morbidity of children and clinical decisions regarding transplantation.

Available research on psychosocial functioning suggests that infants with CHD have temperamental characteristics which may make feeding difficult, a finding which could in part explain the tendency for children with CHD to have abnormal growth. While there is some evidence of problems between parents and infants during feeding, more controlled research is needed in this area.

There are some reports of psychosocial adjustment difficulties later in childhood in the more severe, cyanotic children. Older children may have concerns with autonomy, social anxiety, and feelings of vulnerability. However, mean scores are generally within the normal range when standardized behavioral ratings are reported. In general, the data suggest that the risk of adjustment problems increases when corrective surgery occurs later in childhood or when physical capacity remains limited and cyanosis persists. Available longer-term follow-up studies suggest that, while most patients report fairly good health, there is an increased risk for psychological distress. Studies of family functioning and peer relationships are lacking, particularly as they may impact QL.

After heart transplantation, the majority of survivors appear to be able to return to school and age-appropriate normal physical activities. However, these children may be at risk for psychosocial adjustment problems, as studies have shown increased depression and behavioral problems and decreased social competence. More studies are needed addressing young patients' understanding of transplantation and its implications for them. It is important to note that the post-transplantation regimen is very demanding and that some physical limitations do persist for these patients. One issue of tremendous clinical significance is nonadherence to immunosuppressive therapies, which can be life-threatening. Several reports have attributed deaths in adolescent patients to this problem. More research is needed in this important area, particularly studies of medication adherence both before and after transplantation, as predictions of adherence are critical in clinical decision-making regarding whether or not a patient will receive a transplant.

Cognitive limitations can have obvious and sometimes subtle impacts on QL. Studies of neurodevelopment and cognitive functioning in children with heart disease indicate that, in general, overall functioning falls within the average range, but often is lower than the cognitive functioning in control groups. A number of factors have been associated with poorer cognitive outcomes, including type of CHD (cyanotic or acyanotic), age at surgical repair, type of surgical support technique, use of ECMO, and episodes of cardiac arrest.

Findings have consistently shown that children with cyanotic CHD are at risk for lower intelligence than children with acyanotic CHD, particularly if their disease is severe, their corrective surgery was not done within the first few years of life, and if there was significant CNS involvement. In these studies comparing cyanotic to acyanotic children, the latter had significantly higher IQ scores (on average about 10 points higher). With cyanotic children having a mean IQ of 102, it is surprising that the acyanotic groups generally averaged above 112. This raises the possibility of sampling bias in the control groups. However, without specification of participation rates, this possibility cannot be confirmed.

It appears that corrective surgery confers significant benefits on IQ when conducted at younger ages, presumably due to better oxygenation of the brain during early development. Corrective surgery is now usually performed during infancy, minimizing the impact of chronic hypoxia. Studies have also shown that the type of surgical support techniques used can contribute to risk of adverse cognitive functioning. Use of deep hypothermic circulatory arrest, particularly for arrest times longer than 45 minutes, has been associated with lower cognitive functioning as compared to low-flow cardiopulmonary bypass.

The focus of many studies has been on overall cognitive functioning, possibly obscuring impairment in specific areas of functioning. Research findings suggest that children with CHD may be at increased risk for subtle deficits in cognitive functioning and learning problems, with some evidence of attentional problems and lower levels of academic achievement. When achievement and classroom placement are included, increased rates of need for specialized services and academic weaknesses have often been reported. However, more studies to identify specific areas of cognitive impairment are needed. Such research must account for the effects of school absence on academic achievement and classroom performance, as lower achievement may be secondary to history of school absences related to illness and treatment rather than impaired learning ability.

There have been few controlled studies reported with respect to the neurodevelopmental outcomes of children receiving ECMO or cardiac transplantation. Available findings suggest children treated with ECMO after cardiac surgery may have a general cognitive impairment as well as lateralized deficits of functions performed by the right hemisphere; however, more studies with larger samples and longer follow up intervals are needed. After heart transplantation, children's cognitive development appears to be lower than children with CHD who have not undergone transplantation. However, as a group, overall cognitive functioning of these children falls within normal limits, although subtle cognitive deficits and lowered academic achievement may be observed. There are some findings indicating that children receiving transplantation at older ages do less well than those treated earlier.

There are a number of methodological problems in the research literature on CHD in children. Many study samples are small, raising concerns about sampling bias. As certain cardiac defects are more likely in boys than girls, study groups have often not been equated for gender. When sociodemographic characteristics of study samples are reported, in most cases the sample is predominantly white and in at least the middle range of socioeconomic status. Additionally, samples are often heterogeneous with regard to age of surgical correction, type of surgical procedure, type of cardiac defect, and preoperative health and developmental functioning. A number of studies did not use appropriate control groups, relying instead on comparisons to findings from normative samples. This approach is problematic because without control for having a chronic disease or having frequent contact with health care professionals, group differences cannot necessarily be attributed to CHD.

Very little intervention research addressing quality of life has been reported for children with cardiovascular disease. Current needs for intervention research could include distress associated with medical procedures, psychosocial adjustment, regimen adherence, and academic functioning. For example, interventions to reduce distress associated with diagnostic and evaluative procedures such as catheterization or biopsies are needed. Cassell (1965) reported that children who were prepared for catheterization with puppet play exhibited less behavioral distress during the procedure than children who received no special preparation. A recent clinical report suggests relaxation and imagery techniques without sedation are helpful for pediatric heart transplant patients during endomyocardial biopsy (Bullock & Shaddy, 1993). In a controlled study, Campbell, Kirkpatrick, Berry, and Lamberti (1995) demonstrated that information and coping skills training was effective in promoting recovery from cardiac surgery.

Intervention research targeting social anxiety and social skills is needed, particularly for children who look differently than their peers (e.g., those who are cyanotic, those with pacemakers, or who are cushingoid due to immunosuppressive medications). If more research documents that older children with more severe disease experience feelings of vulnerability and fears of social rejection, they might benefit from interventions to increase their social competence and decrease their fears. Interventions utilizing and/or targeting both family members and peers may be particularly helpful.

The research findings point to several other clinical concerns. Parents should be counseled while their child is still an infant regarding the risk of temperamental difficulties and associated feeding problems during infancy and early childhood, and how to deal effectively with such difficulties. Training in feeding skills could be initiated early and may help prevent growth problems commonly observed among CHD children. Additionally, counseling regarding potential academic difficulties or learning disabilities may be useful, particularly for school-age children with more severe disease. Considering the potential risk for learning delays, psychoeducational strategies should be planned to facilitate optimal academic performance.

Many parents and patients may have unrealistic beliefs about the risk of sudden death, leading to unnecessary restrictions for the child and greater distress for all. However, with the often disabling effects of cyanotic CHD in particular, counseling about reasonable expectations for age-appropriate activities, such as participation in sports, is needed. For older girls anticipating parenthood, counseling is also indicated regarding the significant risks associated with pregnancy.

This review has not addressed the issue of QL in children who may be at risk for development of later cardiovascular disease due to the presence of risk factors such as high blood lipids and blood pressure. For example, children with hypercholesterolemia may suffer adverse effects on QL due to the rigors of adherence to dietary management and various medications, or worry about future disease (Tonstad, 1996). Children with hypertension may require medications that similarly impact adversely on QL. Future empirical work in this area is needed.

CONCLUSIONS

Very few studies have directly addressed the question of QL in children and adolescents with cardiovascular disease. However, a substantial literature has demonstrated that children with cardiac disease are at risk for difficulties in psychosocial and cognitive functioning. Most of this research has focused on congential heart disease. Regarding psychosocial functioning, children with CHD have generally been rated within the normal range on measures of behavioral and emotional functioning, but are at risk for adjustment problems. With surgical repair made later in childhood, however, there seems to be a greater risk for behavioral or emotional difficulties. Future studies should focus on social competence, social anxiety, feelings of vulnerability, and autonomy issues, as these psychological factors may play an important role in the psychosocial adjustment of children with CHD. In addition, studies should address the role of peer and family relationships in children's QL.

Whereas most children with CHD can be expected to function in the normal range of cognitive functioning, a number of studies have shown that children with severe forms of CHD are at risk for lower levels of intellectual functioning and academic achievement. More deficits in cognitive development could be expected when there is more neurological involvement and cyanosis, and surgical repair is done later in childhood. Further studies are needed of specific areas of cognitive functioning that may be adversely affected by cardiac disorders.

There is a particular need for more intervention research to improve QL of these children and their parents. Significant contributions could be made by developing and evaluating interventions to target feeding difficulties in infants, distress associated with medical procedures, academic functioning, social competence and autonomy, and regimen adherence problems for patients after heart transplantation. Furthermore, few studies have addressed the issue of psychosocial or cognitive functioning in children with acquired heart disease. Reseach targetting adherence with prophylactic medical regimens is especially needed, particularly intervention studies to improve regimen adherence.

Advances in medical management and surgical approaches have dramatically increased survival for youngsters with cardiovascular disease. However, more studies are needed to understand the interplay of disease and functional status, psychosocial and cognitive functioning, as well as the role of peer and family relationships, in determining and improving QL in children and adolescents with various types of cardiovascular disease.

References

Addonizio, L.J. (1996). Current status of cardiac transplantation in children. *Current Opinions in Pediatrics, 8,* 520–526.

Aisenberg, R.B., Wolff, P.N., Rosenthal, A., & Nadas, P. (1973). Psychological impact of cardiac catheterization. *Pediatrics, 51,* 1051–1059.

Alpern, D., Uzark, K., & Dick II, M. (1989). Psychosocial responses of children to cardiac pacemakers. *Journal of Pediatrics, 114,* 494–501.

Andrews, A.F., Nixon, C.A., Cilley, R.E., Roloff, D.W., & Bartlett, R.H. (1986). One- to three-year outcome for 14 neonatal survivors of extracorporeal membrane oxygenation. *Pediatrics, 78,* 692–698.

Apley, J., Barbour, R.F., & Westmacott, F. (1967). Impact of congenital heart disease on the family: A preliminary report. *British Medical Journal, 1,* 103–105.

Aram, D.M., Ekelman, B.L., Ben-Shachar, G., & Levinsohn, M.W. (1985). Intelligence and hypoxemia in children with congenital heart disease: Fact or artifact? *Journal of the American College of Cardiology, 6,* 889–893.

Aurer, E.T., Senturia, A.G., Shopper, M., & Biddy, R. (1971). Congenital heart disease and child adjustment. *Psychiatric Medicine, 2,* 210–219.

Backer, C.L., Zales, V.R., Harrison, H., Idriss, F.S., Benson, D., & Mavroudis, C. (1991). Intermediate term results of infant orthotopic cardiac transplantation from two centers. *Journal of Thoracic and Cardiovascular Surgery, 101,* 826–832.

Backer, C.L., Zales, V.R., Idriss, F.S., Lynch, P., Crawford, S., Benson, D.W. Jr., & Mavroudis, C. (1992). Heart transplantation in neonates and children. *Journal of Heart and Lung Transplantation, 11,* 311–319.

Baer, P.E., Freedman, D.A., & Garson, Jr., A. (1984). Long-term psychological follow-up of patients after corrective surgery for tetralogy of fallot. *Journal of the American Academy of Child Psychiatry, 23,* 622–625.

Bailey, L., Gundry, S., Razzouk, A., & Wang, N. (1992). Pediatric heart transplantion: Issues relating to outcome and results. *Journal of Heart and Lung Transplantation, 11,* 267–271.

Baum, D., Beck, R., Kodama, A., & Brown, B. (1980). Early heart failure as a cause of growth and tissue disorders in children with congenital heart disease. *Circulation, 62,* 1145–1151.

Baum, D., & Bernstein, D. (1993). Heart and lung transplantation in children. In I.H. Gessner and B.E. Victoria (Eds.), *Pediatric cardiology: A problem oriented approach* (pp. 245–252). Philadelphia: W.B. Saunders Co.

Baum, M., Chinnock, R., Ashwal, S., Peverini, R., Trimm, F., & Bailey, L. (1993). Growth and neurodevelopmental outcome of infants undergoing heart transplantation. *Journal of Heart and Lung Transplantation, 12,* S211–S7.

Bellinger, D.C., Jonas, R.A., Rappaport, L.A., Wypij, D., Wernovsky, G., Kuban, K.C., Barnes, P.D., Holmes, G.L, Hickey, P.R., Strand, R.D., Walsh, A.Z., Helmers, S.L, Constantinou, J.E., Carranzana, E.J., Mayer, J.E., Hanley, F.L., Castaneda, A.R., Ware, J.H., & Newburger, J.W. (1995). Developmental and neurologic status of children after heart surgery with hypothermic circulatory arrest or low-flow cardiopulmonary bypass. *New England Journal of Medicine, 332,* 549–555.

Bellinger, D.C., Rappaport, L.A., Wypij, D., Wernovsky, G., & Newburger, J.W. (1997). Patterns of developmental dysfunction after surgery during infancy to correct transposition of the great arteries. *Journal of Developmental and Behavioral Pediatrics, 18,* 75–83.

Bellinger, D.C., Wernovsky, G., Rappaport, L.A., Mayer, J.E., Castaneda, A.R., Farrell, D.M., Wessel, D.L., Lang, P., Hickey, P.R., Jonas, R.A., & Newburger, J.W. (1991). Cognitive development of children following early repair of transposition of the great arteries using deep hypothermic circulatory arrest. *Pediatrics, 87,* 701–707.

Bloom, A.A., Wright, J.A., Morris, R.D., Campbell, R.M., & Krawiecki, N.S. (1997). Additive impact of in-hospital cardiac arrest on the functioning of children with heart disease. *Pediatrics, 99*, 390–398.

Bradford, R. (1990). Short communication: The importance of psychosocial factors in understanding child distress during routine X-ray procedures. *Journal of Child Psychology and Psychiatry, 31*, 973–982.

Brandhagen, D., Feldt, R., & Williams, D. (1991). Long-term psychologic implications of congential heart disease: A 25-year follow-up. *Mayo Clinic Proceedings, 66*, 474–479.

Bullock, E.A., & Shaddy, R.E. (1993). Relaxation and imagery techniques without sedation during right ventricular endomyocardial biopsy in pediatric heart transplant patients. *Journal of Heart and Lung Transplantation, 12*, 59–62.

Campbell, L., Kirkpatrick, S., Berry, C., & Lamberti, J. (1995). Preparing children with congenital heart disease for cardiac surgery. *Journal of Pediatric Psychology, 20*, 313–328.

Casey, F.A., Sykes, D.H., Craig, B.G., Power, R., & Mulholland, H.C. (1996). Behavioral adjustment of children with surgically palliated complex congenital heart disease. *Journal of Pediatric Psychology, 21*, 335–352.

Cassell, S. (1965). Effect of brief psychotherapy upon the emotional responses of children undergoing cardiac catherization. *Journal of Consulting and Clinical Psychology, 29*, 1–8.

Castaneda, A.R., Mayer, J.E., Jonas, R.A., Lock, J.E., Wessel, D.L., & Hickey, P.R. (1989). The neonate with critical congenital heart disease: Repair-A surgical challenge. *Journal of Thoracic and Cardiovascular Surgery, 98*, 869–875.

Del Nido, P.J. (1996). Extracorporeal membrane oxygenation for cardiac support in children. *Annals of Thoracic Surgery, 61*, 336–339.

DeMaso, D.R., Beardslee, W.R., Silbert, A.R., & Fyler, D.C. (1990). Psychological functioning in children with cyanotic heart defects. *Developmental and Behavioral Pediatrics, 11*, 289–293.

DeMaso, D.R., Campis, L.K., Wypij, D., Bertram, S., Lipshitz, M., & Freed, M. (1991). The impact of maternal perceptions and medical severity on the adjustment of children with congenital heart disease. *Journal of Pediatric Psychology, 16*, 137–149.

Douglas, J.F., Hsu, D.T., & Addonizio, L.J. (1993). Noncompliance in pediatric heart transplant patients. *Journal of Heart and Lung Transplantation, 12*, S92.

Du Plessis, A.J., Newburger, J., Jonas, R.A., Hickey, P., Naruse, H., Tsuji, M., Walsh, A., Walter, G., Wypij, D., & Volpe, J.J. (1995). Cerebral oxygen supply and utilization during infant cardiac surgery. *Annals of Neurology, 37*, 488–497.

Elkins, R., Knott-Craig, C., McCue, C., & Lane, M. (1997). Congenital aortic valve disease: Improved survival and quality of life. *Annals of Surgery, 225*, 503–511.

Fallon, P., Aparicio, J.M., Elliott, M.J., & Kirkham, F.J. (1995). Incidence of neurological complications of surgery for congenital heart disease. *Archives of Disease in Childhood, 72*, 418–422.

Ferry, P.C. (1987). Neurological sequelae of cardiac surgery in children. *American Journal of Diseases of Children, 141*, 309–312.

Franklin, W.H., Allen, HD., & Fontana, M.E. (1995). Sports, physical activity, and school problems (pp. 673–682). In G. Emmanouilides, T. Riemenschneider, H. Allen, & H. Gutgesell (Eds.), *Moss and Adams' heart disease in infants, children, and adolescents* (Vol. 1) (5th Ed.). Baltimore: Williams & Wilkins.

Fricker, F., Griffith, B., Hardesty, R., Trento, A., Gold, L., Schmeltz, K., et al. (1987). Experience with heart transplantation in children. *Pediatrics, 79*, 138–146.

Friedman, W.F. (1995). Aortic stenosis (pp. 1087–1097). In G. Emmanouilides, T. Riemenschneider, H. Allen, & H. Gutgesell (Eds.), *Moss and Adams' heart disease in infants, children, and adolescents* (Vol. 1) (5th Ed.). Baltimore: Williams & Wilkins.

Fyler, D.C. (1992). Trends. In D.C. Fyler (Ed.), *Nadas' pediatric cardiology* (pp. 273–280). Philadelphia: Hanley & Belfus, Inc.

Fyler, D.C. (Ed.) (1992). *Nadas' pediatric cardiology.* Philadelphia: Hanley & Belfus, Inc.

Garson, A., Williams, R.B., & Redford, T. (1974). Long term follow up of patients with tetralogy of fallot: Physical health and psychopathology. *Journal of Pediatrics, 85*, 429–433.

Gersony, W.M. (1987). The cardiovascular system. In R.E. Behrman & V.C.Vaughan (Eds.), *Nelson textbook of pediatrics* (13th Ed.)(pp. 943–1026). Philadelphia: W.B. Saunders Co.

Glauser, T.A., Rorke, L.B., Weinberg, P.M., & Clancy, R.R. (1990). Acquired neuropathological lesions associated with the hypoplastic left heart syndrome. *Pediatrics, 85,* 991–1000.

Glauser, T.A., Rorke, L.B., Weinberg, P.M., & Clancy, R.R. (1990). Congenital brain anomalies associated with the hypoplastic left heart syndrome. *Pediatrics, 85,* 984–990.

Graham, T.P., Bricker, J.T., James, F.W., & Strong, W.B. (1994). 26th Bethesda conference recommendations for determining eligibility for competition in athletes with cardiovascular abnormalities. *Journal of the American College of Cardiology, 24,* 867–873.

Green, M., & Levitt, E. (1962). Constriction of body image in children with congenital heart diseases. *Pediatrics, 29,* 438–443.

Gudermuth, S. (1975). Mothers' reports of early experiences of infants with congenital heart disease. *Maternal Child Nursing Journal, 4,* 155–164.

Gumbiner, C.H., & Takao, A. (1990). Ventricular septal defect. *The Science and Practice of Pediatric Cardiology, 59,* 1002–1022.

Hofkosh, D., Thompson, A.E., Nozza, R.J., Kemp, S.S., Bowen, A., & Feldman, H.M. (1991). Ten years of extracorporeal membrane oxygenation: neurodevelopmental outcome. *Pediatrics, 87,* 549–555.

Hosenpud, J.D., Novick, R.J., Breen, T.J., Keck, B., & Daily, P. (1995). The registry of the International Society for Heart and Lung Transplantation: Twelfth official report-1995. *Journal of Heart and Lung Transplantation, 14,* 805–815.

Hsu, D., Garofano, R., Douglas, J., Michler, R., Quaegebeur, J., Gersony, W., & Addonizio, L. (1993). Exercise performance after pediatric heart transplantation. *Circulation, 88,* 238–242.

Jemerin, J.M., & Boyce, W.T. (1990). Psychobiological differences in childhood stress response. II. Cardiovascular markers of vulnerability. *Journal of Developmental and Behavioral Pediatrics, 11,* 140–150.

Klein, M.D. (1988). Neonatal ECMO. *TransAmerican Society of Artificial Internal Organs, 34,* 39–42.

Klein, M.D., Shaheen, K.W., Whittlesey, G.C., Pinsky, W.W., & Arciniegas, E. (1990). Extracorporeal membrane oxygenation (ECMO) for the circulatory support of children after repair of congenital heart disease. *Journal of Thoracic and Cardiovascular Surgery, 100,* 498–505.

Kramer, H.H., Awiszus, D., Sterzel, U., van Halteren, A., & Clarsen, R. (1989). Development of personality and intelligence in children with congenital heart disease. *Journal of Child Psychology and Psychiatry, 30,* 299–308.

Kriett, K., & Kaye, M.P. (1990). The registry of the International Society of Heart Transplantation: seventh official report. *Journal of Heart and Lung Transplantation, 9,* 323–330.

Lawrence, K., & Fricker, R. (1987). Pediatric heart transplantation: Quality of life. *Journal of Heart Transplantation, 6,* 329–333.

Linde, L.M., Rasof, B., & Dunn, O.J. (1967). Mental development in congenital heart disease. *Journal of Pediatrics, 71,* 198–203.

Linde, L.M., Rasof, B., & Dunn, O.J. (1970). Longitudinal studies of intellectual and behavioral development in children with congenital heart disease. *Acta Paediatrica Scandinavica, 59,* 169–176.

Lobo, M.L. (1992). Parent-infant interaction during feeding when the infant has congenital heart disease. *Journal of Pediatric Nursing, 7,* 97–105.

Lock, J.E., Keane, J.F., Mandell, V.S., & Perry, S.B. (1992). Cardiac catheterization. In D.C. Fyler (Ed.), *Nadas' pediatric cardiology* (pp. 187–224). Philadelphia: Hanley and Belfus, Inc.

Lott, I.T., McPherson, D., Towne, B., Johnson, D., & Starr, A. (1990). Long-term neurophysiologic outcome after neonatal extracorporeal membrane oxygenation. *Pediatrics, 86,* 343–349.

Mai, F.M., McKenzie, F.N., & Kostuk, W.J. (1990). Psychosocial adjustment and quality of life following heart transplantation. *Canadian Journal of Psychiatry, 35,* 223–227.

Marino, B.L., & Lipshitz, M. (1991). Temperament in infants and toddlers with cardiac disease. *Pediatric Nursing, 17,* 445–448.

Martin, A.B., Bricker, J.T., Fishman, M., Frazier, O.H., Price, J.K., Radovancevic, B., Louis, P.T., Cabalka, A.K., Gelb, B.D., & Towbin, J.A. (1992). Neurologic complications of heart transplantation in children. *Journal of Heart and Lung Transplantation, 11,* 933–942.

Meijboom, F., Szatmari, A., Deckers, J., Utens, E., Roelandt, J., Bos, E., & Hess, J. (1995). Cardiac status and health-related quality of life in the long term after surgical repair of Tetralogy of Fallot in infancy and childhood. *Journal of Thoracic and Cardiovascular Surgery, 110*, 883–891.

Mendoza, J.C., Shearer, L.L., & Cook, L.N. (1991). Lateralization of brain lesions following extracorporeal membrane oxygenation. *Pediatrics, 88*, 1004–1009.

Miller, G., Mamourian, A.C., Tesman, J.R., Baylen, B.G., & Myers, J.L. (1994). Long-term MRI changes in brain after pediatric open heart surgery. *Journal of Child Neurology, 9*, 390–397.

Morris, R.D., Krawiecki, N.S., Wright, J.A., & Walter, L.W. (1993). Neuropsychological, academic, and adaptive functioning in children who survive in-hospital cardiac arrest and resuscitation. *Journal of Learning Disabilities, 26*, 46–51.

Newburger, J.W., Jonas, R.A., Wernovsky, G., Wypij, D., Hickey, P.R., Kuban, C.K., Farrell, D.M., Holmes, G.L., Helmers, S.L.,Constantinou, J., Carrazana, E., Barlow, J.K., Walsh, A.Z., Lucius, K.C., Share, J.C., Wessel, D.L., Hanley, F.L., Mayer, J.E., Castaneda, A.R., & Ware, J.H. (1993). A comparison of the perioperative neurologic effects of hypothermic circulatory arrest versus low-flow cardiopulmonary bypass in infant heart surgery. *New England Journal of Medicine, 329*, 1057–1064.

Newburger, J.W., Silbert, A.R., Buckley, L.P., & Fryler, D.C. (1984). Cognitive function and age at repair of transportation of the great arteries in children. *New England Journal of Medicine, 310*, 1495–1499.

Newburger, J.W. (1992). Kawasaki Syndrome. In D.C. Fyler (Ed.), *Nadas' pediatric cardiology* (319–328). Philadelphia: Hanley & Belfus, Inc.

Nixon, P., Fricker, F., Noyas, B., Webber, S., Orenstein, D., & Armitage, J. (1995). Exercise testing in pediatric heart, heart-lung, and lung transplant recipients. *Chest, 107*, 1328–1335.

Oates, R.K., Simpson, J.M., Turnbull, J.A., & Cartmill, T.B. (1995). The relationship between intelligence and duration of circulatory arrest with deep hypothermia. *Journal of Thoracic and Cardiovascular Surgery, 110*, 786–792.

O'Dougherty, M., Berntson, G.G., Boysen, S.T., Wright, F.S., & Teske, D. (1988). Psychophysiological predictors of attentional dysfunction in children with congenital heart defects. *Psychophysiology, 25*, 305–315.

O'Dougherty, M., Wright, F.S., Garmezy, N., Loewenson, R.B., & Torres, F. (1983). Later competence and adaptation in infants who survive severe heart defects. *Child Development, 54*, 1129–1142.

O'Dougherty, M., Wright, F.S., Loewenson, R.B., & Torres, F. (1985). Cerebral dysfunction after chronic hypoxia in children. *Neurology, 35*, 42–46.

Paris, W., Muchmore, J., Pribil, A., Zuhdi, N., & Cooper, D.K.C. (1994). Study of the relative incidences of psychosocial factors before and after heart transplantation and the influence of posttransplantation psychosocial factors on heart transplantation outcome. *Journal of Heart and Lung Transplantation, 13*, 424–432.

Schumacher, R.E., Palmer, T.W., Roloff, D.W., LaClaire, P.A., & Bartlett, R.H. (1991). Follow-up of infants treated with extracorporeal membrane oxygenation for newborn respiratory failure. *Pediatrics, 87*, 451–457.

Short, B.L., Miller, M.K., & Anderson, K.D. (1987). Extracorporeal membrane oxygenation in the management of respiratory failure in the newborn. *Clinics in Perinatology, 14*, 737–749.

Sigfusson, G., Fricker, F., Bernstein, D., Addonizio, L., Baum, D., Hsu, D., Chin, C., Miller, S., Boyle, G., Miller, J., Lawrence, K., Douglas, J., Friffith, B., Reitz, B., Michler, R., Rose, E., & Webber, S. (1997). Long-term survivors of pediatric heart transplantation: A multicenter report of sixty-eight children who have survived longer than five years. *Journal of Pediatrics, 130*, 862–871.

Silbert, A., Wolff, P.H., Mayer, B., Rosenthal, A., & Nadas, A.S. (1969). Cyanotic heart disease and psychological development. *Pediatrics, 43*, 192–200.

Spieth, L., & Harris, C. (1996). Assessment of health-related quality of life in children and adolescents: An integrative review. *Journal of Pediatric Psychology, 21*, 175–194.

Spurkland, I., Bjornstad, P.G., Lindberg, H., & Seem, E. (1993). Mental health and psychosocial functioning in adolescents with congenital heart disease. A comparison between adolescents born with severe heart defect and atrial septal defect. *Acta Paediatrica, 82*, 71–76.

Starnes, V.A., Bernstein, D., Oyer, P.E., Gamberg, P.L., Miller, J.L., Baum, D., & Shunway, N.E. (1989). Heart transplantation in children. *Journal of Heart and Lung Transplantation, 8,* 20–26.

Stewart, S.M., Kennard, B.D., Waller, D.A., & Fixler, D. (1994). Cognitive function in children who receive organ transplantation. *Health Psychology, 13,* 3–13.

Swain, J.A., McDonald, T.J., Griffith, P.K., Balaban, R.S., Clark, R.E., & Ceckler, T. (1991). Low-flow hypothermic cardiopulmonary bypass protects the brain. *Journal of Thoracic and Cardiovascular Surgery, 102,* 76–84.

Taylor, G.A., Glass, P., Fitz, C.R., & Miller, M.K. (1987). Neurologic status in infants treated with extracorporeal membrane oxygenation: correlation of imaging findings with developmental outcome. *Radiology, 165,* 679–682.

Tindall, S., Tothermel, R.R., Delamater, A., Pinsky, W.W., & Klein, M.D. (in press). Neuropsychological abilities of children with cardiac disease treated with extracorporeal membrane oxygenation. *Developmental Neuropsychology,* in press.

Tonstad, S. (1996). Familial hypercholesterolaemia: A pilot study of parents' and children's concerns. *Acta Paediatrica, 85,* 1307–1313.

Trimm, F. (1991). Physiologic and psychological growth and development in pediatric heart transplant recipients. *Journal of Heart and Lung Transplantation, 10,* 848–855.

Utens, E.M., Verhulst, F.C., Erdman, R.A., Meijboom, F.J., Duivenvoorden, H.J., Bos, E., Roelandt, J.R., & Hess, J. (1994). Psychosocial functioning of young adults after surgical correction for congenital heart disease in childhood: A follow-up study. *Journal of Psychosomatic Research, 38,* 745–758.

Uzark, K.C., Sauer, S.N., Lawrence, K.S., Miller, J., Addonizio, L., & Crowley, D.C. (1992). The psychosocial impact of pediatric heart transplantation. *Journal of Heart and Lung Tranplantation, 11,* 1160–1167.

Vick, G.W., & Titus, J.L. (1990). Defects of the atrial septum including the atrioventricular canal. *The Science and Practice of Pediatric Cardiology, 60,* 1025.

Walsh, E.P., & Saul, J.P. (1992). Cardiac arrhythmias. In D.C. Fyler (Ed.), *Nadas' pediatric cardiology* (pp. 377–434). Philadelphia: Hanley & Belfus, Inc.

Wray, J., Pot-Mees, C., Zeitlin, H., Radley-Smith, R., & Yacoub, M. (1994). Cognitive function and behavioral status in paediatric heart and heart-lung transplant recipients: the Harefield experience. *British Medical Journal, 309,* 837–841.

Wray, J., & Yacoub, M. (1991). Psychosocial evaluation of children after open heart surgery versus cardiac transplantation. In M. Yacoub & J.R. Pepper (Eds.) *Annals of Cardiac Surgery, 90–91* (pp. 50–55). London: Current Science Publications.

Wright, M., & Nolan, T. (1994). Impact of cyanotic heart disease on school performance. *Archives of Disease in Childhood, 71,* 64–70.

Yagel, S. et al. (1997). Congenital heart defects: Natural course and in utero development. *Circulation, 96,* 550–555.

Yang, L., Liu, M., & Townes, B. (1994). Neuropsychological and behavioral status of Chinese children with acyanotic congenital heart disease. *International Journal of Neuroscience, 74,* 109–115.

Zuberbuhler, J.R. (1995). Tetralogy of Fallot. In G. Emmanouilides, T. Riemenschneider, H. Allen, & H. Gutgesell (Eds.), *Moss and Adams' heart disease in infants, children, and adolescents* (Vol. 1) (5th Ed.). Baltimore: Williams & Wilkins.

Chapter 12

CYSTIC FIBROSIS

Robert J. Thompson
Lisa Karlish

Cystic fibrosis (CF) is a genetic disease which affects approximately 1 in 2,000 live births, making it the most common, lethal, congenital disease among the Caucasian population (Boat, Welsh, & Beaudet, 1989). The basic defect of CF occurs in the secretory epithelia which controls the exchange of water, salt, and other solutes between the blood and the external environment. As a result of decreased fluid and increased salt production, mucous secretions of the exocrine glands are dehydrated, making them more viscous than normal (Levitan, 1989). This viscous mucus has a deleterious impact on a number of major organ systems, including the respiratory, digestive, and reproductive systems.

The primary impact of CF is on the lungs and pancreas. Mucous accumulation in the bronchi and bronchioles leads to airway obstruction. In addition, CF patients are susceptible to bacterial infection in the lungs which results in gradual deterioration of pulmonary functioning. It is estimated that chronic respiratory disease causes 90–95% of the morbidity and mortality in patients with CF (Wood, Boat, & Doershuk, 1976).

Pancreatic involvement is estimated to occur in 85% of patients with CF. Pancreatic ducts become blocked, preventing proper secretion of gastric enzymes. This gastric enzyme deficiency results in poor digestion of food, foul-smelling, bulky stools, and poor absorption of undigested nutrients, particularly fats (Matthews & Drotar, 1994). Because of these digestive complications, many CF patients are severely malnourished causing them to be underweight and of small stature. Damage to the pancreas also causes insulin-dependent diabetes mellitus in 4–10% of patients with CF (Fitzsimmons, 1993; Lewiston, 1985).

Because CF patients are now living beyond their teens, into adulthood, the impact of CF on reproductive functioning has become an increasing concern. Males with CF are typically sterile due to obstruction of the epididymis, vas deferens, and seminal vesicles. Females with CF also have impaired fertility due to thick cervical mucus and obstruction of the cervical canal (Koch & Lanng, 1995). Although successful pregnancies have been achieved in women with CF, pregnancy can complicate their health status (Stark, Jelalian, & Miller, 1995).

There currently is no cure for CF and it is ultimately a fatal disease. Consequently, the focus of treatment has been on maximizing life span by preventing pulmonary disease and malnutrition. Advances in treatments have significantly lengthened the life expectancy of individuals with CF. The median age of survival has increased from 10.4 years in 1966 (Orenstein & Wachnowsky, 1985) to 30 years in 1996 (Wilson & Wilson, 1996). However, because of the complexity, involvement, and invasiveness of the typical CF treatment regimen, it can often be as much of a burden to CF patients and their families as the disease itself.

In order to delay lung deterioration, CF patients must undergo extensive pulmonary treatments which serve to reduce bronchiole obstruction and control infections (Orenstein & Wachnowsky, 1985). One such treatment is chest physical therapy (CPT) which involves techniques such as postural draining, manual or mechanical percussion, and directed coughing to loosen the sputum and facilitate its expulsion (Turpin & Knowles, 1993). Typical chest therapy regimens take approximately 20–30 minutes per session, with one to four sessions being prescribed per day (Orenstein & Wachnowsky, 1985). Antibiotic regimens are also central to the preservation of lung functioning through the control of infections. Oral antibiotics are prescribed when there is evidence of increased symptoms. In cases of more severe exacerbations, antibiotics are administered intravenously, typically during a 10–12 day hospital stay (Orenstein & Wachnowsky, 1985).

Gastrointestinal therapy is also an essential component of CF patients' treatment regimen. The goal of this therapy is to maintain proper nutrition to maximize weight gain and growth while minimizing gastrointestinal discomfort. Although in the past, high calorie, low fat diets were typically prescribed, it is now known that with pancreatic enzyme replacement even high fat diets can be tolerated (Orenstein & Wachnowsky, 1985). Thus, physicians now recommend at least normal diets, and in some cases high fat diets, in conjunction with 4 to 10 capsules of replacement enzyme per meal (Koocher, Gudas, & McGrath, 1992; Orenstein & Wachnowsky, 1985). Supplements of vitamins A, D, E, and K are also typically prescribed resulting in a medication regimen that often exceeds 40 pills per day (Orenstein & Wachnowsky, 1985). In addition, invasive nutritional interventions, such as feedings through nasogastric tubes, central intravenous hyperalimentation, and gastronomy tubes, are sometimes necessary to combat malnutrition.

In terms of quality of life, the broad range of manifestations, the progressive course, the daily, lifelong, and intrusive treatment regime, and the ultimate fatality that constitutes CF presents substantial challenges to the child and his or her family. Furthermore, because advances in health care have led to a lengthening of life expectancies for children with CF, the child and their family are confronting the stresses and tasks associated with CF for substantially greater periods of time. As a result, efforts have moved beyond solely increasing the quantity of life of patients with CF, and now include a focus on enhancing adaptation, that is, the process of accommodation that occurs between the developing child and his or her environment as reflected in both duration and quality of life (Thompson & Gustafson, 1996).

Despite this shift of focus to the process of adaptation, the construct of "quality of life" (QL) has not yet been applied to the CF population in an integrative fashion. Rather, assessments of quality of life in patients with CF have typically been limited to one specific domain as opposed to evaluating the patients overall quality of life. This approach has its limitations because not only may quality of life differ across domains, but each domain may carry differential importance based on individual characteristics or other surrounding circumstances (Croog, 1990; Osoba, 1994). Furthermore, clinical research has addressed only a few specific domains: the child's psychological adjustment and social functioning, and the family's overall adjustment. Thus, for the purposes of this chapter, the functional impact of the manifestations of CF and its treatment will be discussed in relation to these three domains.

The purpose of this chapter is to review the existing literature pertaining to quality of life issues in patients with CF, and make suggestions for future directions regarding assessment and intervention in QL. To achieve this goal, we will first discuss the impact of the symptoms of CF and its treatment on the QL domains of psychological, social, and family adjustment. Then, the assessment measures commonly used in evaluating QL in patients with CF will be presented, with a discussion of areas of improvement to follow. Finally, programs designed to improve QL in patients with CF will be discussed, and other potential intervention targets will be suggested.

IMPLICATIONS OF CYSTIC FIBROSIS FOR QUALITY OF LIFE
PSYCHOLOGICAL IMPACT

Both the manifestations of CF and its treatment present the child with a number of stressors which could be detrimental to their QL in the psychological domain. Children with CF must cope with multiple physical abnormalities such as short stature, below average weight, barrel chest, and finger and toe clubbing which differentiates them from healthy peers (Koocher, Gudas, & McGrath, 1990). Both the physical toll of CF and the tremendous time required for treatment regimens such as chest physical therapy have the potential to severely limit the CF patient's ability to engage in normal, everyday childhood activities. Additionally, because many of the chest physical therapy procedures are not self-administered, the independence of patients with CF is compromised, which can be a particularly salient issue during adolescence.

Given these stressors that patients with CF must confront, it seems reasonable to expect that children with CF would have poor psychological adjustment (e.g., lower self-esteem, higher incidence of behavior/emotional problems and psychiatric diagnoses) than healthy peers. Indeed, early studies reported a relatively high frequency of psychological problems in children with CF (e.g., Gayton & Friedman, 1973). However, later studies have not found as high rates of adjustment problems (e.g., Drotar, et al., 1981) which may be largely attributable to the use of multiple informants and empirical measures in the assessment of children's psychological adjustment (Thompson, Merritt, Keith, Murphy, & Johndrow, 1993).

Our research program has conducted a series of studies to assess the frequency and types of disruptions children with CF experience in their psychological QL as reported by themselves and their mothers. In the initial study, children's self-report was used to compare the psychological adjustment of children with CF to the adjustment of psychiatrically referred and non-referred children (Thompson, Hodges, & Hamlett, 1990). The criteria for a major DSM-III (American Psychiatric Association, 1980) diagnosis were met by 77% of the psychiatrically referred children, 58% of the children with CF, and 23% of the non-referred controls. The children with CF were similar to the psychiatrically referred children on the content domains of worry and self-image and on symptoms associated with separation anxiety and over-anxious disorder. Children with CF did not, in general, demonstrate more symptoms of behavioral disturbances such as attention deficit disorder, conduct disorder, oppositional behavior disorders than healthy children. Nor did they differ from healthy peers in the domains of school, friends, family, mood, somatic concerns, anger, depression, and thought disorders. These findings suggest that children with CF are primarily at risk for internalizing, as opposed to externalizing, behavior problems. Furthermore, the internalizing difficulties identified in this study were primarily anxiety based. Although conduct-related externalizing problems were rare (12%), oppositional behavior as reflected by disobedience, provocativeness, and stubbornness occurred relatively frequently (23%). This suggests that when children with CF do act out, it is likely to be reflected in oppositional disorder rather than severe conduct disorder (Thompson, et al., 1990).

Subsequent studies have demonstrated relative consistency regarding both the frequency and types of behavioral and emotional problems demonstrated by children with CF. In a study comparing mother and child report of the psychological adjustment of children with CF, 60% of children met criteria for a behavior problem based on their mother's report and 62% qualified for a DSM-III diagnosis based on self-report (Thompson, Gustafson, Hamlett, & Spock, 1992a). Similarly, in a study of adolescent patients with CF, 51% had a DSM-III diagnosis as per their own report (Thompson, Gustafson, & Gil, 1995). In both studies, diagnoses of anxiety and oppositional behavior disorders were most frequent.

Interestingly, although the overall rates of psychological adjustment problems in children with CF remain stable when assessed long-itudinally, there is considerable variability at the level of the individual as to who is demonstrating behavioral or emotional problems at any given time. In a study assessing psychological adjustment over two time points spanning 12 months, good adjustment was demonstrated by 24% of the children and poor adjustment by 49% across both time points while 27% of the children changed classifications (Thompson, Gustafson, George, & Spock, 1994). In a subsequent longitudinal study assessing adjustment over three time points spanning 2 years, only 31% of children demonstrated the same adjustment classification over the three time points (19% exhibiting consistently good adjustment and 12% demonstrating consistently poor adjustment). Of the remaining children, 44% changed classifications one time and 25% changed classifications both times (Thompson, Gustafson, Gil, Kinney, & Spock, 1999). These findings suggest that there are likely other factors that mediate the relationship between CF and psychological QL. It is important that work be done to identify these mediating factors because they may serve as salient QL intervention targets.

SOCIAL IMPACT

Just as aspects of CF and its treatment may interfere with a child's QL in the psychological domain, these stressors may also negatively affect a child's social QL. As previously mentioned, CF has several physical manifestations such as short stature, below average weight, barrel chest, and finger and toe clubbing. These physical abnormalities may stand as a barrier to the acceptance of the child with CF into the peer world. Excessive coughing and gastrointestinal symptoms, such as flatulence, likely cause the child significant social embarrassment. Furthermore, limitations on their activity level and frequent hospitalizations can prevent the child having adequate access to social opportunities.

Unfortunately, there has not yet been much empirical investigation regarding the peer relations of children with CF. It does appear that children with CF do have concerns about their social functioning. For example, when adolescents were asked to identify problems related to their CF which concern them, many of the problems they identified were social in nature. Girls tended to indicate problems in social relationships such as friends and romantic relationships, while boys described concerns about gaining weight presumably because of the social connotations physical size has for males (Stark, Jelalian, & Miller, 1996). However, it is unknown as to whether these concerns are greater than that of the typical, healthy adolescent. Furthermore, there has been no examination of the peer status of children with CF as evaluated by their healthy peers. Such work is sorely needed.

FAMILY IMPACT

Not only does CF influence the quality of life of the individual child, but it also has repercussions for the QL of the entire family system. The parents' time is likely to be consumed with administering treatment procedures and helping their child with managing their CF symptoms. The time and effort these tasks require can be an inordinate strain on the primary care giver and may also interfere with other family relationships. Finances are also likely to be a stressor as the average yearly cost in health care for CF patients is nearly $40,000, with this figure rising sharply in the end stages of the disease (Cystic Fibrosis Foundation, 1995). Parents must also prepare themselves and their child for the eventual fatality of the child's disease. Indeed, a recent review indicated that the most commonly cited concerns by parents of children with CF included the difficulty of the treatment regimen, the terminal nature of CF, disruptions in intrafamilial relationships, financial difficulties, and lack of information about the disease provided by health care providers (Ievers & Drotar, 1996).

As would be expected, the stresses that CF presents for family members have been found to negatively affect their own QL. Comparative studies indicate that parents of children with CF experience higher levels of general and illness-specific stress than parents of physically healthy children (Ievers & Drotar, 1996). Mothers of children with CF exhibit elevated levels of psychological distress, parenting stress, family role strain, and depression (Ievers & Drotar, 1996; Quittner, DiGirolomo, Michel, & Eigen, 1992; Thompson, Gustafson, Hamlett, & Spock, 1992b). For example, in a study of mothers of children with CF ages 7–17, 34% of mothers met case criteria for poor adjustment (as evidenced by a Global Severity Index or two of the nine symptom dimensions on the SCL-90-R falling above the 90th percentile) (Thompson, et al., 1992b). Furthermore, there is evidence that CF differentially influences the family based on the interactions among characteristics of the illness, child, and family. This suggests a need to consider family QL in relation to specific dimensions of childhood illness, including illness phase, developmental stage of the child and family, and concomitant alterations in family roles (Quittner, et al., 1992).

Although the impact of CF on the QL of the family system is of concern in and of itself, it becomes particularly important when considering the subsequent effects of family functioning on other aspects of the child's QL. Family functioning and maternal adjustment have been found to be significantly associated with child QL domains such as psychological adjustment and even health status. In a study examining the relationship between family functioning and health indices, family functioning variables such as family stress, family resources, and parental coping were found to account for significant portions of the variance in changes in both pulmonary functioning and height and weight (Patterson, McCubbin, & Warwick, 1990). Family members' psychological adjustment also accounts for changes in the behavioral adjustment of children with CF. Thompson et al. (1992b) found that when assessed longitudinally, decreases in maternal anxiety accounted for significant improvements in both internalizing and externalizing symptoms in their children. Similarly, the impact of CF on the family was shown to be associated with behavioral and emotional symptomatology in CF children while no such relationship was found between symptomatology and illness severity. Thus, good family functioning may buffer the child from the impact of CF, while poor family functioning may amplify the effects of illness-related stress (Pumariega,

Pearson, & Seiheimer, 1993). Taken together, these findings suggest that intervening at the level of the family may have multiple benefits for the QL of both the family and the child.

QUALITY OF LIFE MEASUREMENT FOR CYSTIC FIBROSIS

As previously indicated, an integrative definition of QL has not yet been applied to the CF population. Rather, the QL of CF patients has largely been examined in a domain specific way, for example, as psychological adjustment or social functioning. As such, there have been few traditionally defined QL measures either developed for or applied to this population. Instead, the measures typically used are those most applicable to the domain of interest and are often not specific to a pediatric population. Although this has been a useful starting point, there is significant room for the development of measures that are more directly related to QL issues within the CF population. We will consider measures of disease, psychological, and family impact.

MEASUREMENT OF DISEASE IMPACT

Schwachman rating system

The most frequently used assessment tool for evaluating QL in terms of disease status has been the Schwachman rating system (Schwachman & Kulczycki, 1958). With the Schwachman rating system, the clinician assesses child functioning in four areas: activity, pulmonary physical findings and cough, growth and nutrition, and chest X-ray film findings. Total scores range from 20 to 100 with higher scores indicating better functioning and lesser severity. Based on their total score, patients are classified as: poor (<55), mild (55–70); good (71–85); and very good (86–100).

Despite the widespread use of this scoring system, concerns about its limitations have been raised. Although this scale has been shown to be predictive of longevity and pulmonary functioning, they are slow to capture the results of short-term medical interventions (Eigen, et al., 1987). It has been advocated that a measurement of integrated function that would permit the assessment of several organ systems at one time should be developed (Eigen, et al., 1987).

Quality of well-being scale

One health status measure which has attempted to address these limitations of the Schwachman rating system is the Quality of Well-being scale (QWB, Kaplan & Anderson, 1988). The QWB was developed as a general health status measurement, has been validated in the general population, and has been applied to several disease populations, including CF (see Chapter 4 for a more detailed description). This scale consists of a fifteen minute interview in which a trained interviewer asks the child and/or parent questions about the child's level of functioning in three domains: mobility, physical activity, and social activity. In addition to evaluating functioning, patients are classified as having any of 22 symptoms which might impair functioning. Using a preferential weighting system, the combination of functioning and symptoms are placed on a continuum ranging from 0.0 (dead) to 1.0 (optimal functioning).

This scale has been shown to have utility in rating the health status of CF patients. The QWB is significantly associated with traditional measures of pulmonary functioning yet is also sensitive to other problems associated with the disease and its treatment (Orenstein, Nixon, Ross, & Kaplan, 1989). Additionally, the QWB has been shown to be able to track changes in the general well-being of CF patients over time and to detect changes associated with pulmonary exacerbation and its treatment (Orenstein, Pattishall, Nixon, Ross, & Kaplan, 1990). However, this scale is more difficult to use than scales such as the Schwachman and requires more extensive training for administration.

MEASUREMENT OF PSYCHOLOGICAL IMPACT

The QL of children with CF in the psychological domain has been conceptualized in numerous ways including self-esteem, specific symptoms (e.g., anxiety, depression), behavioral and emotional problem syndromes (e.g., internalizing or externalizing disorders) and psychiatric diagnoses (e.g., overanxious disorder). Methods for assessing children's adjustment include checklists, questionnaires, and diagnostic clinical interviews completed by children or their parents.

It must be noted that evidence has converged to indicate that comprehensive assessment of psychological adjustment of children requires multiple informants and measures (Edelbrock, Costello, Dulcan, Conover, & Kalas, 1986). Indeed, several specific factors have been identified as influencing the degree of concordance between parent and child assessment of children's adjustment. One such factor is child age, with parent–child agreement being higher for adolescents than for children (Edelbrock, et al., 1986). The type of behavioral problems exhibited by the child is another factor that affects concordance. In general, agreement is higher for externalizing symptoms than for internalizing symptoms (Hodges, Gordon, & Lennon, 1990). The impact of parental distress on their perceptions of child adjustment has also been identified as a contributing factor to low agreement between parent and child report (Webster-Straton, 1990). Because CF children and their parents typically demonstrate the types of adjustment problems that are likely to make concordance rates low, we have found it essential to gather both parent and child reports regarding children's psychological adjustment. Specifically, we have found two instruments to have considerable clinical utility in assessing CF children's psychological QL: the Missouri Child Behavior Checklist (MCBC), which is a parent completed measure, and the Child Assessment Schedule (CAS), which is completed by the child.

Missouri Child Behavior Checklist

The Missouri Child Behavior Checklist (MCBC; Sines, Pauker, Sines, & Owen, 1969) is a parent-completed measure which consists of 77 items. On this instrument, parents indicate (yes–no) as to whether their child has demonstrated the behavior described in the last 6–12 months. The MCBC yields scores across seven domains: aggression, activity level, sleep disturbance, inhibition, somatic complaints, depression, inhibition, and sociability. Factor analysis of a large sample of children with developmental delays, chronic illnesses, and psychiatric problems has previously demonstrated that from these scales, three factors emerge: Externalizing, Internalizing, and Sociable (Thompson, Kronenberger, & Curry, 1989). Furthermore, hierarchical cluster analysis of these three factor scores has identified seven behavior pattern profiles in which children can be classified. Four of these profiles are problem patterns (i.e., Internal, External, Mixed Internal and External, and Undifferentiated Disturbance profiles) and three profiles are problem-free patterns (i.e., Low Social Skills, Problem Free, and Sociable profiles) (Thompson et al., 1989).

Although the MCBC is useful in identifying behavioral and emotional adjustment problems in children with CF, it is not specifically tailored towards addressing the psychological issues raised by the challenges of the disease. Thus, while this measure certainly assesses general psychological adjustment, it is impossible to determine whether problems in adjustment are related to their health condition or other factors. Also, the use of physical symptomatology as an indicator of internalizing problems (i.e., somatization scale) may be problematic with children with CF because of their presentation of numerous, biologically based health problems.

Child Assessment Schedule

The Child Assessment Schedule (CAS; Hodges, Kline, Stern, Cytryn, & McKnew, 1982) is a semi-structured interview for latency aged and adolescent children. Questions are organized around 11 topics including school, friends, activities/hobbies, family, fears, worries/anxieties, self-image, mood, physical complaints, expression of anger, and reality testing. Many of the questions are designed to be open-ended, thus, this instrument can yield very rich data. In addition, the CAS yields information about the presence, onset, and duration of psychiatric symptomatology which allows for a diagnosis based on DSM-III-R criteria.

Similar to the MCBC, the problem with using the CAS as a psychological QL measure for CF is the lack of specificity of the measure to the parameters of the disease. However, the CAS is not quite as limited as the MCBC in this regard due to its open-ended format.

MEASUREMENT OF FAMILY IMPACT

Family Environment Scale

The Family Environment Scale (Moos, 1974) is a 90-item, true–false measure that is typically completed by parents. It yields ten subscales across three dimensions. The relationship dimension assesses interpersonal relationships within the family and is comprised of the cohesion, expressiveness, and conflict subscales. The personal growth dimension assesses the family's goal orientation and is comprised of the independence, achievement orientation, intellectual-cultural orientation, active recreational orientation, and moral-religious emphasis. The system maintenance dimension assesses the structure of the family and is comprised of two subscales, organization and control. A family relationship index is derived from a composite of the cohesion, expressiveness, and conflict scales. A more recent factor analysis has yielded 3 factors: Supportive, Conflicted, and Controlling.

This measure is well validated and has been shown to have good psychometric properties. However, as with the measures discussed assessing psychological QL, this measure has not been tailored towards a CF or even a chronic illness population. Thus, while it does provide a tool by which the family functioning of children with CF can be compared to the family functioning of healthy children or other chronically ill populations, it does not give information about how the characteristics of the disease and its treatment affect the QL of the family.

Impact of Illness on the Family Scale

The Impact of Illness on the Family Scale (Stein & Reissman, 1980), is a 29-item scale which assesses the degree of burden and stress experienced by the family of a chronically ill child. From this scale, a total score and four subscales are derived, including financial functioning, social and family functioning, personal strain, and general mastery. Higher total Impact of Illness on Family scores have been associated with a mother's perception that her child is difficult to care for, poor functioning and psychological adjustment on the part of the child, increased number of hospitalizations, the mother's report that the illness has affected her life, and increased psychiatric symptoms on the part of the child (Stein & Jessop, 1985).

Cystic Fibrosis Role Strain Index

The Cystic Fibrosis Role Strain Index (Quittner et al., 1992), was designed to assess the impact that caring for a child with CF has upon parental roles. The scale consists of a brief structured interview and 14 true/false items, and was developed from the Questionnaire on Resources and Stress (Holroyd, 1974). Items from the scale assess the respondents responsibility for treatment, the availability of spouse, assistance with caretaking, and extent to which they perceived their time to be limited by caretaking demands. Although this measure has not been subject to rigorous psychometric validation, the authors report an internal consistency of .72. Furthermore, this measure was shown to be significantly correlated with mothers' reports of depression (Quittner, et al., 1992).

FUTURE DIRECTIONS FOR MEASURES OF QUALITY OF LIFE

What emerges from this review of QL assessment measures for the CF population is the lack of specificity of the measures used regarding the stresses and challenges inherent to the disease and its treatment. Within the CF population, QL has been approached in a domain specific way, therefore there are no measures designed to assess the patient's general QL across domains. Even within domains, the measures typically used assess general functioning within that particular area, but do not address functioning relative to the impact of the disease. Thus, it appears that developing measures with greater specificity to the illness demands of CF is the next step in QL assessment. Additionally, it would be useful to develop a method for assessing the overall QL of CF patients across domains while still preserving the rich data yielded by a multidimensional approach to QL.

Along with greater measurement specificity, several other measurement issues need to be taken into account in developing future QL measures for CF. For one, the way in which the child's developmental level interacts with illness demands must be taken into consideration. Children with CF must cope with their illness throughout their lifespan. The changing developmental tasks with which they are faced are likely to make different aspects of an illness salient at different points of the child's life. For example, the impact of CF on children's social activities and peer relationships is not likely to affect the child's overall QL until the child is at the stage in which peers take central importance. Likewise, the limitations the treatment of CF places on a child's autonomy from their parents is likely to have greater significance during adolescence, when a child is expected to be establishing independence.

Secondly, QL measurements for CF should be sensitive to the phases and course of the disease. Although CF is a chronic disease, it is also characterized by periods of exacerbations as well as progressive deterioration. Shifts in disease phase are likely to influence those aspects of quality of life most salient to the individual as well as their perceptions of their own QL. Additionally, these phases of illness interact with the child's stage of development to create unique patterns of what might be considered good and poor QL. In support of this, Rolland (1993) has postulated a model in which QL is a function of a three-way "goodness of fit" among family life phase, illness phase, and family functioning style.

Thus, the measurement issues relevant to quality of life in CF track the evolution of the construct of QL with both general aspects that cut across chronic illnesses and variations specific to CF. The multi-dimensionality and dynamic interrelationship among dimensions as a function of individual development, family life course, and phases of illness are particularly salient aspects of quality of life for those confronting CF. Correspondingly, QL measurement for CF needs to become more differentiated and tailored in an effort to reflect these interactions among disease phase, family life phase, and developmental levels.

PROGRAMS TO IMPROVE QUALITY OF LIFE
IMPROVING HEALTH CARE AND HEALTH STATUS

For the most part, research has not yet moved to the level of controlled intervention studies aimed at improving the QL of children with CF and their families. The work that has been done has been focused on improving QL through decreasing the burdens of treatment and enhancing patients' health status.

Heart-lung transplantation is increasingly being used in the management of end-stage lung disease. Stark, Jelalilan, and Miller (1995) summarize a number of studies indicating that patients with CF who survive lung transplantation experience improved pulmonary functioning, increased weight, increased exercise capacity, and improved quality of life in terms of mental status, fewer hospitalizations, and return to age appropriate activities. Survival rates for patients with CF who have had lung transplants are estimated at 67% for one year and 64% at three years (Whitehead, et al., 1995), with organ rejection and infection being the primary complications of transplantation (Sheppard, 1995).

Advancements have also been made in the development of techniques and alternate procedures that allow the patient to receive the benefits of typical treatments while minimizing some of the burden. Mechanical percussion vests and individually administered techniques such as positive expiratory pressure have allowed patients with CF to maintain the benefits of chest physical therapy (CPT) with less sacrifice of their independence (Ramsey & Marshall, 1995; Turpin & Knowles, 1993). Exercise regimens are increasingly advocated as an adjunctive and/or alternative method to CPT to loosen mucus and clear obstructions from the lungs (Orenstein, Henke, & Cherny, 1983). For many adolescent and adult CF patients, daily exercise may be preferred over conventional CPT because it does not require parental involvement and appears to others to be in service of overall health rather than disease management (Turpin & Knowles, 1993). Patients are also being taught to administer antibiotics intravenously at home, which reduces their number of hospital stays (Aalderen, et al., 1995). Such home treatments have been shown to be overwhelmingly preferred by patients with CF as it allows them to remain in their own home and causes minimal disruption to family life (Bramwell, et al., 1995). Furthermore, home care has been shown to be significantly less expensive than hospital care (Bramwell, et al., 1995). Additional empirical investigation is necessary to determine the specific benefits these treatment alternatives have on the QL of CF patients.

Other more formal intervention programs have been developed to more directly enhance QL by targeting the health status of CF patients. In a series of studies, Stark and colleagues have demonstrated the effectiveness of parent training intervention regarding behavioral child management strategies to motivate children to consume adequate calories (Stark et al., 1990, 1993, 1994, 1996). Critical family behavior during mealtimes, such as high rates of parental coaxing and ineffective parental commands, were associated with poorer consumption. Parents were taught to use differential attention and contingent privileges, to set realistic behavior expectations at mealtimes, and to introduce non-preferred foods. Interventions led to more effective parental attention to appropriate eating behaviors, less attention to disruptive behavior, and more caloric intake.

Another intervention program designed to enhance QL through improving health status was a three-month supervised running program targeting exercise conditioning and cardiopulmonary fitness (Orenstein et al., 1981). The conditioning program consisted of three meetings each week that had four phases: warm-up, jog-walk, cool down, and "fun". In comparison to the non-exercise group, the exercise group had significantly improved exercise tolerance and peak oxygen consumption, significantly lower heart rates for submaximal work, and increased respiratory muscle endurance.

IMPROVING BEHAVIORAL CORRELATES OF QUALITY OF LIFE

Although research regarding other domains of QL (e.g., psychological, social, family functioning) has not progressed to the intervention trial stage, conceptual models have delineated correlates of QL domains which provides an empirical basis for efforts to enhance the QL of CF patients. More specifically, this research delineates three interrelated intervention targets: compliance, maternal adjustment, and child and adolescent adjustment.

The importance of adherence to the goal of improving quality of life is well recognized. "If health compliance behaviors can be promoted and maintained, the likelihood of a child living a more normal life, in spite of chronic illness, is greatly increased" (Krasnegor, 1993, p. 357). There is considerable evidence for the effectiveness of behavioral strategies in improving adherence (Epstein & Cluss, 1982). In addition, the change to a more family centered approach to treatment and corresponding tailoring of a consensual medical regime affords the opportunity to improve adherence by developing treatment plans that are consistent with family life priorities and social stresses. For example, analysis of 1,200 critical incidents elicited from 223 patients with CF and their families led to a description of three basic typologies of non-adherence: inadequate knowledge, psychosocial resistance, and educated non-adherence (Koocher, McGrath, & Gudas, 1990). This typology can be helpful in targeting intervention efforts to the specific needs of each patient and family. In a related study, perceived compliance was related to age, socioeconomic level, regimen component, and levels of optimism and child knowledge of the disease (Gudas, Koocher, & Wypij, 1991). Also necessary to fostering adherence are efforts to determine the efficacy and specific benefits of the various disease symptoms components of treatment.

In terms of improving the QL of the family system, particularly mothers, the transactional stress and coping model (Thompson & Gustafson, 1996) indicates that efforts should be directed at decreasing maternal perceptions of daily stress, increasing use of adaptive as opposed to palliative coping methods, and increasing family supportiveness. Such an intervention would not only serve to improve mothers adjustment, but would also positively impact the psychological QL of the child as it has been shown that there is a reciprocal relationship between maternal and child adjustment. Other programs have been developed to increase family support and positive family interactions around the management of chronic illness such as the multifamily group intervention for children with diabetes (Satin, La Greca, Zigo, & Skyler, 1989).

In terms of the social/psychological QL of the child, improving perceptions of self-worth and increasing peer support are salient intervention targets. In particular, there is support from studies of other child chronic illnesses, that perceived social support from classmates is a significant predictor of depressive symptomatology and self-esteem (Varni, Rubenfeld, Talbot, & Setoguchi, 1989a, 1989b). In turn, a number of effective social skills training programs have been developed (Varni, Katz, Colegrove, & Dolgin, 1993) and can be modified for the specific characteristics of CF.

FUTURE DIRECTIONS

In 1989, the CF gene was identified which raised the hope of discovering a cure (Levitan, 1989). Since then, an additional 150 mutations have been identified but a cure has remained elusive. Consequently, as with other chronic childhood illnesses, research and clinical care must continue to address the challenges of increasing life expectancy while intensifying the focus on enhancing QL. The dual goals of extending the duration of life and improving QL requires a biopsychosocial approach because of the interrelationship of biological, psychosocial, and developmental processes on child and family functioning. Stated another way, biological and psychosocial processes are mediators of the health outcomes of life expectancy and QL. The goals of care within a biopsychosocial framework for chronic childhood illness have been clearly articulated and are applicable to CF:

> To confine the consequences of the biologic disorder to its minimum manifestation, to encourage normal growth and development, to assist the child in maximizing potential in all possible areas, and to prevent or diminish the behavioral and social consequences (Stein & Jessop, 1984, pp. 193–194).

Consistent with employing a biopsychosocial approach, additional effort needs to be directed toward enhancing adaptation of children and their families to the stresses and tasks associated with CF. Adaptation is a continuous process of accommodation to internal and external, biological and social-ecological, and developmental and detrimental changes. This focus on the positive process of adaptation will require that researchers and health care providers further commit to family-centered health care that is designed to foster empowerment of families. The goal is to enable, that is, proactively create opportunities for children and their families, to acquire competencies to become better able to solve problems, meet their needs, and achieve their aspirations (Dunst, Trivette, Davis, & Cornwell, 1988). Some of the research on correlates of adjustment, for example, stress processing, support eliciting social skills, and effective parenting, fits nicely within the competency and skill development approach.

We have argued that adaptation to chronic illness can be fostered by minimizing the impact of the illness on normal developmental processes and family functioning (Thompson & Gustafson, 1996). Maintaining as normal a life as possible, in spite of chronic illness, allows the child to remain involved with peers and engaged in developmental tasks which preserves opportunities for skill acquisition and self-esteem. Similar benefits of normalization apply to family members as well.

One of the most important goals for the next phase of research is to link the efforts of symptom management/disease control to normalization through functional status. Functional status is one of the domains of QL recognized by the World Health Organization and refers to the individual's ability to engage in developmentally appropriate activity, work roles, and leisure activity (Spieth & Harris, 1996). In children, functional status has been shown to be more strongly related to other nonmedical aspects of QL than has disease severity (Stein & Jessop, 1984; Wallander, Varni, Babani, Barris, De Haan, & Wilcox,

1989). To achieve this linkage, research needs to focus on delineating developmentally sensitive indicators of normalization, around which degrees of deviation can be measured. It will be essential that such measures of normalization based functional status include both objective and subjective parameters.

It is also essential that the effectiveness of commonly used treatments, as well as new interventions, be scientifically established. There are two needs. First, since "few physiological markers for the disease have been correlated with longevity or can be used to indicate successful management, either short-term or long-term" (Eigin, Clark & Wolle, 1987, p. 1501), physiological measures that are clinically relevant to the natural course of the disease must be developed. Second, given the impact on the child and family, the individual and comparative effectiveness of therapies must be established. For example, the scientific basis for even the most common therapies has not yet been established. The optimal number of chest physical therapy treatments over what period of time has not been empirically determined (Stark, Jelalian, & Miller, 1995). Similarly, a specific efficacious antibiotic treatment regimen has not been empirically established (Eigen, Clark & Wolle, 1987).

Once treatment effectiveness has been empirically established for various regimen components and objective and subjective measures of normalization-based functional status have been derived, research on adherence and adaptation can proceed on a much firmer basis. The foci of enhancing adaptation and adherence are the acquisition of specific knowledge and skills to manage tasks in ways that are tailored to the specific needs, aspirations, and life situations of the child and family. To enhance QL, the child, family and care providers must be informed about what activities and skills will make a difference.

References

van Aalderen, W.M.C., Mannes, G.P.M, Bosma, E.S., Roorda, R.J., & Heymans, H.S.A. (1995). Home care in cystic fibrosis patients. *European Respiratory Journal, 8,* 172–175.

Boat, T.F., Welsh, M.J., & Beaudet, A.L. (1989). Cystic Fibrosis. In C.L. Scriver, A.L. Beaudet, W.S. Sly, & D. Valle (Eds.), *The metabolic bases of inherited disease* (pp. 2469–2680). New York: McGraw-Hill.

Bramwell, E.C., Halpin, D.M.G., Duncan-Skingle, F., Hodson, M.E., & Geddes, D.M. (1995). Home treatment of patients with cystic fibrosis using the 'Intermate': The first year's experience. *Journal of Advanced Nursing, 22,* 1063–1067.

Croog, S.H. (1990). Current issues in conceptualizing and measuring QOL. *Proceedings of NIH Workshop, Quality of Life Assessment: Practice, Problems, and Promise* (pp. 11–20). Bethesda, MD, NIH.

Cystic Fibrosis Foundation (1995). *Homeline.* Bethesda, MD: Cystic Fibrosis Services, Inc.

Drotar, D., Doershuk, C.F., Stern, R.C., Boat, T.F., Boyer, W., & Matthews, L. (1981). Psychosocial functioning of children with cystic fibrosis. *Pediatrics, 67,* 338–343.

Dunst, C.J., Trivette, C.M., Davis, M., & Cornwell, J. (1988). Enabling and empowering families of children with health impairments. *Children's Health Care, 17,* 71–81.

Edelbrock, C., Costello, A.J., Dulcan, M.K., Conover, N.C., & Kalas, K. (1986). Parent-child agreement on child psychiatric symptoms assessed via structured interview. *Journal of Child Psychology and Psychiatry, 27,* 181–190.

Eigen, H., Clark, N.M., & Wolle, J.M. (1987). Clinical-behavioral aspects of cystic fibrosis: Directions for future research. *American Review of Respiratory Diseases, 136,* 1509–1513.

Epstein, L.H., & Cluss, P.A. (1982). A behavioral medicine perspective on adherence to long-term medical regimens. *Journal of Consulting and Clinical Psychology, 59,* 950–971.

FitzSimmons, S.C. (1993). The changing epidemiology of cystic fibrosis. *Journal of Clinical Psychology, 48,* 99–103.

Gayton, W.F., & Friedman, S.B. (1973). Psychosocial aspects of cystic fibrosis. *American Journal of Disabled Children, 126,* 859.

Gudas, L.J., Koocher, G.P., & Wypij, D. (1991). Perceptions of medical compliance in children and adolescents with cystic fibrosis. *Journal of Developmental and Behavioral Pediatrics, 12,* 236–242.

Hodges, K., Gordon, Y., & Lennon, M.P. (1990). Parent-child agreement on symptoms assessed via a clinical research interview for children: The Child Assessment Schedule (CAS). *Journal of Child Psychology and Psychiatry, 31,* 427–436.

Hodges, K., Kline, J., Stern, L., Cytryn, L., & McKnew, D. (1982). The development of a child assessment interview for research and clinical use. *Journal of Abnormal Child Psychology, 10,* 173–189.

Holroyd, J. (1974). The Questionnaire on Resources and Stress: An instrument to measure family response to a handicapped family member. *Journal of Community Psychology, 2,* 92–94.

Ievers, C.E., & Drotar, D. (1996). Family and parental functioning in cystic fibrosis. *Developmental and Behavioral Pediatrics, 17,* 48–55.

Kaplan, R.M., & Anderson, J.P. (1988). The quality of well-being scale: Rationale for a general quality of live measure. In S. Walker and R. Rosser (Eds.), *Quality of life: Assessment and application.* London: MTP Press.

Koch, C., & Lanng, S. (1995). Other organ systems. In M.E. Hodson & D.M. Geddes (Eds.), *Cystic Fibrosis* (pp. 295–314). London: Chapman & Hall.

Koocher, G.P., Gudas, L.J., & McGrath, M.L. (1992). Behavioral aspects of cystic fibrosis. In M. Wolraich & D.K. Routh (Eds.), *Advances in developmental and behavioral pediatrics* (Vol. 10, pp. 195–220). Greenwich, CT: JAI Press.

Koocher, G.P., McGrath, M.L., & Gudas, L.J. (1990). Typologies of nonadherence in cystic fibrosis. *Journal of Developmental and Behavioral Pediatrics*, 11, 353–358.

Krasnegor, N.A. (1993). Epilogue: Future research directions. In N.A. Krasnegor, L. Epstein, S.B. Johnson, & S.J. Yaffe (Eds.), *Developmental aspects of health compliance behavior* (pp. 355–358). Hillside, NJ: Erlbaum.

Levitan, I.B. (1989). The basic defect in cystic fibrosis. *Science*, 244, 1423.

Lewiston, N.J. (1985). Cystic fibrosis. In N. Hobbs & J.M. Perrin (Eds.), *Issues in the care of children with chronic illness* (pp. 196–213). San Francisco: Jossey-Bass.

Matthews, L.W., & Drotar, D. (1984). Cystic fibrosis: A challenging long-term chronic disease. *Pediatric Clinics of North America*, 31, 133–152.

Moos, R.H., & Moos, B.S. (1981). *Family Environment Scale manual*. Palo Alto, CA: Consulting Psychologist Press.

Orenstein, D., Franklin, B., Doershuk, C., Hellerstein, H., Germann, K., Horowitz, J., & Stern, R. (1981). Exercise conditioning and cardiopulmonary fitness in cystic fibrosis. *Chest*, 80, 392–398.

Orenstein, D.M., Pattishall, E.N., Nixon, P.A., et al. (1990). Quality of well-being before and after antibiotic treatment of pulmonary exacerbation in patients with cystic fibrosis. *Chest*, 98, 1081.

Orenstein, D.M., Henke, K., & Cherny, F. (1983). Exercise in cystic fibrosis. *Physician and Sports Medicine*, 11, 57–63.

Orenstein, D.M., Nixon, P., Ross, E.A., & Kaplan, R.M. (1989). The quality of well-being in cystic fibrosis. *Chest*, 95, 344–347.

Orenstein, D.M., & Wachnowsky, D.M. (1985). Behavioral aspects of cystic fibrosis. *Annals of Behavioral Medicine*, 7, 17–20.

Osoba, D. (1994). Lessons learned from measuring health-related quality of life in oncology. *Journal of Clinical Oncology*, 12, 608–616.

Patterson, J.M., Hamilton, I.M., McCubbin, H.I., & Warwick, J.W. (1990). The impact of family functioning on health changes in children with cystic fibrosis. *Social Science Medicine*, 31, 159–164.

Pumariega, A.J., Pearson, D.A., & Seilheimer, D.K. (1993). Family and childhood adjustment in cystic fibrosis. *Journal of Child and Family Studies*, 2, 109–118.

Quittner, A.L., DiGirolomo, A.M., Michel, M., & Eigen, H. (1992). Parental response to cystic fibrosis: A contextual analysis of the diagnostic phase. *Journal of Pediatric Psychology*, 17, 683–704.

Ramsey, B., & Marshall, S. (1995). Pediatrics. In M.E. Hodson & D.M. Geddes (Eds.), *Cystic fibrosis*. London: Chapman & Hall Medical.

Rolland, J.S. (1993). Mastering family challenges in serious illness and disability. In F. Walsh (ed.), *Normal family processes* (2nd ed.). New York: The Guilford Press.

Satin, W., La Greca, A.M., Zigo, M.A., & Skyler, J.S. (1989). Diabetes in adolescence: Effects of multifamily group intervention and parent simulation of diabetes. *Journal of Pediatric Psychology*, 14, 259–275.

Sheppard, M.N. (1995). The pathology of cystic fibrosis. In M.E. Hodson & D.M. Geddes (Eds.), *Cystic fibrosis* (pp. 131–150). London: Chapman & Hall.

Shwachman, H., & Kulczycki, L.L. (1958). Long-term study of one hundred and five patients with cystic fibrosis. *American Journal of Diseases of Children*, 96, 6–15.

Sines, J.O., Pauker, J.D., Sines, L.K., & Owen, D.R. (1969). Identification of clinically relevant dimensions of children's behavior. *Journal of Consulting and Clinical Psychology*, 33, 728–734.

Spieth, L.E., & Harris, C.V. (1996). Assessment of health-related quality of life in children and adolescents: An integrative review. *Journal of Pediatric Psychology*, 21, 175–193.

Stark, L.J., Jelalian, E., & Miller, D.L. (1995). Cystic fibrosis. In M.C. Roberts (Ed.), *Handbook of pediatric psychology*. New York: The Guilford Press.

Stark, L.J., Knapp, L., Bowen, A.M., Powers, S.W., Jelalian, E., Evans, S., Passero, M.A., Mulvihill, M.M., & Hovell, M. (1993). Behavioral treatment of calorie consumption in children with cystic fibrosis: Replication with two year follow-up. *Journal of Applied Behavior Analysis*, 26, 435–450.

Stark, L.J., Mulvihill, M.A., Powers, S.W., Jelalian, E., Kearing, K., Creveling, S., Brynes-Coins, B., Miller, D.L., Harwood, I., Passero, M.A., Light, M., & Hovell, M. (1994). *Increased calorie intake and weight gain in children with cystic fibrosis receiving behavioral treatment versus wait list controls*. Manuscript submitted for publication.

Stark, L.S., Spieth, L., Opipari, L., Quittner, A.L., Jelalian, E., Lapey, A., Khaw, K.T., Higgins, L., Duggan, C.P., & Stallings, V.A. (1996). The efficacy of behavioral intervention: Parent training vs. nutrition education. *Pediatric Pulmonology, 13* (suppl.):S17.2, 203–204.

Stark, L.J., Spirito, A.J., & Hobbs, S.A. (1990). The role of behavior therapy in cystic fibrosis. In A. Gross & R. Drabman (Eds.), *Handbook of clinical behavioral pediatrics* (pp. 253–265). New York: Plenum Press.

Stein, R.E.K., & Jessop, D.J. (1984). Relationship between health status and psychological adjustment among children with chronic conditions. *Pediatrics, 73,* 169–174.

Stein, R., & Reissman, C.K. (1980). The development of an impact-on-family scale: Preliminary findings. *Medical Care, 18,* 465–472.

Thompson, R.J., Jr., & Gustafson, K.E. (1996). *Adaptation to chronic childhood illness.* Washington D.C.: American Psychological Association.

Thompson, R.J., Jr., Gustafson, K.E., George, L., & Spock, A. (1994). Change over a 12-month period in the psychological adjustment of children and adolescents with cystic fibrosis. *Journal of Pediatric Psychology, 19,* 189–204.

Thompson, R.J., Jr., Gustafson, K.E., & Gil, K. (1995). Psychological adjustment of adolescents with cystic fibrosis of sickle cell disease and their mothers. In J. Wallander & L. Siegel (Eds.), *Advances in pediatric psychology: II. Behavioral perspectives on adolescent health* (pp. 232–247). New York: Guilford Press.

Thompson, R.J., Jr., Gustafson, K.E., Gil, K., Kinney, T.R., & Spock, A. (1999). Change in the psychological adjustment of children with cystic fibrosis or sickle cell disease and their mothers. *Journal of Clinical Psychology in Medical Settings, 6,* 373–392.

Thompson, R.J., Jr., Gustafson, K.E., Hamlett, K.W., & Spock, A. (1992a). Psychological adjustment of children with cystic fibrosis: The role of child cognitive processes and maternal adjustment. *Journal of Pediatric Psychology, 17,* 741–755.

Thompson, R.J., Jr., Gustafson, K.E., Hamlett, L.K., & Spock, A. (1992b). Stress, coping, and family functioning in the psychological adjustment of mothers of children with cystic fibrosis. *Journal of Pediatric Psychology, 17,* 573–585.

Thompson, R.J., Jr., Hodges, K., & Hamlett, K.W. (1990). A matched comparison of adjustment in children with cystic fibrosis and psychiatrically referred and non-referred children. *Journal of Pediatric Psychology, 15,* 745–759.

Thompson, R.J., Jr., Kronenberger, W., & Curry, J.F. (1989). Behavior classification system for children with developmental, psychiatric, and chronic medical problems. *Journal of Pediatric Psychology, 14,* 559–575.

Thompson, R.J., Jr., Merritt, K.A., Keith, B.R., Murphy, L.B., & Johndrow, D.A. (1993). The role of maternal stress and family functioning in maternal distress and mother-reported and child-reported psychological adjustment of non-referred children. *Journal of Clinical Child Psychology, 22,* 78–84.

Turpin, S.V., & Knowles, M.R. (1993). Treatment of pulmonary disease in patients with cystic fibrosis. In P.B. Davie (Ed.), *Cystic Fibrosis.* New York: Marcel Dekker, Inc.

Varni, J.W., Katz, E.R., Colegrove, R., Jr., & Dolgin, M. (1993). The impact of social skills training on the adjustment of children with newly diagnosed cancer. *Journal of Pediatric Psychology, 18,* 751–767.

Varni, J.W., Rubenfeld, L.A., Talbot, D., & Setoguchi, Y. (1989a). Determinants of self-esteem in children with congenital/acquired limb deficiencies. *Journal of Developmental and Behavioral Pediatrics, 10,* 13–16.

Varni, J.W., Rubenfeld, L.A., Talbot, D., & Setoguchi, Y. (1989b). Family functioning, temperament, and psychologic adaptation in children with congenital/acquired limb deficiencies. *Pediatrics, 84,* 323–330.

Wallander, J.L., Varni, J.W., Babani, L., Banis, H.T., DeHaan, C.B., & Wilcox, K.T. (1989). Disability parameters: Chronic strain and adaptation of physically handicapped children and their mothers. *Journal of Pediatric Psychology, 14,* 23–42.

Webster-Stratton, C. (1990). Stress: A potential description of parent perceptions and family interactions. *Journal of Clinical Child Psychology, 19,* 302–312.

Whitehead, B.F., Rees, P.G., Sorensen, K., Bull, C., Fabre, J., de Leval, M.R., & Elliot, M.J. (1995). Results of heart-lung transplantation in children with cystic fibrosis. *European Journal of Cardiothoracic Surgery, 9,* 1–6.

Wilson, J.M., & Wilson, C.B. (1996). *Cystic Fibrosis: Pointing to the medicine of the future.* Paper presented at the North American Cystic Fibrosis Conference. Orlando, FL.

Wood, R.E., Boat, T.F., & Doershuk, C.F. (1976). State of the art of cystic fibrosis. *American Review of Respiratory Disease, 113,* 833–878.

Chapter 13

HEADACHES

Johannes H. Langeveld
Jan Passchier

Quality of life (QL) research in juvenile headache patients represents an integrative approach to the study of headache impact on the lives of children and adolescents. In contrast to separate investigations, QL assessment offers a comprehensive approach to the study of sickness impact, in which the quality of the major aspects of the subject's life is assessed together.

The authors of this chapter adhere the position that QL should be perceived as a multidimensional concept, which encompasses psychological and social well-being, physical, role, and social functioning, health perception and pain (Stewart et al., 1989; Aaronson et al., 1991). Spilker's multi-level model of QL (Spilker, 1996) is an approach that further clarifies the authors' position. Three levels of QL are described: (1) the individual's overall satisfaction with life and one's general sense of personal well-being; (2) broad domains of QL (e.g., physical, psychological, and social domains); (3) specific components of each domain (e.g., among the specific components of the psychological domain are anxiety and depression).

As can be derived from data from the 1988 US National Health Survey (Newacheck & Taylor, 1992), the impact of frequent or severe headache on the QL of children and adolescents is salient. There are several reasons to measure QL in young headache patients. Firstly, from a public health point of view (population level), there is a need to study the impact of the headaches on general health and one's ability to function actively in society in order to stimulate health care in a rational way. Secondly, headache is a subjective experience with few, if any, objective symptoms. In routine laboratory investigations, no abnormalities are found. Therefore, in addition to an objective effect evaluation, studies on the effects of headache and its treatment on the lives of young subjects should also include subjective measures. This evaluation should be systematic and reproducible. Accordingly, in treatment effect studies (at the group level), the inclusion of valid and reliable QL measurements will result in a more comprehensive evaluation of the effects of headache and its treatment. Thirdly, to select a proper treatment, the clinician facing children and adolescents with frequent headache or migraine may want to survey the impact of the disorder on the subject's quality of life (at an individual level) systematically. Subsequently, an adequate treatment can be chosen and its effect be evaluated by quality of life measurement.

This chapter will begin by presenting the characteristics and prevalence of primary headache in children and adolescents. It will then review some causal and maintaining factors in juvenile headache. Then, studies on the effects of headache on QL are presented and discussed. Finally, suggestions to improve QL research with this patient group are given.

CHARACTERISTICS OF MIGRAINE AND TENSION-TYPE HEADACHE

All headaches discussed in this chapter refer to the criteria of the International Headache Association (Headache Classification Committee of the IHS, 1988). Despite their limitations (Solomon, Lipton, & Newman, 1992), the IHS criteria are considered a major advance in the field of headache classification (Lipton, Silberstein, & Stewart, 1994). To obtain high interobserver reliability in headache diagnosis, well-defined criteria are required. The IHS criteria satisfy this requirement (Granella et al., 1994).

In children, few headaches are associated with structural lesions (McGrath & Humphreys, 1989). Following the IHS criteria, headaches not associated with structural lesions are migraine, tension-type headache, and cluster headache. As cluster headache is a condition that very seldomly occurs in children and adolescents (Nappi & Russell, 1993), in this chapter the description of headache conditions is restricted to migraine and tension-type headache.

MIGRAINE

Pediatric migraine is an idiopathic recurring headache disorder manifesting in attacks lasting from 2 to 72 hours. Typical characteristics of migraine-type headache are unilateral location, pulsating quality, moderate or severe intensity, aggravation by routine physical activity, and associated nausea, photo-, and phonophobia.

A typical migraine attack can be divided into different stages; a pre-headache, headache, and post-headache phase. Although, strictly speaking, a migraine diagnosis should not be applied until a subject has experienced five attacks, a migraine attack can also occur as infrequently as once in a lifetime. On the other hand, some migraine subjects experience several attacks a week. The duration of attack varies from attack to attack and from subject to subject. In any migrainous subject, a migraine attack can vary from a fragment of the clinical spectrum to one in which all phases occur (Campbell, 1990). Besides the headache, migraine can be accompanied by a wide spectrum of symptoms. Vague symptoms like mood changes, increased thirst or a sensation of lethargy can occur before the attack. An aura may precede a migraine attack, which is a sensation that forewarns the actual attack. Visual or sensory auras are most common. The most frequently reported visual aura is a 'scintillating hemianopic phenomenon that spreads across the visual field' (Campbell, 1990). As sensory auras, positive- (tingling) and negative phenomena (numbness) are described. A variety of autonomic disturbances may accompany a migraine attack, i.e., nausea, vomiting, skin pallor, changes in the cardiovascular system, fluid, electrolyte disturbances, and respiratory manifestations. More rare disturbances accompanying a migraine attack are: motor disturbances, disturbances of language, and cognitive disturbances. Headache in migraine usually has a gradual onset.

The diagnosis of migraine in children is often problematic for the following reasons: (1) non-specific headache symptoms are presented at an early stage of the disorder; (2) specific migraine symptoms are often absent in children; (3) the children's stage of intellectual development hampers a subtle report of headache symptoms; (4) in children with migraine, nausea, vomiting, and abdominal pain are often more prominent than in adults, especially in younger children (McGrath & Unruh, 1987); (5) headache in children is often inextricably linked with wide-ranging psycho-social problems (Hockaday, 1988; Hockaday, & Barlow, 1993). Though in adult migraine patients head pain is most often reported to occur unilaterally, head pain in migrainous children is often not (Hockaday, 1988). However, it is difficult to detect whether or not a headache is unilateral in children, and especially in small children. Since in pediatric patients, the actual duration of migraine attacks is commonly much shorter than in adults, Winner et al. (1995) propose a revision of the IHS criteria so that a migraine attack only requires a minimum of thirty minutes duration. Furthermore, Winner et al. propose modifications relating to duration, location, quality of intensity, and symptoms related to photophobia and phonophobia.

The differences in severity, duration and symptoms between attacks and the variations in the duration of the attack-free periods complicate the measurement of quality of life at one moment only. Therefore, to obtain representative QL data, measurements at more points in time are required.

Tension-type headache can be classified into two subtypes. An *episodic* tension type headache diagnosis requires at least ten previous headache episodes that last from thirty minutes to seven days. These headaches should have at least two of the following characteristics: (1) a pressing/ tightening character, (2) mild or moderate intensity, (3) occurring bilateral, and (4) not aggravated by routine physical activity. The headaches should not be accompanied by vomiting, nausea, photophobia, or phonophobia. For a *chronic* tension-type headache diagnosis the subject should suffer from headache more than fifteen days a month (180 days a year) and more than six months.

Tension-type headache is generally described and defined by the following clinical picture (Rapoff, Walsh, & Engel, 1988):

"The headache is almost continuous or daily, varying in severity, and has primarily a nonthrobbing quality, which may be described as an ache, pressure or tightness, and usually a frontal location, although vertex and occiput are other possible sites. Gastro-intestinal and neurological symptoms are lacking" (page 163).

In children with tension-type headache, the typical pallor and behavioral change of the child with migraine are not seen, and the parent is usually only aware of headache if informed by the child (Hockaday & Barlow, 1993).

PREVALENCE OF HEADACHE

Headache in children is extremely common. In a stratified 4% sample of the entire Amsterdam population between ten and seventeen years, only 12% of the subjects mentioned absence of headache during the past year (Passchier & Orlebeke, 1985). In a study on 8993 children in the age from seven to fifteen years, Bille (1962) found that 58% of the boys and 59% of the girls were familiar with headache. Frequent no-migraine headache was found in 5.9% of the boys and 7.7% of the girls. The prevalence of migraine was 3.3% for boys and 4.4% for girls. Other studies showed a migraine prevalence in schoolchildren from 2% (Stang & Osterhaus, 1993) to 10.6% (Abu-Arefeh & Russell, 1994). Differences in prevalence rates may be due to differences in employed migraine criteria and procedure of data aggregation. It is estimated that 10% to 15% of adult migraineurs experience an aura with some attacks. In children and adolescents the prevalence of auras accompanying a migraine attack is also high (Abu-Arefeh & Russell, 1994; Raieli et al., 1995). The prevalence of frequent no-migraine headache and migraine increases with age (Abu-Arefeh & Russell, 1994; Bille, 1962; Sillanpaa, Piekkala, & Kero, 1991). Sillanpaa et al. (1991), in a study of school children in Finland, found that 37% of the children had experienced headache by the age of seven. By the age of fourteen this number had risen to 69%. The prevalence of migraine was found to increase from 2.7% by the age of seven to 10.6% at the age of fourteen. Passchier & Orlebeke (1985) reported that the number of adolescents from twelve to seventeen years of age who suffer each week from one or more headaches is about 15%.

CAUSAL, TRIGGERING AND MAINTAINING FACTORS IN PRIMARY HEADACHE

Most children familiar with primary headache and their parents will make an effort to reduce the frequency, duration and intensity of the children's headache attacks. To do so, the children may refrain from known causal, triggering and maintaining factors. As such, the headache may hamper the children's functional status. Consequently, this avoidance behavior could result in increased levels of stress, which may have an impact on their psychological functioning. The best-known triggering factor in migraine is the experience of stress. Several studies following a prospective study design, including the use of a diary, show that more stress occurs the day before a migraine attack (Passchier & Andrasik, 1993). In youngsters too, epidemiological and clinical findings suggest that experience of stress elicits migraine (Andrasik, Holroyd, & Abell, 1979; Egermark-Eriksson, 1982; Maratos, & Wilkinson, 1982; Passchier & Andrasik, 1993). Also, Passchier and Orlebeke (1985) demonstrated that most young headache subjects, when asked for the cause of their headache, attribute a major causal effect to stress. In a prospective study on no-migraine headache and psychosocial factors in college students, Labbe, Murphy, and O'Brien (1997) found that perception of stress was one of the best predictors of a headache attack. Migraine and no-migraine headache subjects seem to tolerate lower levels of stress. In children and adolescents, a lower tolerance of stress will affect role functioning at school, psychological functioning, and overall satisfaction with life.

EFFECTS OF HEADACHE ON SEPARATE QUALITY OF LIFE DOMAINS

Since only one study can be identified in which the QL of young headache and migraine subjects as a whole is compared systematically with no headache controls (Langeveld et al., 1996; Langeveld, Koot, &

Passchier, 1997), investigations are presented that study the effects of headache or migraine on one or more specific QL domains in children and adolescents. Effects of headache on the QL domains of psychological functioning and well-being, physical functioning, role and social functioning will be presented.

PSYCHOLOGICAL FUNCTIONING, WELL-BEING AND PHYSICAL FUNCTIONING IN YOUNG HEADACHE SUBJECTS

Compared with no-headache controls, juvenile subjects who are familiar with headache or migraine, report a maladaptive behavioral/psychological functioning (Andrasik & Passchier, 1993). Also Passchier and Knippenberg (1991) indicate that children with migraine or chronic headache show impairment in their psychological well-being. Several studies suggest that headache or migraine in children results in distinct psychological consequences: Engström (1992) found that juvenile subjects (9–18 years) with headache score higher on anxiety, compared with subjects with irritable bowel syndrome or healthy control subjects. Further, juvenile headache subjects present higher scores on depression than healthy controls. Andrasik et al. (1988) performed a study in which children experiencing recurrent headache or migraine were compared with no-headache peer controls matched for age, sex, and social class. Children with migraine revealed higher scores on all scales measuring depression and somatic complaints; adolescent headache sufferers also revealed increased levels of trait anxiety. Larsson (1988), in a cross-sectional study comparing a non-clinical sample of adolescents with recurrent headache with a group of matched head-ache-free controls, found more psychological distress and somatic symptoms in subjects with recurrent headache than in their headache free counterparts. Also Wisniewski, Naglieri, and Mulick (1988) showed that, compared with no-headache controls, juvenile subjects who are familiar with headache report more somatic complaints. As Bree, Passchier, and Emmen (1990) demonstrated, they generally evaluate their health as less satisfactory.

Cunningham et al. (1987) performed a study in which they compared children with migraine with a "pain" control group and with a "no-pain" control group. The amount of pain experienced by the children in the migraine group and the "pain" group was controlled. Children with headache were found to present a similar pattern of behavioral and personality characteristics as children with musculo-skeletal pain. Both study groups showed a greater incidence of internalizing behavior problems and somatic complaints compared with the "no-pain" group. Furthermore, both pain groups were observed to be less happy. Cunningham et al. suggest that the personality and behavioral features of children with migraine may not be characteristic of pediatric migraine patients, but instead result from the common chronic pain experience.

Frequent headache or migraine does not seem to affect cognitive functioning (Leijdekker et al., 1990) or intellectual development. Bille (1962), in his classical study on Swedish primary school pupils, showed that children with migraine did not have marks above or below their peers without headache or migraine. Neither did they show any differences in other cognitive and intellectual tasks.

ROLE AND SOCIAL FUNCTIONING IN YOUNG HEADACHE SUBJECTS

Role and social functioning at school

Migraine causes significantly reduced school attendance. Collin, Hockaday, and Waters (1985) reported that over a time span of twelve weeks, the prevalence of school absence due to headache for children five to nineteen years of age was 3.7%. Based on data from the 1989 US National Health Survey, Stang and Osterhaus (1993) estimated for children aged six to seventeen years in the USA that 10% of school-aged migraineurs missed at least one day at school over a two-week period because of migraine; nearly 1% missed four days. Data from the 1988 US National Health Survey demonstrate that regarding number of annual school absence days in children and adolescents with chronic disorders, only asthma had a significantly greater impact than frequent or severe headache (Newacheck & Taylor, 1992). For comparison, the average number of annual school absence days due to frequent or severe headaches was 3.3, for asthma this number was 4.6. However, headache subjects reported more bother caused by their disorder than asthma subjects. Of the subjects with frequent or severe headache, 57% experienced a great deal of bother by their disorder, whereas 34% of the children with asthma reported a great deal of bother. Apparently, though asthma leads to more school absence days, frequent or severe headache is more disturbing.

Role and social functioning in the family

Caring for a child with a physical disease puts a strain on the child's family. School absence and frequent somatic complaints due to frequent headache or migraine may lead to what Breslau, Strauch, and Mortimer

(1982) describe as "perceived role restriction" in the parents. They define perceived role restriction as "the extent to which a person feels unable to pursue one's own personal interests due to the responsibilities involved with raising a child with a chronic physical condition" (Wallander, 1994, p. 621). Perceived role restriction is not found to be related to the objective aspects of the child's disability. Rather, it is related to the extent to which the child's family perceives social support from their social network. Therefore, though severe headache or migraine is not regarded as a disabling physical disease, it may lead to a perceived role restriction in the family to the same degree as disabling diseases. As such, it can be expected that the QL related to the young headache patients' role functioning in his or her family will be decreased. However, this has so far not been studied in families with children with migraine or other headache complaints.

STUDIES ON OVERALL QUALITY OF LIFE IN HEADACHE AND MIGRAINE PATIENTS

This section will begin with a summary of the present knowledge on overall QL in adult headache patients and will then present and discuss findings from the only study known to be performed on QL in adolescent headache subjects.

QUALITY OF LIFE STUDIES IN ADULTS WITH HEADACHE

The number of studies comparing the quality of life of adult headache patients with other patient groups and no-headache controls is limited. Following a general assessment approach, Solomon, Skobieranda, and Gragg (1993), using the generic Medical Outcomes Study Short Form Health Survey (SF-20), showed that the QL of adult chronic headache patients is significantly worse than the QL (i.e., physical-, social-, and role-functioning, and mental health) of patients with major chronic medical conditions such as arthritis and diabetes. These authors also showed that quality of life differs among headache diagnoses in adults (Solomon, et al., 1994). Social functioning was poorer for cluster and tension-type headache than for migraine. Further, Solomon et al. (1994) demonstrated that a significantly higher percentage of tension-type headache patients have a poor health associated with mental health than patients with migraine. They defined poor health associated with mental health as the lowest 19% of scores in the general population on five items of the SF-20 which survey "general mood or affect in the past eight weeks". In line with this study, Passchier et al. (1996) showed that tension headache patients are at least equally impaired in QL as migraine patients. However, they conclude that the impairment is mainly present in tension-type headache and migraine patients who visit the doctor for their complaints. Concerning migraine headache patients, Osterhaus, and Townsend (1991) showed that these patients' physical functioning and health perception scores were similar to those of patients suffering of arthritis, gastro-intestinal disorders and diabetes. Yet, role functioning, social functioning, pain, and mental health scores were lower in migraineurs than in other chronic diseases. In a study on the health status of migraine patients, Essink-Bot et al. (1995) demonstrated that the health status of migraineurs is significantly impaired in comparison with a control group. The largest differences between migraine sufferers and controls were observed in the domains of pain, role limitations, household work, social functioning, home-life, vitality, energy, overall health, and valuation of own health. Following a disease-specific approach in adult migraine subjects, Santanello et al. (1995) showed a significantly decreased QL during a migraine attack compared with a migraine-free period. Thus, even between attacks, the QL of a migraine patient seems poorer than in healthy controls. Yet, during a migraine attack the migraine patients' QL seems even poorer than in a migraine free period.

No studies could be identified that studied the effect of tension headache on overall QL in adults.

QUALITY OF LIFE IN CHILDREN AND ADOLESCENTS WITH MIGRAINE OR OTHER HEADACHES

To assess QL in juvenile subjects with headache, a generic or a disease-specific QL instrument can be applied. To date, no studies in children and adolescents have been reported in which the QL of headache or migraine subjects is compared with the QL in no-headache controls, employing a purely generic QL instrument. Following an approach that combines a generic and a disease-specific approach, Langeveld et al. (1996) describe the findings of a study in which the QL of migraine and no-migraine in juvenile headache subjects is compared with the QL in no-headache controls. Since the instrument that they used is to date the only QL questionnaire developed for youngsters with chronic headache or migraine, it is described in more detail below.

Quality of Life in Adolescents: The QLH-Y Questionnaire

The Quality of Life Headache in Youth (QLH-Y) (Langeveld et al.,1996; Langeveld, Koot, & Passchier, 1997) was developed as a QL measurement scale for adolescents between twelve and eighteen years of age with chronic headaches or migraine. The four QL domains of psychological functioning, functional status, physical symptoms and social functioning are covered by 69 multiple choice items. Two visual analogue scales assess the QL domains of satisfaction with life in general and health perception. The QLH-Y combines five generic modules with one specific module related to headache or migraine. This single headache-specific module questions the impact of the subjects' headache on different aspects of their functional status. In the other modules, subjects are not asked to make causal inferences about their QL (e.g., "To what degree do you feel anxious, *due to your headache*"), but are asked to make statements about their QL unrelated to their headache (e.g., "Last week, I was feeling ..."). Completion of the questionnaire usually takes 15 to 20 minutes. All subscales, except two of the three Social Functioning subscales showed a coefficient of internal consistency (Cronbach's alpha) of above .70, which was considered satisfactory (Nunnally, 1978). To obtain proxy measurements of the subjects' QL, a preliminary parent version of the QLH-Y was developed (QLH-P). The reliability of the questionnaire for juveniles is supported by satisfying test-retest correlations and adolescent–parent agreement. The median of 1-week test-retest subscale score correlations (intra class correlations) was 0.59, of the 2-week test-retest correlations 0.59, and of the 6-month test-retest correlations 0.47. The median of the parent–youth agreements (intra class correlations between the subscale scores on the QLH-Y and QLH-P) was 0.36.

Findings with the QLH-Y supporting its validity

Compared with no headache controls, subjects familiar with migraine or no-migraine headaches reported a lower QL regarding all relevant QL domains. They reported poorer physical functioning, psychological functioning, and social functioning. Further, they showed a lower satisfaction with life in general and with health. However, compared with no-migraine headache subjects, migraine subjects only presented minor differences in their QL: Migraine subjects reported somewhat more fatigue and stress compared with no-migraine headache subjects.

Following a multiple-measurement design including a headache diary, the QL domains of functional status, psychological functioning, satisfaction with life in general and health perception showed fluctuations that ran parallel to those in actual presence of headache before QL registration. Fluctuations in headache activity in young headache patients measured by a headache diary was found to be related to fluctuations in the subjects' functional status, psychological functioning, overall satisfaction with life and health perception. QL was diminished in case of a higher level of preceding headache activity.

CONCLUSION AND RECOMMENDATIONS

In this chapter, it was shown that QL research is relevant for juvenile headache patients. Several studies on the effects of headache and migraine on separate QL domains, and one that presents an overall picture, were discussed. Studies on separate QL domains and overall QL show more anxiety, depression, social problems, and less school attendance, school functioning, and satisfaction with health and life in general in youngsters with recurrent headache than in their healthy counterparts. Youngsters with recurrent headache do not show typical diagnosis-related patterns in the way their QL is affected (e.g., migraine versus no-migraine primary headache). While young headache patients experience a poorer QL even between attacks, their QL scores also vary in the predicted direction with their headache attacks. As was expected, the ability to perform school tasks was most affected by the subjects' headache. All studies presented in this chapter point at the serious effect of migrainous and non-migrainous chronic headache on the life of the young patient. The study of QL contributes to a better understanding of this effect.

Future study in the QL of young headache subjects may have various focuses: (1) To reach more conclusive results regarding the quality of life in young chronic headache or migraine patients, studies including higher numbers of subjects are requested. In these studies, the quality of life of young headache subjects should be compared with healthy controls and with subjects with chronic diseases. (2) Though completion of the QLH-Y is not especially time consuming, the development of a shorter QL measurement scale than the QLH-Y is desirable. A shorter measurement scale will be easier to administrate and will therefore result in a higher response rate. Shortening of the QLH-Y might be an option. (3) The QLH-Y was developed to be used on a target population of adolescents between twelve and eighteen years of age. In younger subjects, a proxy-measurement might be preferred, preferably completed by one of the parents. Regarding the QLH-Y, a preliminary parent version is already available. Such a proxy-measurement might be combined with a diary in which, in a few simple questions, the subjects are asked to evaluate some core aspects of their QL. (4) Another method to improve the exploration of the effects of severe headache and migraine on the QL of children and adolescents might be to include well-validated, domain specific, measurement scales in future treatment effect studies. This may result in a more detailed evaluation of the effects of headache and its treatment on these specific domains. (5) Studies in adults suggest that patients can be differentiated into subpopulations according to their help-seeking behavior (Passchier et al., 1996). Headache patients who consult a physician show generally more problems with their QL than those who do not. Future studies might classify those youngsters with chronic headache who have a low QL due to their headaches from those who lead a rather unaffected life. Such a classification can provide clues about the patients who need additional support and those who have sufficient resources.

References

Aaronson, N.K., Meyerowitz, B.E., Bard, M., Bloom, J.R., Fawzy, F.I., Feldstein, M., Fink, D., Holland, J.C., Johnson, J.E., Lowman, J.T., Patterson, B., & Ware, J.E. (1991). Quality of life research in oncology. *Cancer, 67,* 839–843.

Abu-Arefeh, I., & Russell, G. (1994). Prevalence of headache and migraine in schoolchildren. *British Medical Journal, 309,* 765–769.

Andrasik, F., Holroyd, K., & Abell, T. (1979). Prevalence of Headache Within a College Student Population: A Preliminary Analysis. *Headache, 19,* 384–387.

Andrasik, F., Kabela, E., Quinn, S., Attanasio, V., Blanchard, E.B., & Rosenbaum, E.L. (1988). Psychological functioning of children who have recurrent migraine. *Pain., 34,* 43–52.

Andrasik, F., & Passchier, J. (1993). Tension-type headache, cluster headache, and miscellaneous headaches: Psychological aspects. In J. Olesen, P. Tfelt-Hansen, & K.M.A. Welsh (Eds.), *The headaches* (pp. 489–492). New York: Raven Press.

Bille, B. (1962). Migraine in School Children. *Acta Paediatrica, 51,* Supplement, chapter 4: 33–55.

Bree, M. van der, Passchier, J., & Emmen, H. (1990). Influence of quality of life and stress coping behaviour on headaches in adolescent male students: An explorative study. *Headache, 30,* 165–168.

Breslau, N., Strauch, K., & Mortimer, E. (1982). Psychological distress in mothers of disabled children. *American Journal of Diseases in Children, 136,* 682–686.

Campbell, J.K. (1990). Manifestations of migraine. *Neurologic Clinic, 8,* 841–855.

Collin, C., Hockaday, J.M., & Waters, W.E. (1985). Headache and school absence. *Archives of Disease and Childhood, 60,* 245–247.

Cunningham, S.J., McGrath, P.J., Ferguson, H.B., Humphreys, P., D'Astous, J., Latter, J., Goodman, J.T., & Firestone, P. (1987). Personality and behavioral characteristics in pediatric migraine. *Headache, 27,* 16–20.

Egermark-Eriksson, I. (1982). Prevalence of headache in Swedish schoolchildren. A questionnaire survey. *Acta Paediatrica Scandinavica, 71,* 135–140.

Engström, I. (1992). Mental health and psychological functioning in children and adolescents with inflammatory bowel disease: A comparison with children having other chronic illnesses and with healthy children. *Journal of Child Psychiatry, 33,* 563–582.

Essink-Bot, M., van Royen, L., Krabbe, P., Bonsel, G.J., & Rutten, F.F. (1995). The impact of migraine on health status. *Headache, 35,* 200–206.

Granella, F., D'Alessandro, R., Manzoni, G.C., Cerbo, R., D'Amato, C.C., Pini, L.A., Savi, L., & Zanferrari, C. (1994). International Headache Society classification: Interobserver reliability in the diagnosis of primary headaches. *Cephalalgia, 14,* 16–20.

Headache Classification Committee of the IHS (1988). Classification and Diagnostic Criteria for Headache Disorders, Neuralgias and Facial Pain. *Cephalalgia, 8 (Suppl. 7),* 1–96.

Hockaday, J. (1988). Definitions, clinical features and diagnosis of childhood migraine. In J. Hockaday (Ed.), *Childhood migraine* (pp. 5–9). London: Butterworth.

Hockaday, J.M., & Barlow, C.F. (1993). Headache in children. In J. Olesen, P. Tfelt-Hansen, & K.M.A. Welsh (Eds.), *The headaches* (pp. 795–808). New York: Raven Press.

Labbe, E.E., Murphy, L., & O'Brien, C. (1997). Psychosocial factors and prediction of headaches in college adults. *Headache, 37,* 1–5.

Langeveld, J.H., Koot, H.M., & Passchier, J. (1997). Headache Intensity and quality of life in adolescents: How are changes in headache Intensity in adolescents related to changes in experienced quality of life? *Headache, 37,* 37–42.

Langeveld, J.H., Koot, H.M. Loonen, M.C. Hazebroek, A.A.J.M., & Passchier, J. (1996). A quality of life instrument for adolescents with chronic headache. *Cephalalgia, 16,* 183–196.

Larsson, B. (1988). The role of psychological, health-behaviour and medical factors in adolescent headache. *Developmental Medicine and Child Neurology, 30,* 616–625.

Leijdekker, M.L.A., Passchier, J., Goudswaard, P., Menges, L.J., & Orlebeke, J.F. (1990). Migraine patients cognitive impaired? *Headache, 30,* 352–358.

Lipton, R.B., Silberstein, S.D., & Stewart, W.F. (1994). An update on the epidemiology of migraine. *Headache, 34,* 319–328.

Maratos, J., & Wilkinson, M. (1982). Migraine in children: A medical and psychiatric study. *Cephalalgia, 2,* 179–187.

McGrath, P.J., & Humphreys, P. (1989). Recurrent headaches in children and adolescents: Diagnosis and treatment. *Pediatrician, 16,* 71–77.

McGrath, P.J. (1987). Headache. In P. McGrath (Ed.), *Pain in children and adolescents* (pp. 181–220). Amsterdam: Elsevier Science Limited.

Nappi, G., & Russell, D. (1993). Tension-type Headache, cluster headache, and miscellaneous headaches. In J. Olesen, P. Tfelt-Hansen, & K.M.A. Welsh (Eds.), *The headaches* (pp. 577–589). New York: Raven Press.

Newacheck, P.W., & Taylor, W. (1992). Childhood chronic illness: Prevalence, severity, and impact. *American Journal of Public Health, 82,* 364–371.

Nunnally, J.C. (1978) *Psychometric theory.* New York: McGraw-Hill.

Osterhaus, J., & Townsend, R. (1991). The quality of life of migraineurs: A cross sectional profile. *Cephalalgia, 11 (suppl.),* 103–104.

Passchier, J., & Andrasik, F. (1993). Migraine: Psychological factors. In J. Olesen, P. Tfelt-Hansen, & K.M.A. Welsh (Eds.), *The headaches* (pp. 233–240). New York: Raven Press.

Passchier, J., Boo, M. de, Quaak, H.Z.A., & Brienen, J.A. (1996). Health related quality of life of migraine and tension headache patients is related to the emotional components of their pain. *Headache, 36,* 556–560.

Passchier, J., & van Knippenberg, F.C.E. (1991). Relevance and limitations of Quality of Life measurements in juvenile patients with chronic headaches. In V. Gallai and V. Guidetti (Eds.), *Juvenile headache: Etiopathogenesis, clinical diagnosis and therapy: Proceedings* (pp. 449–455). Amsterdam: Excerpta Medica Elsevier.

Passchier, J., & Orlebeke, J.F. (1985). Headache and stress in school children: An epidemiological study. *Cephalalgia, 5,* 167–176.

Raieli, V., Raimondo, D., Cammalleri, R., & Camarde, R. (1995). Migraine headaches in adolescents: A student population-based study in Monreale. *Cephalalgia, 15,* 5–15.

Rapoff, M., Walsh, D., & Engel, J.M. (1988). Assessment and management of chronic pediatric headaches. *Issues in Comprehensive Pediatric Nursing, 11,* 159–178.

Santanello, N.M., Hartmaier, S.L., Epstein, R.S., & Silberstein, S.D. (1995). Validation of a new Quality of Life questionnaire for acute migraine headache. *Headache, 35,* 330–337.

Sillanpaa, M., Piekkala, P., & Kero, P. (1991). Changes in the prevalence of migraine and other headaches during the first seven school years. *Headache, 31,* 15–19.

Solomon, G.D., Skobieranda, F.G., & Gragg, L.A. (1993). Quality of life and well-being of headache patients: Measurement by the Medical Outcomes Study instrument. *Headache, 33,* 351–358.

Solomon, G.D., Skobieranda, F.G., & Gragg, L.A. (1994). Does Quality of Life differ among headache diagnoses? Analyses using the Medical Outcomes Study Instrument. *Headache, 34,* 143–147.

Solomon, S., Lipton, R.B., & Newman, L.C. (1992). Evaluation of chronic daily headache: Comparison to criteria for chronic tension type headache. *Cephalalgia, 12,* 365–368.

Spilker, B. (1996). *Quality of life and pharmacoeconomics in clinical trials* (2nd ed.) (pp. 1–11). Philadelphia: Lippincott-Raven Publishers.

Stang, P.E., & Osterhaus, J.T. (1993). Impact of migraine in the United States: Data from the National Health Interview Survey. *Headache, 33,* 29–35.

Stewart, A.I., Greenfield, S., Hays, R.D., Wells, K., Rogers, W.H., Berry, S.D., & McGlynn, Jr., J.E.W. (1989). Functional status and well-being of patients with chronic conditions: Results from the Medical Outcome Studies. *JAMA, 262,* 907–913.

Wallander, J.L. (1994). Perceived role restriction and adjustment of mothers of children with chronic physical disability. *Journal of Pediatric Psychology, 20,* 619–632.

Winner, P., Martinez, E., Mate, L., & Bello, L. (1995). Classification of pediatric migraine: Proposed revisions to the IHS criteria. *Headache, 35*, 407–410.

Wisniewski, J.J., Naglieri, J.A., & Mulick, J.A. (1988). Psychosomatic properties of a children's psychosomatic checklist. *Journal of Behavioral Medicine, 11*, 497–507.

Chapter 14

INSULIN-DEPENDENT DIABETES MELLITUS

Suzanne Bennett Johnson
Amy R. Perwien

There are two types of diabetes mellitus: (1) juvenile or Type I or insulin-dependent diabetes mellitus (IDDM), which is typically diagnosed in childhood and is the focus of this chapter, and (2) adult or Type II or non-insulin dependent diabetes (NIDDM) which usually occurs in later adulthood. Although IDDM onset can occur at any age, its peak incidence appears to be around puberty. Prevalence data suggest that in the US and European countries, IDDM is one of the more common chronic diseases of childhood. In the US, the risk of developing IDDM is much greater than that of pediatric AIDS, cystic fibrosis, muscular dystrophy, rheumatoid arthritis, and childhood cancer. International comparisons indicate that IDDM prevalence is highest in Scandinavian countries, lower in the US and non-Scandinavian European countries, and lowest in Asian countries (LaPorte, Matsushima, & Chang, 1995).

PICTURE AND TREATMENT

Recent evidence suggests that IDDM is an autoimmune disease in which the body attacks and destroys its own insulin-producing islet cells within the pancreas. Overt diabetes occurs only when sufficient numbers of islet cells have been destroyed. However, the mechanism that triggers this autoimmune process is unknown (Thai & Eisenbarth, 1993). Genetic factors are clearly implicated since relatives of IDDM patients are at greatly increased risk of developing the disease themselves. Nevertheless, only about 1 child in 25 who is a brother or sister of an IDDM patient will actually develop diabetes before age 30. Further, the concordance rate among monozygotic twin pairs is less than 50% (Harris, 1995). Other factors, in addition to some type of genetic predisposition, seem to be involved in the development of this disease. Nevertheless, islet cell antibodies appear to predate disease onset by months or even years and are currently being used in large scale screening programs as a predictive marker of who will develop IDDM in the future (Riley et al., 1990; Schatz et al., 1994).

At the time of diagnosis, the child presents with fatigue, thirst, hunger, frequent urination, and weight loss despite excessive eating. Without insulin, the child has been literally "starving" despite eating large quantities of food. The child's high levels of circulating blood glucose cannot be utilized and the body responds as if it is in a state of starvation by breaking down body fats into fatty acids. The liver converts the fatty acids to ketone bodies, which can be used by peripheral tissues. However, since insulin also inhibits fat breakdown, fatty acids and ketones soon begin to accumulate. The body's attempt to eliminate this glucose and ketone build-up results in frequent urination and excessive thirst; dehydration can easily result. When the kidney cannot effectively eliminate the high levels of ketones entering the blood stream, ketosis or ketoacidosis occurs. This is a very serious condition which, if left untreated, produces coma and ultimately death (Davidson, 1991).

IDDM is a chronic disease for which there is no cure. To survive, the patient with IDDM must acquire insulin by one or more daily injections for the rest of his or her life. Three types of insulin are commonly used: short-acting (Lispro, Regular or Semilente), intermediate-acting (NPH or Lente) and long-acting (Ultralente). They vary in absorption rate, time of maximal action, and duration of action. Lispro is the shortest acting insulin with a rapid onset of only 15 minutes, a peak effect of 1.5 hours and an effect duration of 3 hours. It is usually taken immediately before a meal. Other short-acting insulins are typically taken 30–45 minutes before eating because they begin working slightly later than Lispro, with peak effects around 2 hours post-injection and a 5–6 hour effect duration. Intermediate-acting insulins have even more delayed effects; initial effects occur 1 to 3 hours post injection and peak effects at 8 hours, with a 20 hour effect duration. Ultralente is the most long-acting, with initial effects at 2–4 hours, peak effects at 16 hours, and an effect duration of 32–36 hours. Different types of insulin are usually combined and injected before a meal. The short-acting insulins help handle the glucose produced by the meal while the intermediate- and long-acting insulins help maintain insulin availability throughout the day (Saudek, Rubin, & Shump, 1997).

Although patients attempt to maintain their blood glucose within the normal range, even combining types of insulin does not guarantee normoglycemia. In the healthy person without diabetes, the pancreas produces insulin in response to blood glucose (e.g., after eating), maintaining blood glucose within a constant and relatively narrow range (80–120 mg/dl). Unfortunately, current methods of insulin replacement by injection do not mimic the sensitivity of the normal human pancreas. If the patient with IDDM eats too much, given the available supply of insulin, hyperglycemia (excessively high blood glucose levels) will result. If the patient eats too little, given the available supply of insulin, hypoglycemia (excessively low blood glucose levels) will occur. Hypoglycemia (also called insulin shock), can lead to relatively rapid cognitive disorientation, convulsions, and coma. Consequently the patient is told to eat small amounts frequently throughout the day. Three small meals and two or three snacks, to be consumed at regular intervals, are recommended.

Exercise, considered beneficial because it improves insulin action, may also result in hypoglycemia if insufficient calories are consumed. Illness and stress may impair insulin action, leading to hyperglycemia. Because of the interacting influences of diet, exercise, illness, emotional state, and insulin action, blood glucose variability is to be expected. As a consequence, blood glucose levels must be monitored several times a day in order to manage hypo- or hyperglycemic episodes appropriately, should they occur. Home blood glucose monitoring is accomplished by obtaining a small sample of blood, from a finger stick, that is placed on a reagent strip. The strip is inserted into a computerized meter that "reads" the strip and reports the results. Home blood glucose monitoring, although now widely accepted in the US and Europe, is a relatively new phenomenon. It is the product of technological advances that permit reliable and accurate blood glucose measurement in the home environment. Prior to these developments, urine glucose tests were the usual method of monitoring blood glucose. However, since urine glucose tests are an indirect measure of blood glucose, they are far less sensitive.

Diabetes also takes its toll over time. Fifteen to twenty years after diagnosis, many patients develop one or more complications including retinopathy (often leading to blindness), nephropathy (often leading to kidney failure), peripheral vascular disease (often leading to leg or foot amputations), and atherosclerotic heart disease (often leading to cardiac arrest or stroke). However, recently published results of the Diabetes Complications and Control Trial (DCCT) provide evidence that maintaining "tight" glycemic control, with blood glucose levels in the near normal range, can significantly delay the onset and slow the progression of eye disease (retinopathy), kidney disease (nephropathy), and nerve disease (neuropathy) (DCCT Research Group, 1993). Side effects associated with the intensive therapy required to produce the near normal blood glucose levels of "tight" glycemic control, included weight gain and increased severe hypoglycemia. Nevertheless, the DCCT Research Group currently recommends that most patients with IDDM, including adolescent patients, intensify their diabetes management in an effort to maintain near normal blood glucose levels.

OVERVIEW OF CHAPTER

There has been an increasing realization that traditional medical outcome measures do not completely capture the impact of diseases and health care interventions especially from the patient's point of view (Jenkinson, 1994). The term "quality of life", or "QL," has been adopted to capture those aspects of health, functional status, and well-being that go beyond the traditional outcomes of death and physiologic measures of disease activity (Guyatt, Feeny, & Patrick, 1993). The heightened interest in QL measurement has been related to the realization that traditional morbidity and mortality measures do not provide a full picture of disease impact and the effects of new medical treatments (Jenkinson, 1994).

Despite the agreement that QL is an important, multidimensional construct, operational definitions of the term vary. Domains commonly assessed include disease and treatment-related symptoms, functional status, psychological functioning, and social-role functioning (Aaronson et al., 1991; Schipper, Clinch, & Olweny, 1996). Each of these four domains will be briefly summarized below, as they relate to children and adolescents with IDDM and their families. Then developmental issues that are important to QL assessment in IDDM childhood populations will be discussed, emphasizing both the changing needs of the child and the changing demands of the disease itself. Next measurement of QL in IDDM youth will be addressed; both generic and disease-specific measurement strategies will be covered. Programs designed to improve QL in this patient population will be described. Finally, we conclude by describing critical gaps in our current knowledge base, highlighting future directions in greatest need of empirical attention.

QUALITY OF LIFE AND INSULIN-DEPENDENT DIABETES MELLITUS

Disease and treatment related symptoms

This domain includes the unpleasant physical feelings associated with a disease and its treatment. Poorly controlled IDDM may be associated with fatigue, weight loss, thirst, bed-wetting and frequent urination.

Acute pain may occur when injecting insulin or conducting a finger stick for blood glucose testing. Hypoglycemia is associated with headaches, confusion and in severe cases, seizures and coma. Behavioral changes such as poor concentration, irritability, and tearfulness have also been found to occur relatively frequently in children (McCrimmon et al., 1995). The long-term complications of IDDM result in a variety of significant symptomatology (e.g., blindness, gastrointestinal pain, diarrhea, impotence, loss of physical sensation in the feet, orthostatic hypotension, angina). However, since these complications occur 10–15 years post-diagnosis, most children and adolescents do not experience them until they are adults.

FUNCTIONAL STATUS

Functional status generally refers to a person's ability to perform a variety of age-appropriate activities assumed to reflect physical health including self-care activities, mobility, physical activities, role activities, and leisure activities (Eisen et al., 1979). Spieth and Harris (1996) recently noted that functional status has received the bulk of attention in the QL literature which has focused primarily on medically ill adults. Although many diabetes-related complications (e.g., blindness, kidney failure, leg amputations) have marked effects on functional status, they occur many years after diabetes onset and are rarely seen in children and adolescents. Consequently, this QL domain may have limited relevance to youth with IDDM. Diabetes per se does not preclude a child from participating in most age-appropriate activities. However, in some cases, it can serve as a barrier. For example, exercise-induced hypoglycemia is a risk and youngsters are instructed to ingest sufficient calories and to monitor their blood glucose levels before or during exercise. Although schools usually allow youngsters to participate in school sports (and their health providers encourage them to do so), some organizations (e.g., private summer camps) do not want to take the risk of caring for a child with diabetes. Obtaining a driver's license, a major milestone of adolescence, is another example. Since hypogly-cemia can result in significant cognitive impairment, most states require physician approval before issuing a license to a person with diabetes. While hypoglycemia certainly impacts a patient's functional status, its effects are acute. Available measures of functional status, developed for medically ill adults, have focused on chronic, rather than acute, effects and consequently have limited or no relevance to youngsters with IDDM.

PSYCHOLOGICAL FUNCTIONING

Psychological status includes both affective (psychological attitudes and behaviors) and cognitive (alertness, confusion, or impaired thought and concentration) components (Patrick & Erickson, 1993).

Affective and behavioral functioning

Affective components most frequently addressed in IDDM samples include depression, anxiety, and worry. Kovacs et al. (1997) followed youths diagnosed with diabetes over a 10-year period. IDDM appeared to be associated with an elevated risk of psychiatric disorders, with depression being the most common. However, the authors noted that the highest risk period for a psychiatric disorder was during the first year after diagnosis. After an initial period of distress, most patients adjusted remarkably well. In fact, studies reporting higher levels of depression in children with diabetes compared to normative data are the exception (Nelms, 1989) rather than the rule (Brown et al., 1991; Grey, Cameron, & Thurber, 1991; Kuttner, Delamater, & Santiago, 1990; Mullins et al., 1995; Schoenherr et al., 1992). Studies examining anxiety also suggest that children and adolescents with diabetes are generally within the normal range (Kovacs et al., 1990b; LaGreca et al., 1995b). However, children with diabetes may be particularly susceptible to the development of specific fears, namely fear of hypoglycemia (Green, Wysocki, & Reineck, 1990; White et al., 1989). Estimates of the frequency of severe hypoglycemia, which is generally defined as an event requiring assistance from others or resulting in a coma or convulsion, range between 4.8 and 17.9 events/100 patient-years (Davis et al., 1997; Rovet, Ehrlich, & Hoppe, 1988). It should come as no surprise that family experiences with seizures or severe loss of consciousness is associated with increased fear of hypoglycemia in both parents and children (Marrero et al., 1997). For some, this leads to deliberate maintenance of high blood glucose levels and/or over-treatment of hypoglycemic symptoms (Cox et al., 1987; Marrero et al., 1997).

Standardized parent-report measures of the child's internalizing and externalizing symptoms have often substantiated the general psychological health of children with diabetes (Brown et al., 1991; Schoenherr et al., 1992; Wallander et al., 1988; Wertlieb, Hauser, & Jacobson, 1986), although there are occasional reports of increased adjustment problems (Rovert, Ehrlich, & Hoppe, 1987; Sterling, & Friedman, 1996).

While children and adolescents with diabetes often perform within the normal range on general measures of psychological adjustment, some studies have documented an increased risk for eating disorders, particularly bulimia (Neumark-Sztainer et al., 1996; Rodin et al., 1985). It is generally accepted that eating disorder behaviors, such as binge-eating or food restriction, will disrupt a patient's glycemic control. Further, the necessity of closely monitoring food intake for individuals with IDDM may potentiate disordered eating characteristics. More controversial is whether the IDDM patient population suffers from an increased prevalence of eating disorders per se (Peveler et al., 1992; Pollock, Kovacs, & Charron-Prochownik, 1995; Striegel-Moore, Nicholson, & Tamborlane, 1992).

Cognitive functioning

Cognitive functioning in children and adolescents with diabetes has been explored by a growing number of studies (see Holmes, O'Brien, & Greer, 1995; Rovet et al., 1993; Ryan, 1990, for reviews). In summarizing the literature on the impact of diabetes on intellectual functioning, Rovet et al. (1993) noted that, as a general rule, children who develop diabetes at an early age (before 6 years) appear to have more deficits than do children who develop diabetes later. Young children may be particularly vulnerable to the cognitive effects of glucose deregulation because they are still undergoing brain growth and development (Holmes, O'Brien, & Greer, 1995). For this reason, tight glycemic control is not recommended for young children (Ryan et al., 1985). Although most youngsters with IDDM manifest average intelligence, difficulties with decision-making efficiency and attention can occur in any child during hypoglycemia (Gschwend et al., 1995; Reich et al., 1990; Ryan et al., 1990). Further studies are needed to address the cumulative or enduring cognitive effects of hypoglycemia. Nevertheless, the preponderance of the evidence suggests that hypoglycemia may result in later cognitive impairment, particularly in children who develop IDDM before 6 years of age (Bjorgaas et al., 1997; Golden et al., 1989).

SOCIAL-ROLE FUNCTIONING

In children, social functioning is often examined in relation to interactions with peers, but may also include relationships with family members and teachers (Spieth & Harris, 1996).

Peer relationships

Despite limited research, peer relationships are clearly relevant to children and adolescents with diabetes. In an analogue study, Royal and

Roberts (1987) found that IDDM was one of the most "acceptable" of chronic diseases or disabilities in childhood (i.e., most healthy children reported that they would like to have a child with IDDM as a friend). Indeed, children with diabetes are described as socially competent and, in some cases, more pro-social than their physically healthy peers (Ferrari, 1984; Nassau & Drotar, 1995; Sterling & Friedman, 1996). However, adolescents may use parent and peer support in different ways, with tangible support for daily diabetes care activities coming predominantly from family members and emotional support coming from peers. Girls, in particular, report more support from friends (LaGreca et al., 1995a).

Family relationships

IDDM places numerous demands upon a family, as parents attempt to manage the child's illness while providing a home environment supportive of normal growth and development. Mothers may be particularly affected as they most often serve as the child's primary caretaker (Hauenstein et al., 1989; Kovacs et al., 1985; Wysocki et al., 1989). Good diabetes management occurs in families that are organized but flexible, with low family conflict and frequent diabetes-specific supportive behaviors (Bobrow, AvRuskin, & Siller, 1985; Hanson et al., 1992a, 1992b, 1995; Hauser et al., 1990; Miller-Johnson et al., 1994; Schafer et al., 1983; Schafer, McCaul, & Glasgow, 1986; Wysocki et al., 1989). Sibling relationships could be affected, although this has been the subject of little empirical research. Data from a population survey (Cadman, Boyle, & Offord, 1988) and a multi-site collaborative study (Sahler et al., 1994) suggest that there is an increased prevalence of behavioral and emotional problems in siblings of chronically ill youngsters compared to siblings of well children; nevertheless, the majority of chronically ill youngsters' siblings are well adjusted. Little research of this type has focussed specifically on the siblings of youngsters with IDDM. However, research that examines sibling adjustment, rather than sibling roles within the family, may miss subtle illness-related differences in parental disciplinary practices such as family chore assignment and the relative time parents spend with each child.

School functioning

Fowler, Johnson, and Atkinson (1985) examined school achievement test scores and frequency of school absences in children with 11 different chronic health conditions. Although children with diabetes had fewer absences compared to children with most other conditions, they ranked fourth lowest in school achievement. Further, compared to healthy youngsters, the available literature suggests that children with diabetes are absent from school about twice as often (Holmes et al., 1992; Ryan, Longstreet, & Morrow, 1985) and show a tendency toward worse school performance (Rovet et al., 1993). Consistent with these findings, Holden et al. (1997) reported that children with diabetes viewed themselves as less scholastically competent. Several factors may underlie these findings. School absences, the acute effects of hypoglycemia, or the longer term effects of poor glycemic control on the developing brain may all compromise the school performance of youngsters with IDDM.

DEVELOPMENTAL ISSUES

Like all children, youngsters with IDDM face a variety of challenges as they progress from childhood, through adolescence, to young adulthood. These challenges are complicated by a disease that changes over time, presenting unique additional stresses. To adequately understand the QL issues facing this population, we must place them within a context that includes both the changing needs of the developing child and the changing demands of the disease itself. Although the special issues relevant to the development of the child and the development of the disease are described separately below, they are often experienced as simultaneous challenges by children and families.

DEVELOPMENT OF THE CHILD

Although IDDM can be diagnosed at any time from birth to adulthood, each developmental period presents its own special challenges. For the youngster who develops IDDM during adolescence, the special needs of infants, toddlers, preschoolers and elementary school children will not be relevant. In contrast, the infant with diabetes must meet the demands of every developmental period within the context of diabetes.

Infants and toddlers with IDDM are difficult to manage because erratic eating behavior places them at risk for hypoglycemia and their lack of language makes communication difficult between parent and child. The parent cannot "explain" why shots and finger sticks are necessary. Finicky and irregular eating, so common in toddlers, places the child at risk for hypoglycemia, heightening parental anxiety. Since the child cannot tell a parent about an impending hypoglycemic episode, the parent may feel impelled to constantly monitor the child. Some parents may delay taking the baby's bottle away. Others may continue to let the baby sleep in the parents' room, delaying the move to a crib in the child's own room. Mothers often complain of being exhausted because the baby has never learned to sleep through the night. Parents may have difficulty letting the baby cry, fearing the child is hyper- or hypoglycemic. Time away from the baby is nonexistent, as baby sitters don't have the training to care for an infant or toddler with diabetes and parents are so uncomfortable leaving the child with others that they may fail to train someone to offer assistance.

By the time the child is a preschooler, the child is more verbal and socially interactive, raising new challenges. The child is now invited to birthday parties and wants to participate in various holiday events which are invariably associated with a myriad of sugary delights (e.g., going trick-or-treating on Halloween; finding candy canes on the Christmas tree; sharing candy hearts on Valentine's day; looking for a basket from the Easter bunny). For the first time, the child may realize that he or she is different from other children and the "differentness" seems defined by pain (finger sticks and injections) and deprivation (no or limited candy or other sweets). If the child begins day care or preschool, the parents must educate the day care workers or preschool teachers how to care for the child's diabetes. Parents may feel anger or helpless when a preschool or day care center indicates that it would prefer not to admit their child. Or, if the child is admitted, the parent may worry that the setting cannot appropriately care for the child. Day care or preschool settings also expose the child to a wide variety of acute, infectious diseases. Ear infections, colds, flu, stomach and intestinal disorders are all common and easily transferred from one child to another. Acute illness episodes present special problems for the child with diabetes. Illness can interfere with insulin action, raising blood glucose levels. Upset stomachs may make it difficult to assure sufficient caloric and fluid intake, increasing the risk of hypoglycemia and/or dehydration.

For those children who do not attend day care or preschool, elementary school is their first exposure to large groups of youngsters in an educational setting. In the US, as a result of the Education for All Handicapped Children Act of 1975, educational services are guaranteed to school-aged children with IDDM. However, parents must educate school personnel about diabetes management. Occasionally the school will offer a more restrictive approach, such as providing home bound instruction, which contrasts sharply with parent and health care provider preferences. Or, schools will constantly call parents, at the first sign of any medical problem; for working parents, this can be extremely disruptive. During the elementary school years, children often have the first opportunity to spend a night with a friend, to join a sports team, or participate in Scouts. These opportunities expand the number of supervising adults who must be educated to respond appropriately to the child's diabetes but also increase the risk of rejection because of the child's diabetes (e.g., a child may not be invited to attend a friend's sleep-over because the friend's parent does not feel comfortable taking responsibility for the child's diabetes).

By adolescence, the youngster is primarily responsible for his or her own diabetes care. Although adolescents have the cognitive capacity to understand diabetes and its management better than younger children, this rarely translates into more adherent behavior. In fact, poor adherence has been repeatedly documented in IDDM adolescents (Christensen et al., 1983; Hanson et al., 1992b, 1995; Ingersoll et al., 1986; Jacobson et al., 1987, 1990; Johnson et al., 1986, 1990, 1992; Lorenz, Christensen, & Pichert, 1985; Miller-Johnson et al., 1994). Both parents and adolescents become less rule-oriented about diabetes care during this developmental period, and parents supervise their children less (Johnson, 1995). Adolescents' preference for a more chaotic life-style, increased opportunities for experimentation and risk-taking behavior, their tendency to deny bad outcomes, and an increased self-consciousness and desire to "fit-in" with peers, may further contribute to poor diabetes care. Biologically, puberty is associated with increased insulin resistance in all youngsters, presenting special problems for the adolescent with IDDM (Amiel et al., 1986; Blethen et al., 1981; Bloch, Clemons, & Sterling, 1987; Cutfield et al., 1990). Consequently, for both social and biological reasons, IDDM is particularly difficult to manage during this developmental period.

While the concerns and needs of children and adolescents with diabetes have been the focus of considerable commentary, issues relevant to the transition from adolescence to young adulthood have received far less attention. Young adults with IDDM appear to marry and work at rates similar to their healthy peers (Cowie & Eberhardt, 1995; Jacobson et al., 1997; Tebbi et al., 1990). However, they may report lower general well-being, particularly in terms of health-related fears and feelings of depression (Tebbi et al., 1990), and a lower sense of self-competence (Jacobson et al., 1997; Lloyd et al., 1992). Several investigators have documented more social isolation or less social support in young people with IDDM (16–25 years of age) compared to healthy peers (Lloyd et al., 1993; Wysocki et al., 1992). No longer buffered by the self-protective denial of adolescence, the fears and concerns of young adults with this disease may be justified. Some are experiencing early signs of diabetic complications (Wysocki et al., 1992). Many decide not to have children (Ahlfield, Soler, & Marcus, 1985; Lloyd et al., 1993). Others report difficulties obtaining/maintaining employment or being rejected for health or disability insurance (Lloyd et al., 1992; Robinson et al., 1993; Tebbi et al., 1990). Based on data from the Children's Hospital of Pittsburgh IDDM registry in the United States, 48% of IDDM patients experience work limitations by age 45 and persons with IDDM are seven times more likely to report work disability than their non-diabetic siblings (Harris, 1995).

DEVELOPMENT OF THE DISEASE

Developmental challenges experienced by children and adolescents are further complicated by the changing nature of IDDM, a progressive incurable disease with increasing complications over time. IDDM diagnosis is often associated with mild distress in children and parents which typically dissipates within 6 months (Grey et al., 1995; Kovacs et al., 1985, 1986; Northam et al., 1996); mothers appear more affected than fathers. However, as might be expected, initial reaction to IDDM diagnosis is predictive of psychological adaptation many years later (Kovacs, et al., 1990a, 1990b); those children who developed an adjustment disorder at the time of diagnosis are more likely to develop a new psychiatric disorder in subsequent years (Kovacs, Ho, & Pollock, 1995).

Once the child is diagnosed and begins to receive insulin, he or she often enters a "honeymoon" period during which some endogenous insulin production occurs, making management of the disease relatively easy (Davidson, 1991). Although adherence with the diabetes regimen appears best at the time of diagnosis, it often deteriorates thereafter (Jacobson et al., 1990). During the "honeymoon" period, such lapses in diabetes care may go undetected. However, one to two years after diagnosis, complete pancreatic failure occurs (Davidson, 1991) with an associated deterioration in glycemic control (Grey et al., 1995). At this point, patients and families may experience renewed distress as health providers apply increased pressure to improve the youngster's diabetes management (Grey et al., 1995).

Over the course of diabetes, there are certain periods that place increasing demands on the patient and family: the time of diagnosis; the end of the "honeymoon" period when complete pancreatic failure occurs; the onset of puberty when insulin resistance increases; initial signs of diabetes complications; and times of deteriorating functional status due to complications as well as the additional treatment demands the management of complications requires. In addition, there are acute events that further complicate the management of the disease, such as illness, which can impede insulin action, and severe hypoglycemic events, which place children and families on high alert trying to prevent subsequent episodes. How the child and family manage these events is a product of both the specific demands of the disease at a specific point in time and the developmental needs and abilities of the child at the same point in time.

MEASURING QUALITY OF LIFE IN INSULIN-DEPENDENT DIABETES MELLITUS PATIENTS

There are two general types of QL measures: generic and specific. Generic measures purport to be broadly applicable across disease type and severity, across different medical or health interventions, and across demographic and cultural subgroups (Patrick & Deyo, 1989). Consequently, they are considered most useful when decisions or comparisons have to be made for large groups of patients with disparate conditions and backgrounds. In contract, specific measures are designed to assess the QL for a particular diagnostic group (e.g., IDDM) and are presumed to be more sensitive to changes within a homogenous patient group, permitting assessment of QL issues of particular relevance to a specific medical condition (McSweeny & Creer, 1995).

USE OF GENERIC QUALITY OF LIFE MEASURES WITH INSULIN-DEPENDENT DIABETES MELLITUS PATIENTS

Several generic measures have been used in QL studies of adults with IDDM; the most frequent being the Medical Outcomes Study Short-Form 36 (SF-36). This measure has been used to examine the validity of disease specific measures (Boyer & Earp, 1997; DCCT Research Group, 1988), the impact of intensive insulin therapy (DCCT Research Group, 1996), the relationship between QL, demographic, and disease characteristics (Jacobson, DeGroot, & Samson, 1994; Nerenz et al., 1992), and the impact of organ transplantation (Piehlmeier et al., 1996). In adolescents, the Psychosocial Adjustment to Illness Scale (PAIS) has been used to examine the construct validity of a disease specific QL measure (Diabetes Quality of Life Measure, DQL) (Jacobson and the DCCT Research Group, 1994).

The Quality of Well Being Scale (QWB), which classifies individuals according to mobility, physical activity, social activity, and symptom/problem complex, has been suggested for use in individuals with diabetes to capture the different effects of the illness and its treatment including the impact of poor control, side-effects of treatment, and benefits of treatment (Kaplan, 1994). However, because complications are much less frequent in children with diabetes compared to adults with the disease, the QWB scales examining mobility, physical activity, and social activity may not be sensitive to differences in QL in younger patients.

Several generic QL measures have been specifically developed for use with children, but have yet to be systematically studied or applied to children and adolescents with diabetes. For example, the RAND Health Status Measure for Children conceptualizes child health as a four-component construct: physical functioning, mental health, social relations, and overall health (Eisen et al., 1979). Although all four components appear relevant to youngsters with IDDM, some of the specific items (such as those relating to mobility) may not be as applicable. Further, as Eisen et al. (1980) originally noted, the purpose of the instrument was to measure changes in children's health status as a result of changing health care financing arrangements. Thus, the measure may not be sensitive to differences or changes in IDDM health status per se.

The Functional Status Measure II (FS II) is another generic measure developed for use with children (Stein & Jessop, 1990) but not yet used with children who have IDDM. It assesses children's behavioral responses to illness that interfere with normal social role performance. The mood and energy components of the FS II appear to be potentially relevant to children with IDDM, while the communication and self-care scales seem less relevant. Further, psychological functioning, considered important to the well-being of children and adolescents with IDDM, is only minimally addressed in an age-appropriate manner by the FS II. Thus, the instrument may be more useful for younger children with diabetes than older school-age children or adolescents with the disease.

The Dartmouth Primary Care Cooperative Information Project chart system (COOP) provides a very brief generic assessment of QL relevant to adults or adolescents (Nelson et al., 1996; Wasson et al., 1994).

There are no published COOP data with youth who have IDDM. Although the concepts addressed, physical fitness, emotional feelings, school work, and social support, appear appropriate for adolescents with IDDM, the brevity of the instrument may reduce its sensitivity to changes in disease state.

Two measures appear particularly promising for assessing QL in youngsters with IDDM: the Child Health and Illness Profile-Adolescent Edition (CHIP-AE; Starfield et al., 1993, 1995) and the Child Health Questionnaire (CHQ; Landgraf, Abetz, & Ware, 1996). The CHIP-AE, a self-report measure appropriate for 11–17 year-olds, examines physical and emotional discomfort, activity limitations, satisfaction with health, self-esteem, medical and psychosocial disorders, achievement (academic and work performance), and environmental and behavioral factors that may influence health (e.g., family characteristics and risk behaviors). The CHQ, designed for both school-aged children and adolescents, examines physical, emotional, and social well-being. Both the CHIP-AE and CHQ appear promising for youngsters with IDDM because of the variety of relevant areas they address in the physical, functional status, psychological, and role-functioning domains. The CHQ has the further advantage of offering an assessment for a wider age range of youth. While no published data are yet available for IDDM populations, the CHQ has been employed in samples of children with chronic conditions including asthma, epilepsy, and juvenile rheumatoid arthritis (Landgraf et al., 1996). The CHIP-AE has been used with secondary school students and has yet to be tested in samples of children with chronic illnesses.

DISEASE-SPECIFIC QUALITY OF LIFE MEASURES

Of the disease-specific measures, the Diabetes Quality of Life measure (DQL), which was developed for use in the DCCT (DCCT Research Group, 1988), has been used by a variety of investigators (Chantelau et al., 1997; DCCT Research Group, 1996; Jacobson et al., 1994; Lloyd et al., 1992; Nathan et al., 1991; Parkerson et al., 1993; Selam et al., 1992). Also available is the Quality of Life: Status and Change (QLsc) measure which addresses several domains: physical; psychological; social, activity/behavioral; religious; and economic (Hanestad, 1993; Hanestad & Albrektsen, 1992). To date, the QLsc has enjoyed somewhat limited use; administration has been primarily to adults attending Norwegian diabetes clinics.

Diabetes Quality of Life (DQL)

The Diabetes Quality of Life (DQL), the most frequently used diabetes QL measure in the US, includes four rationally-derived subscales: Satisfaction, Impact, Worry-Diabetes Related, and Worry-Social Vocational (DCCT Research Group, 1988). In addition to 46 core items, there are 13 additional items for use with adolescent populations. Responses to DQL items are made using a five-point Likert scale with the Satisfaction subscale rated from "very satisfied" to "very dissatisfied" and the Impact and Worry subscales rated from "no impact" or "never worried" to "always affected" or "always worried."

The reliability and validity of the DQL was initially assessed in a study of conventionally treated IDDM adolescents (n = 56) and adults (n = 192) (DCCT Research Group, 1988); study participants were similar to DCCT patients in age, duration of IDDM, and complication status (Jacobson & the DCCT Research Group, 1994). A more recent study conducted by Jacobson et al. (1994) examined the psychometric properties of the DQL in a more heterogeneous group of outpatient adults with IDDM (n = 111) or NIDDM (n = 129). Internal consistency reliability estimates for the DQL total score and subscale scores were similar across studies; coefficient α ranged from .83–.92 for the Total score, .86–.88 for the Satisfaction subscale, .77–.85 for the Impact subscale, .66–.77 for the Worry-Diabetes Related subscale, and .47–.87 for the Worry-Social/Vocational subscale. For the adolescents, internal consistency estimates ranged from .66 (Worry-Diabetes Related) to .92 (DQL total) (DCCT Research Group, 1988). One-week test-retest reliability coefficients ranged from r = .88 to r = .92 in the adolescent sample (DCCT Research Group, 1988). Although factor analysis studies of the DQL have yet to be published, correlations between the DQL subscales indicated small to moderate between-scale associations (ranging from r = .26 to r = .68), suggesting a simpler underlying structure.

The DQL Total, Satisfaction, and Impact scores have exhibited significant associations with other more generic measures of QL (DCCT Research Group, 1987; 1988). The DQL Worry subscale correlates most highly with measures of psychological distress (Jacobson & the DCCT Research Group, 1994). DQL scores have also exhibited a significant relationship to severity of diabetes complications, number of complications, and treatment regime (insulin, oral agents, and diet/exercise alone) (Jacobson et al., 1994; Lloyd et al., 1992). Further, the

DQL scores appeared to be sensitive to change in patients undergoing kidney or combined kidney/pancreas transplantation (Nathan et al., 1991) and in patients receiving an implantable insulin pump (Selam et al., 1992). With the exception of the original 1988 psychometric study conducted by the DCCT Research Group, all of these studies involved adult patients only, highlighting the need for validity work with children and adolescent samples.

Eiser et al. (1992) and Wysocki et al. (1992) did use the DQL in samples of young adults (15–25 years) with IDDM. Eiser et al. (1992) replaced the two DQL questions addressing "sex life" with questions concerning "friendships with the opposite sex." Based on some preliminary factor analytic work, Eiser et al. (1992) regrouped the DQL items into three subscales: general impact; social satisfaction; and diabetes satisfaction. In their sample, diabetes satisfaction was greater with longer disease duration, better clinic attendance, and better glycemic control. Complementing this latter findings, impact was great with poorer glycemic control. Women also reported greater impact than men. However, social satisfaction was unrelated to any of the disease variables. Further, no subscale was related to patient age, diabetes knowledge, or insulin regimens (twice-daily vs. multiple injections). Wysocki et al. (1992) analyzed the total DQL score, not the subscale scores, and found their young adult sample experienced poorer QL than the adolescents studied in the DCCT.

A revised version of the DQL was developed by Ingersoll and Marrero (1991) for use with older children and adolescents. The authors dropped items of limited relevance to youth (e.g., "How often do you worry about whether you will be denied insurance?") and added items related to school life and peers. This measure was then field tested on a small sample of 11 to 15 year-old patients. Based on these results, the wording of questions was further simplified and readability improved. The revised measure included 17 Diabetes Life Satisfaction items, 26 Disease Impact items, 13 Disease-Related Worry items, and a general self-rating of overall health. Internal consistency for the revised scales ranged between $\alpha = .82$ to $\alpha = .85$. The three scales correlated with each other ($r = .45$ to $r = .58$) and to the self-rating of overall health ($r = .42$ to $r = .45$). None of the scales were related to age or current level of glycemic control, but longer disease duration was associated with greater disease impact, a finding opposite to that reported by Eiser et al. (1992). While the Ingersoll and Marrero (1991) revised version of the DQL appears promising for use in children and adolescents, data on the test-retest reliability, factor structure, and validity of the measure are not available at this time.

PROGRAMS DESIGNED TO IMPROVE QUALITY OF LIFE IN INSULIN-DEPENDENT DIABETES MELLITUS PATIENTS

Intervention programs for patients with diabetes are almost always designed to improve glycemic control, rather than impact QL per se. However, by improving glycemic control, the patient's QL is presumed to improve as well. The DCCT was the largest trial of this type.

Because pancreatic islet cell destruction begins well before the development of overt diabetes, individuals can now be identified in the pre-diabetic state. This makes diabetes prevention trials possible. The Diabetes Prevention Trial — Type 1 (DPT-1, 1994) (American Diabetes Association, 1998b; Bloomgarten, 1997) is the first large prevention trial to be conducted in the US Although the goal is to prevent IDDM, or at least delay its onset, the patients' QL is presumed to be positively affected as well.

THE DIABETES COMPLICATIONS AND CONTROL TRIAL (DCCT)

At the time of the Diabetes Complications and Control Trial (DCCT's) inception in 1982, diabetologists believed that maintaining tight glycemic control, with blood glucose values near normal, would prevent, delay, or minimize the serious complications associated with IDDM. The DCCT tested this hypothesis with over 1400 volunteers (aged 13–39 years) in 29 different centers across the US. The volunteers were randomized to either intensive therapy designed to achieve tight control or conventional therapy. Intensive therapy consisted of three or more injections per day (or the use of an insulin pump), four or more blood glucose tests per day, daily insulin adjustment by the patient, and weekly provider contact. Conventional therapy represented usual care at that time: one or two insulin injections per day, daily blood or urine glucose testing, and a clinic visit every 3 months. Within 6 months, the intensive therapy patients exhibited significantly improved glycemic control compared to the conventional therapy patients. Further, the intensive therapy patients were able to maintain their improved glycemic control over the course of the study. Most importantly, intensive therapy was associated with marked reductions in risk for all of the major complications of diabetes: eye disease (76% reduced risk); kidney disease (50% reduced risk); nerve disease (60% reduced risk); and cardiovascular disease (35% reduced risk). The reduced risk was so substantial that the trial was terminated a year early (DCCT Research Group, 1993). The National Diabetes Information Clearinghouse has subsequently published and widely disseminated the DCCT results to patients, health providers, and the public (NDIC, 1994).

Although IDDM is typically diagnosed in childhood, most (86%) of the volunteers who participated in the DCCT were adults. An analysis of the adolescent participants indicated that their glycemic control was poorer than that of adult participants throughout the study, although intensive therapy improved glycemic control in both adolescents and adults (DCCT Research Group, 1994). However, improved glycemic control came with a cost. Intensive therapy was associated with an increased incidence of severe hypoglycemia. The rate of severe hypoglycemia (measured in events per 100 patient years) was significantly higher for adolescents (85.7) than adults (56.9). Weight gain was also a problem; five years of intensive therapy resulted in a mean gain of 4.6 kg over and above any weight gain associated with conventional therapy (DCCT Research Group, 1993). Among adolescents, 48% treated with intensive therapy became overweight compared to 28% treated with conventional therapy (DCCT Research Group, 1994). Despite the multiple demands of intensive therapy and the associated increased risk of hypoglycemia and weight gain, there was no evidence of poorer QL as measured by the DQL (DCCT Research Group, 1996). The reduced risk of retinopathy, nephropathy, neuropathy and cardiovascular disease associated with intensive therapy led the DCCT Research Group to recommend intensive therapy for both adults and adolescents (DCCT Research Group, 1994). For the DCCT Research Group, QL issues surrounding the development of diabetic complications *in the future* outweighed the costs (e.g., increased hypoglycemia and weight gain) associated with intensive therapy.

However, it is important to point out that volunteers in the DCCT were a select sample of highly motivated, predominantly adult, patients. It remains to be seen how many IDDM patients can manage the rigors of intensive therapy and successfully achieve the same tight glycemic control accomplished in the DCCT, with little or no reduction in current QL. Without tight glycemic control, any future QL benefits will be lost, making the multiple demands of intensive therapy, as well as the increased hypoglycemia and weight gain associated with its use, appear more costly.

The rigors of intensive therapy may prove particularly difficult for children and adolescents. Indeed, intensive therapy is not recommended for children less than two years old and should be undertaken only with extreme caution in children two to seven years of age because hypoglycemia may impair normal brain development (American Diabetes Association, 1998a). Adolescents are known to be less adherent with their diabetes management than younger children (Johnson, 1995) and may have particular difficulty accepting the rigors of intensive therapy. Further, they may be particularly concerned about the weight gain associated with its use (Striegel-Moore, 1993). During adolescence, the severe hypoglycemic episodes associated with intensive therapy are not only embarrassing but become life-threatening as the adolescent experiences increased freedom and responsibilities (e.g., decreased parental supervision, opportunity to drive a car). Clearly QL issues associated with intensive therapy need to be carefully monitored in all patients with diabetes, but particularly in children and adolescents.

THE DIABETES PREVENTION TRIAL (DPT-1)

The Diabetes Prevention Trial (DPT-1) is a multicenter clinical trial currently being conducted in the US. Relatives of persons with IDDM who volunteer are initially screened; those positive for islet cell autoantibodies are further tested to determine risk for IDDM. Those at high risk are then offered random assignment to either a trial of twice daily insulin injections (preceded by 4 days of continuous insulin infusion requiring hospitalization) or no treatment. Those at inter-mediate risk are offered random assignment to a trial of oral insulin or an oral placebo. All those randomized are monitored every six months to determine possible progression towards diabetes (Diabetes Prevention Trial Type 1, 1994). Although the prevention or delay of IDDM onset is presumed to improve participants' *future* QL, the current impact of the DPT-1 protocol is not being assessed. Previous research suggests that notification of a person's at-risk status induces clinically significant anxiety in both the at-risk person and in family members (Johnson et al., 1990; Johnson & Tercyak, 1995). Although this initial anxiety usually dissipates over time, children who cope with the news with high levels of avoidant and wishful thinking, are more likely to remain anxious. Mothers who cope by blaming themselves for their child's at-risk status are also more likely to remain anxious (Johnson, 1997). Further, findings from a study of families who participated in a previous nonrandomized prevention trial using subcutaneous insulin, suggest that significant difficulties adhering to the DPT-1 treatment regimen are likely (Tercyak, Johnson, & Schatz, 1997). Clearly, prevention trials can and probably do impact patients' and families' QL; it is unfortunate that such issues are currently receiving relatively little attention.

CRITIQUE AND FUTURE DIRECTIONS

QL assessment in populations of children and youth with IDDM is in its infancy. In this section, we highlight those areas most deserving of increased attention.

Although there has been a greater realization that traditional medical outcome measures do not completely capture the impact of diseases and health care interventions, the IDDM literature remains dominated by a focus on physiologic measures of disease activity (e.g., measures of glycemic control) rather than QL. When QL is addressed, adults rather than children or adolescents are typically the focus of study. Adults with diabetes far outnumber children with IDDM and adults are the primary victims of the serious complications of diabetes retinopathy, neuropathy, nephropathy, and cardiovascular disease. However, most adults are diagnosed with NIDDM, a different disease with different symptoms than IDDM experienced by children. Consequently, the adult diabetes QL literature is not always relevant to children and the specific QL concerns of children and adolescents need to be more clearly addressed.

Although IDDM is usually diagnosed in childhood, it is interesting to note that the most widely used IDDM-specific QL measure (the DQL) was developed with adults, although some adolescent items were included. Nevertheless, almost all of the available psychometric data on this measure was collected from adult samples. Further, the DQL does not assess the usual domains addressed by QL instruments: disease and treatment-related symptoms, functional status, psychological functioning, and social-role functioning. Instead, four rationally-derived subscales are offered: satisfaction, impact, worry-diabetes related, and worry-social vocational. This may make it difficult to place DQL results within the context of the larger QL literature. Further, the appropriateness of the DQL as an assessment measure for IDDM youth needs to be clarified.

Disease-specific QL measures are presumed to be more sensitive to changes within a particular diagnostic group. However, the contribution of the DQL over and above that offered by more generic QL measures remains to be seen. Although there are a number of good generic QL measures appropriate for children, to our knowledge, no study has used these generic measures with IDDM children nor has the relative utility of generic and disease-specific QL measures in IDDM childhood populations been compared.

Nevertheless, there is a large literature that bears on the traditional QL domains as they relate to youth with IDDM. This literature can serve as a guide to those issues that appear particularly salient with this population. Yet, this literature is limited by a tendency to focus on measures of psychopathology rather than measures that permit a more continuous assessment of impact and adjustment. To the extent that QL is viewed as a continuous, rather than a categorical (good versus bad) construct, the available literature may underestimate the more subtle effects IDDM, and its management, may have on children and families. Consequently, the next generation of QL measures should address the full continuum of potential disease impact from severe limitations, to moderate effects, to subtle consequences, to possible positive effects of living with such a disease.

Since the larger QL literature has focused primarily on adults, it has emphasized the patient's point of view. Children live in families and the child's illness affects every family member, although some family members may be more effected than others. Consequently QL assessments designed for use with chronically ill childhood populations need to go beyond the child's perceptions to include the perceptions of those so intimately involved in the child's daily care.

Children also change as they grow and develop, making QL issues somewhat different at each developmental period. For many diseases, including IDDM, the disease itself changes over time, adding new challenges and further complexity. Because the QL literature has focussed primarily on adults (often with relatively permanent functional diabetes), developmental issues so important to children have received little or no attention. QL measurement strategies that are sensitive to the changing demands and needs of the developing child who is living with a changing disease, need to be developed.

The traditional physiologic measures of disease activity and glycemic control currently in use with IDDM populations offer a useful, but very limited, view of the disease and its treatment. QL assessment in children with IDDM has yet to receive the attention it deserves. Until we can offer a more sophisticated approach to this important issue, the broader needs of children living with this disease and their families will continue to be misunderstood and inadequately addressed.

References

Aaronson, N., Meyerowitz, B., & Bard, M. (1991). Quality of life research in oncology: Past achievements and future priorities. *Cancer, 67*, 839–843.

Ahlfield, J., Soler, N., & Marcus, S. (1985). The young adult with diabetes: Impact of the disease on marriage and having children. *Diabetes Care, 8*, 52–56.

American Diabetes Association. (1998a). Implications for the Diabetes Control and Complications Trial. *Diabetes Care, 21*, suppl. 1, S89–S90.

American Diabetes Association. (1998b). Prevention of type 1 diabetes mellitus. *Diabetes Care, 21*, suppl. 1, S83.

Amiel, S., Sherwin, R., Siminson, D., Lauritano, A., & Tamborlane, W. (1986). Impaired insulin action in puberty: A contributing factor to poor glycemic control in adolescents with diabetes. *New England Journal of Medicine, 315*, 215–219.

Bjorgaas, M., Gimse, R., Vik, T., & Sand, T. (1997). Cognitive function in Type 1 diabetic children with and without episodes of severe hypoglycemia. *Acta Paediatrica, 86*, 148–153.

Blethen, S., Sargeant, D., Whitlow, M., & Santiago, J. (1981). Effect of pubertal stage and recent blood glucose control on plasma somatomedin C in children with insulin-dependent diabetes. *Diabetes, 30*, 868–872.

Bloch, C., Clemons, P., & Sterling, M. (1987). Puberty decreases insulin sensitivity. *Journal of Pediatrics, 110*, 481–487.

Bloomgarden, Z. (1997). American Diabetes Association annual meeting, 1997: Obesity, diabetes prevention, and type 1 diabetes. *Diabetes Care, 20*, 1913–1917.

Bobrow, E., AvRuskin, R., & Siller, J. (1985). Mother-daughter interaction and adherence to diabetes regimens. *Diabetes Care, 8*, 146–151.

Boyer, J.G., & Earp, J.L. (1997). The development of an instrument for assessing the QL of people with diabetes: Diabetes-39. *Medical Care, 35*, 440–453.

Brown, R.T., Kaslow, N.J., Sansbury, L., Meacham, L., & Culler, F.L. (1991). Internalizing and externalizing symptoms and attributional style in youth with diabetes. *Journal of the American Academy of Child and Adolescent Psychiatry, 30*, 921–925.

Cadman, D., Boyle, M., & Offord, D. (1988). The Ontario Child Health Study: Social adjustment and mental health of siblings of children with chronic health problems. *Journal of Developmental and Behavioral Pediatrics, 13*, 11–16.

Changelau, E., Schiffers, T., Schutze, J., & Hansen, B. (1997). Effect of patient-selected intensive therapy on QL. *Patient Education and Counseling, 30*, 167–173.

Christensen, N., Terry, R., Wyatt, S., Prichert, J., & Lorenz, R. (1983). Quantitative assessment of dietary adherence in patients with insulin dependent diabetes mellitus. *Diabetes Care, 6*, 245–250.

Cowie, C., & Eberhardt, M. (1995). Sociodemographic characteristics of persons with diabetes (pp. 85–116). In M. Harris (Ed.), *Diabetes in America* (pp. 37–46) (NIH Publication No. 95–1468). Bethesda, MD: U.S. Department of Health and Human Services, National Institutes of Health.

Cox, D.J., Irvine, A., Gonder-Frederick, L., Nowacek, G., & Butterfield, J. (1987). Fear of hypoglycemia: Quantification, validation, and utilization. *Diabetes Care, 10*, 617–621.

Cutfield, W., Bergman, R., Menon, R., & Sperling, M. (1990). The modified minimal model: Applications to measurement of insulin sensitivity in children. *Journal of Clinical Endocrinology and Metabolism, 70*, 1644–1650.

Davidson, M.B. (Ed.) (1991). *Clinical diabetes mellitus: A problem-oriented approach.* New York: Thieme Medical Publications.

Davis, E.A., Keating, B., Byrne, G.C., Russell, M., & Jones, T.W. (1997). Hypoglycemia: Incidence and clinical predictors in a large population-based sample of children and adolescents with IDDM. *Diabetes Care, 20*, 22–25.

Diabetes Control and Complications Trial Research Group (1987). Diabetes Control and Complications Trial (DCCT): Design and methodological considerations for the feasibility phase. *Diabetes Care, 10*, 1–19.

DCCT Research Group (1994). Effect of intensive diabetes treatment on the development and progression of long-term complications in adolescents with insulin-dependent diabetes mellitus: Diabetes Control and Complications Trial. *The Journal of Pediatrics, 125*, 177–188.

DCCT Research Group (1996). Influence of intensive diabetes treatment on quality-of-life outcomes in the Diabetes Control and Complications Trial. *Diabetes Care, 19*, 195–203.

DCCT Research Group (1988). Reliability and validity of a diabetes quality-of-life measure for the Diabetes Control and Complications Trial (DCCT). *Diabetes Care, 11*, 725–732.

DCCT Research Group (1993). The effect of intensive treatment of diabetes on the development and progression of long-term complications in insulin-dependent diabetes mellitus. *New England Journal of Medicine, 329*, 977–986.

Diabetes Prevention Trial-Type 1. (1994). *Protocol*. National Institute of Diabetes and Digestive and Kidney Diseases, National Institutes of Health.

Egger, M., Gschwend, S., Smith, G.D., & Zuppinger, K. (1991). Increasing incidence of hypoglycemic coma in children with IDDM. *Diabetes Care, 14*, 1001–1005.

Eisen, M., Donald, C.A., Ware, J.E., & Brook, R.H. (1980). *Conceptualization and measurement of health for children in the health insurance study*. Santa Monica, CA: The RAND Corporation, R-2313-HEW.

Eisen, M., Ware, J.E., Donald, C.A., & Brook, R.H. (1979). Measuring components of children's health status. *Medical Care, 17*, 902–921.

Eisen, C., Flynn, M., Green, E., Havermans, T., Kirby, R., & Sandeman, D. (1992). Quality of life in young adults with type 1 diabetes in relation to demographic and disease variables. *Diabetic Medicine, 9*, 375–378.

Ferrari, M. (1984). Chronic illness: Psychosocial effects on siblings. I. Chronically ill boys. *Journal of Child Psychology and Psychiatry, 25*, 459–476.

Fowler, M.G., Johnson, M.P., & Atkinson, S.S. (1985). School achievement and absence in children with chronic health conditions. *Journal of Pediatrics, 106*, 683–687.

Golden, M.P., Ingersoll, G.M., Brack, C.J., Russell, B.A., Wright, J.C., & Huberty, T.J. (1989). Longitudinal relationship of asymptomatic hypoglycemia to cognitive function in IDDM. *Diabetes Care, 12*, 89–93.

Green, L.B., Wysocki, T., & Reineck, B.M. (1990). Fear of hypoglycemia in children and adolescents with diabetes. *Journal of Pediatric Psychology, 15*, 633–641.

Grey, M., Cameron, M., Lipman, T., & Thurber, F. (1995). Psychosocial status of children with diabetes in the first 2 years after diagnosis. *Diabetes Care, 18*, 1330–1336.

Grey, M., Cameron, M., & Thurber, F. (1991). Coping and adaptation in children with diabetes. *Nursing Research, 40*, 144–149.

Gschwend, S., Ryan, C., Atchison, J., Arslanian, S., & Becker, D. (1995). Effects of acute hyperglycemia on mental efficiency and counterregulatory hormones in adolescents with insulin dependent diabetes mellitus. *Journal of Pediatrics, 126*, 178–184.

Guyatt, G.H., Feeny, D.H., & Patrick, D.L. (1993). Measuring health-related QL. *Annals of Internal Medicine, 118*, 622–629.

Hanestad, B.R. (1993). Self-reported QL and the effect of different clinical and demographic characteristics in people with type 1 diabetes. *Diabetes Research and Clinical Practice, 19*, 139–149.

Hanestad, B.R., & Albrektsen, G. (1991). Quality of life, perceived difficulties in adherence to a diabetes regimen, and blood glucose control. *Diabetic Medicine, 8*, 759–764.

Hanestad, B.R., & Albrektsen, G. (1992). The stability of QL experience in people with type 1 diabetes over a period of a year. *Journal of Advanced Nursing, 17*, 777–784.

Hanson, C., DeMcGuire, M., Schinkel, A., & Henggeler, S. (1992a). Comparing social learning and family systems correlates of adaptation in youths with IDDM. *Journal of Pediatric Psychology, 17*, 555–572.

Hanson, C., DeMcGuire, M., Schinkel, A., & Koltermen, O. (1995). Empirical validation for a family-centered model of care. *Diabetes Care, 18*, 1347–1356.

Hanson, C., Henggeler, S., Harris, M., Cigrang, J., Schinkel, A., Rodrigue, J., & Klesges, R. (1992b). Contributions of sibling relations to the adaptation of youths with insulin-dependent diabetes mellitus. *Journal of Consulting and Clinical Psychology, 60*, 104–112.

Harris, M. (1995). Summary (pp. 1–13). In M. Harris (Ed.), *Diabetes in America* (pp. 37–46) (NIH Publication No. 95–1468). Bethesda, MD: U.S. Department of Health and Human Services, National Institutes of Health.

Hauenstein, E., Marvin, R., Snyder, A., & Clarke, W. (1989). Stress in parents of children with diabetes mellitus. *Diabetes Care, 12*, 18–19.

Hauser, S., Jacobson, A., Lavori, P., Wolfsdorf, J., Herskowitz, R., Milley, J., & Bliss, R. (1990). Adherence among children and adolescents with insulin-dependent diabetes mellitus over a four-year longitudinal follow-up: II. Immediate and long-term linkages to family milieu. *Journal of Pediatric Psychology, 15*, 527–542.

Holden, E., Chmielewski, D., Nelson, C., & Kager, V. (1997). Controlling for general and disease-specific effects in child and family adjustment to chronic childhood illness. *Journal of Pediatric Psychology, 22*, 15–27.

Holmes, C.S., Dunlap, W.P., Chen, R.S., & Cornwell, J.M. (1992). Gender differences in the learning status of diabetic children. *Journal of Consulting and Clinical Psychology, 60*, 698–704.

Ingersoll, G.M., & Marrero, D.G. (1991). A modified quality-of-life measure for youths: Psychometric properties. *The Diabetes Educator, 17*, 114–118.

Ingersoll, G.M., Orr, D., Herrold, A., & Golden, M. (1986). Cognitive maturity and self-management among adolescents with insulin-requiring diabetes mellitus. *Journal of Pediatrics, 108*, 620–623.

Jacobson, A.M., & DCCT Research Group (1994). The Diabetes Quality of Life Measure. In C. Bradley (Ed.), *Handbook of psychology and diabetes: A guide to psychological measurement in diabetes research and management* (pp. 65–87). Chur, Switzerland: Harwood Academic Publishers.

Jacobson, A., DeGroot, M., & Samson, J.A. (1994). The evaluation of two measures of QL in patients with type I and type II diabetes. *Diabetes Care, 17*, 267–274.

Jacobson, A., Hauser, S., Lavori, P., Wolfsdorf, J., Herskowtiz, R., Milley, J., Bliss, R., Gelfand, E., Wertlieb, D., & Stein, J. (1990). Adherence among children and adolescents with insulin dependent mellitus over a four year longitudinal follow-up. I. The influence of patient coping and adjustment. *Journal of Pediatric Psychology, 15*, 511–526.

Jacobson, A., Hauser, S., Willett, J., Wolfsdorf, J., Dvorak, R., Herman, L., & DeGroot, M. (1997). Psychological adjustment to IDDM: 10-year follow-up of an onset cohort of child and adolescent patients. *Diabetes Care, 20*, 811–818.

Jacobson, A., Hauser, S., Wolfsdorf, J., Houlihan, J., Milley, J., Herskowtiz, R., Wertlieb, D., & Watt, E. (1987). Psychological predictors of compliance in children with recent onset diabetes mellitus. *Journal of Pediatrics, 110*, 805–811.

Jenkinson, C. (1994). Quality of life measurement: Does it have a place in routine clinical assessment? *Journal of Psychosomatic Research*, 38, 377–381.

Johnson, S.B. (1997). Behavioral and psychological issues in the prevention of Type 1 diabetes. Invited presentation, Annual meeting of the American Diabetes Association, Boston, MA.

Johnson, S.B. (1995). Managing insulin dependent diabetes mellitus: A developmental perspective. In J. Wallander & L. Siegel (Eds.), *Adolescent health problems: Behavioral perspectives* (pp. 265–288). New York: Guilford Press.

Johnson, S.B., Freund, A., Silverstein, J., Hansen, C., & Malone, J. (1990). Adherence-health status relationships in childhood diabetes. *Health Psychology, 9*, 606–631.

Johnson, S.B., Kelly, M., Henretta, J., Cunningham, W., Tomer, A., & Silverstein, J. (1992). A longitudinal analysis of adherence and health status in childhood diabetes. *Journal of Pediatric Psychology, 17*, 537–553.

Johnson, S.B., Riley, W., Hansen, C., & Nurick, M. (1990). Psychological impact of islet cell-antibody screening: Preliminary results. *Diabetes Care, 13*, 93–97.

Johnson, S.B., Silverstein, J., Rosenbloom, A., Carter, R., & Cunningham, W. (1986). Assessing daily management of childhood diabetes. *Health Psychology, 5*, 545–564.

Johnson, S.B., & Tercyak, K. (1995). Psychological impact of islet cell antibody screening for IDDM on children, adults, and their family members. *Diabetes Care, 18*, 1370–1372.

Kaplan, R.M. (1994). Using quality of life information to set priorities in health policy. *Social Indicators Research, 33*, 121–163.

Kovacs, M., Brent, D., Steinberg, T., Paulauskas, S., & Reid, J. (1986). Children's self-reports of psychological adjustment and coping strategies during the first year of insulin-dependent diabetes mellitus. *Diabetes Care, 9*, 472–479.

Kovacs, M., Finkelstein, R., Feinberg, R., Crouse-Novak, M., Paulauskas, S., & Pollack, M. (1985). Initial psychological responses of parents to the diagnosis of insulin-dependent diabetes mellitus in their children. *Diabetes Care, 8*, 568–575.

Kovacs, M., Ho, V., & Pollock, M. (1995). Criterion and predictive validity of the diagnosis of adjustment disorder: A prospective study of youths with new-onset insulin-dependent diabetes mellitus. *American Journal of Psychiatry, 152*, 523–528.

Kovacs, M., Iyengar, S., Goldston, D., Obrosky, D., Stewart, J., & Marsh, J. (1990). Psychological functioning among mothers of children with insulin-dependent diabetes mellitus: A longitudinal study. *Journal of Consulting and Clinical Psychology, 58*, 189–195.

Kovacs, M., Obrosky, D.S., Goldston, D., & Drash, A. (1997). Major depressive disorder in youths with IDDM: A controlled prospective study of course and outcome. *Diabetes Care, 20*, 45–51.

Kuttner, M.J., Delamater, A.M., & Santiago, J.V. (1990). Learned helplessness in diabetic youths. *Journal of Pediatric Psychology, 15*, 581–594.

La Greca, A., Auslander, W., Greco, W., Spetter, D., Fisher, E., & Santiago, J. (1995a). I get by with a little help from my family and friends: Adolescents' support for diabetes care. *Journal of Pediatric Psychology, 20*, 449–476.

La Greca, A.M., Swales, T., Klemp, S., & Madigan, S. (1995b). Adolescents with diabetes: Gender differences in psychosocial functioning and glycemic control. *Children's Health Care, 24*, 61–78.

Landgraf, J.M., Abetz, L.N., & Ware, J.E. (1996). Measuring health outcomes in pediatric populations: Issues in psychometrics and application. In B. Spilker (Ed.), *Quality of life and pharmacoeconomics in clinical trials: Second edition* (pp. 793–802). Philadelphia, PA: Lippincott-Raven Publishers.

LaPorte, R.E., Matsushima, M., & Chang, Y. (1995). Prevalence and incidence of insulin-dependent diabetes. In M. Harris (Ed.), *Diabetes in America* (pp. 37–46) (NIH Publication No. 95–1468). Bethesda, MD: U.S. Department of Health and Human Services, National Institutes of Health.

Lloyd, C.E., Matthews, K.A., Wing, R.R., & Orchard, T.J. (1992). Psychosocial factors and complications of IDDM. *Diabetes Care, 15*, 166–172.

Lloyd, C., Robinson, N., Andrews, B., Elston, M., & Fuller, J. (1993). Are the social relationships of young insulin-dependent diabetic patients affected by their condition? *Diabetic Medicine, 10*, 481–485.

Lloyd, C., Robinson, N., & Fuller, J. (1993). Education and employment experiences in young adults with type 1 diabetes mellitus. *Diabetic Medicine, 9*, 661–666.

Lorenz, R., Christensen, N., & Prichert, J. (1985). Diet-related knowledge, skill, and adherence among children with insulin-dependent diabetes mellitus. *Pediatrics, 75*, 872–876.

McCrimmon, R.J., Gold, A.E., Deary, I.J., Kelnar, C.J.H., & Frier, B.M. (1995). Symptoms of hypoglycemia in children with IDDM. *Diabetes Care, 18*, 858–861.

McSweeny, A.J., & Creer, T.L. (1995). Health-related qualityof-life assessment in medical care. *Disease-a-Month, 41*, 1–71.

Marrero, D.S., Guare, J.C., Vandagriff, J.L., & Fineberg, N.S. (1997). Fear of hypoglycemia in the parents of children and adolescents with diabetes: Maladaptive or healthy response? *The Diabetes Educator, 23*, 281–286.

Miller-Johnson, S., Emery, R., Marvin, R., Clarke, W., Lovinger, R., & Martin, M. (1994). Parent-child relationships and the management of insulin-dependent diabetes mellitus. *Journal of Consulting and Clinical Psychology, 62*, 603–610.

Mullins, L.L., Chaney, J.M., Hartman, V.L., Olson, R.A., Youll, L.K., & Reyes, S. (1995). Child and maternal adaptation to cystic fibrosis and insulin-dependent diabetes mellitus: Differential patterns across disease states. *Journal of Pediatric Psychology, 20*, 173–186.

Nassau, J., & Drotar, D. (1995). Social competence in children with IDDM and asthma: Child, teacher, and parent reports of children's social adjustment, social performance, and social skills. *Journal of Pediatric Psychology, 20,* 187–204.

Nathan, D.M., Fogel, H., Norman, D., Russell, P.S., Tolkoff-Rublin, N., Delmonico, F.L., Auchinloss, H., Camuso, J., & Cosimi, A.B. (1991). Long-term metabolic and quality of life results with pancreatic/renal transplantation in insulin-dependent diabetes mellitus. *Transplantation, 52,* 85–91.

NDIC. (1994). *Diabetes Control and Complications Trial (DCCT).* Bethesda MD: US Department of Health and Human Services, NIH Publications No. 94–3874.

Nelms, B.C. (1989). Emotional behaviors in chronically ill children. *Journal of Abnormal Child Psychology, 17,* 657–668.

Nelson, E.C., Wasson, J.H., Johnson, D.J., & Hays, R.D. (1996). Dartmouth COOP functional health assessment charts: Brief measures for clinical practice. In B. Spilker (Ed.), *Quality of life and pharmacoeconomics in clinical trials:* Second edition (pp. 161–168). Philadelphia, PA: Lippincott-Raven Publishers.

Nerenz, D.R., Repasky, D.P., Whitehouse, F.W., & Kahkonen, D.M. (1992). Ongoing assessment of health status in patients with diabetes mellitus. *Medical Care, 30,* MS112–MS124.

Neumark-Sztainer, D., Story, M., Toporoff, E., Cassuto, N., Resnick, M., & Blum, R. (1996). Psychosocial predictors of binge eating and purging behaviors among adolescents with diabetes mellitus. *Journal of Adolescent Health, 19,* 289–296.

Northam, E., Anderson, P., Adler, R., Werther, G., & Warne, G. (1996). Psychosocial and family functioning in children with insulin-dependent diabetes at diagnosis and one year later. *Journal of Pediatric Psychology, 21,* 699–717.

Parkerson, G.R., Connis, R.T., Broadhead, W.E., Patrick, D.L., Taylor, T.R., & Tse, C.J. (1993). Disease-specific versus generic measurement of health-related QL in insulin-dependent diabetic patients. *Medical Care, 31,* 629–639.

Patrick, D.L., & Deyo, R.A. (1989). Generic and disease-specific measures in assessing health status and QL. *Medical Care, 27,* S217–S232.

Patrick, D.L., & Erickson, P. (1993). *Health status and health policy: Allocating resources to health care.* New York, NY: Oxford University Press.

Peveler, R.C., Fairburn, C.G., Boller, I., & Dunger, D. (1991). Eating disorders in adolescents with IDDM: A controlled study. *Diabetes Care, 15,* 1356–1360.

Piehlmeier, W., Bullinger, M., Kirchberger, I., Land, W., & Landgraf, R. (1996). Evaluation of the QL of patients with insulin-dependent diabetes mellitus before and after organ transplantation with the SF 36 Health Survey. *European Journal of Surgery, 162,* 933–940.

Pollock, M., Kovacs, M., & Charron-Prochownik, D. (1995). Eating disorders and maladaptive dietary/insulin management among youths with childhood-onset insulin-dependent diabetes mellitus. *Journal of the American Academy of Child and Adolescent Psychiatry, 34,* 291–296.

Reich, J.N., Kaspar, C., Puczynski, M.S., Puczynski, S., Cleland, J.W., Dell'Angela, K., & Emanuele, M.A. (1990). Effect of a hypoglycemic episode on neuropsychological functioning in diabetic children. *Journal of Clinical and Experimental Neuropsychology, 12,* 613–626.

Riley, W., Maclaren, N., Krischer, J., Spillar, R., Silverstein, J., Schatz, D., Schwartz, S., Malone, J., Shah, S., Vadheim, C., & Rotter, J. (1990). A prospective study of the development of diabetes in relatives of patients with insulin-dependent diabetes. *New England Journal of Medicine, 323,* 1167–1172.

Robinson, N., Stevens, L., & Protopapa, L. (1993). Education and employment for young people with diabetes. *Diabetic Medicine, 10,* 983–989.

Robinson, N., Yateman, L., Protopapa, L., & Bush, L. (1989). Unemployment and diabetes. *Diabetic Medicine, 6,* 797–803.

Rodin, G.M., Daneman, D., Johnson, L.E., Kenshole, A., & Garfinkel, P. (1985). Anorexia nervosa and bulimia in female adolescents with insulin dependent diabetes mellitus: A systematic study. *Journal of Psychiatric Research, 19,* 381–385.

Rovet, J., Ehrlich, R., & Hoppe, M. (1987). Behaviour problems in children with diabetes as a function of sex and age of onset of disease. *Journal of Child Psychology and Psychiatry, 28,* 477–491.

Rovet, J.F., Ehrlich, R.M., & Hoppe, M. (1988). Specific intellectual deficits in children with early onset diabetes mellitus. *Child Development, 59*, 226–234.

Rovet, J.F., Ehrlich, R.M., Czuchta, D., & Akler, M. (1993). Psychoeducational characteristics of children and adolescents with insulin dependent diabetes mellitus. *Journal of Learning Disabilities, 26*, 7–22.

Royal, G., & Roberts, M. (1987). Students' perceptions of and attitudes toward disabilities: A comparison of twenty conditions. *Journal of Clinical Child Psychology, 16*, 122–132.

Ryan, C.M. (1990). Neuropsychological consequences and correlates of diabetes in childhood. In C.S. Holmes (Ed.), *Neuropsychological and behavioral aspects of diabetes* (pp. 58–84). New York, NY: Springer-Verlag.

Ryan, C.M., Atchison, J., Puczynski, S., Puczynski, M., Arslanian, S., & Becker, D. (1990). Mild hypoglycemia associated with deterioration of mental efficiency in children with insulin dependent diabetes mellitus. *Journal of Pediatrics, 117*, 32–38.

Ryan, C.M., Longstreet, C. & Morrow, L. (1985). The effects of diabetes mellitus on the school attendance and school achievement of adolescents. *Child: Care, Health, and Development, 11*, 229–240.

Ryan, C., Vega, A., & Drash, A. (1985). Cognitive deficits in adolescents who developed diabetes early in life. *Pediatrics, 75*, 921–927.

Sahler, O., Roghmann, K., Carpenter, P., Mulhern, R., Dolgin, M., Sargent, J., Barbarin, O., Copeland, D., & Zeltzer, L. (1994). Sibling adaptation to childhood cancer collaborative study: Prevalence of sibling distress and definition of adaptation levels. *Journal of Developmental and Behavioral Pediatrics, 15*, 353–366.

Saudek, C., Rubin, R., & Shump, C. (1997). *The Johns Hopkins guide to diabetes for today and tomorrow*. Baltimore, MD: Johns Hopkins University Press.

Schafer, L., Glasgow, R., McCaul, K., & Dreher, M. (1983). Adherence to IDDM regimens: Relationship to psychosocial variables and metabolic control. *Diabetes Care, 6*, 493–498.

Schafer, L., McCaul, K., & Glasgow, R. (1986). Supportive and nonsupportive family behaviors: Relationships to adherence and metabolic control in persons with Type 1 diabetes. *Diabetes Care, 9*, 179–185.

Schatz, D., Krischer, J., Horne, G., Riley, W., Spillar, R., Silverstein, J., Winter, W., Muir, A., Derovanesian, D., Shah, S., Malone, J., & Maclaren, N. (1994). Islet cell antibodies predict insulin-dependent diabetes in United States school age children as powerfully as unaffected relatives. *Journal of Clinical Investigation, 93*, 2403–2407.

Schipper, H., Clinch, J.J., & Olweny, C.L.M. (1996). Quality of life studies: Definitions and conceptual issues. In B. Spilker (Ed.), *Quality of life and pharmacoeconomics in clinical trials:* Second edition (pp. 11–23). Philadelphia, PA: Lippincott-Raven Publishers.

Schoenherr, S.J., Brown, R.T., Baldwin, K., & Kaslow, N.J. (1992). Attributional styles and psychopathology in pediatric chronic-illness groups. *Journal of Clinical Child Psychology, 21*, 380–387.

Selam, J.L., Micossi, P., Dunn, F.L., Nathan, D.M. & Implantable Insulin Pump Trial Study Group (1992). Clinical trial of programmable implantable insulin pump for Type I diabetes. *Diabetes Care, 15*, 877–884.

Spieth, L.E., & Harris, C.V. (1996). Assessment of health-related quality of life in children and adolescents: An integrative review. *Journal of Pediatric Psychology, 21*, 175–194.

Starfield, B., Bergner, M., Ensminger, M., Riley, A., Ryan, S., Green, B., McGauhey, P., Skinner, A., & Kim, S. (1993). Adolescent health status measurement: Development of the Child Health and Illness Profile. *Pediatrics, 91*, 430–435.

Stein, R.E., & Jessop, D.J. (1990). Functional status II. *Medical Care, 28*, 1041–1055.

Sterling, C., & Friedman, A. (1996). Empathic responding in children with chronic illness. *Children's Health Care, 25*, 53–69.

Striegel-Moore, R. (1993). Etiology of binge eating: A developmental perspective. In C. Fairburn & T. Wilson (Eds.), *Binge eating: Nature, assessment, and treatment* (pp. 285–292). New York: Guilford.

Striegel-Moore, R.H., Nicholson, T.J., & Tamborlane, W.V. (1992). Prevalence of eating disorder symptoms in preadolescent and adolescent girls with IDDM. *Diabetes Care, 15,* 1361–1367.

Tebbi, C., Bromberg, C., Sills, I., Cukierman, J., & Piedmonte, M. (1990). Vocational adjustment and general well-being of young adults with IDDM. *Diabetes Care, 13,* 99–103.

Tercyak, K., Johnson, S.B., & Schatz, D. (1997). Patient and family perceptions of the use of subcutaneous insulin to prevent IDDM: Implications for future prevention trials. *Diabetes, 46,* supplement 1, Abstract No. 54, pg. 14A.

Thai, A., & Eisenbarh, G. (1993). Natural history of IDDM. *Diabetes Reviews, 1,* 1–14.

Wallander, J.L., Varni, J.W., Babani, L., Banis, H.T., & Wilcox, K.T. (1988). Children with chronic physical disorders: Maternal reports of their psychological adjustment. *Journal of Pediatric Psychology, 13,* 197–212.

Wasson, J.H., Kairys, S.W., Nelson, E.C., Kalishman, N., & Baribeau, P. (1994). A short survey for assessing health and social problems of adolescents. *Journal of Family Practice, 38,* 489–494.

Wertlieb, D., Hauser, S.T., & Jacobson, A.M. (1986). Adaptation to diabetes: Behavior symptoms and family context. *Journal of Pediatric Psychology, 11,* 463–479.

White, N.H., Johnson, P.D., Wolf, F.M., & Anderson, B.J. (1989). Behaviors aimed at avoiding hypoglycemia in adolescents with IDDM. *Diabetes, 38,* 8A.

Wysocki, R., Hough, B., Ward, K., & Green, L. (1992). Diabetes mellitus in the transition to adulthood: Adjustment, self-care, and health status. *Developmental and Behavioral Pediatrics, 13,* 194–201.

Wysocki, T., Huxtable, K., Linscheid, T., & Wayne, W. (1989). Adjustment to diabetes mellitus in preschoolers and their mothers. *Diabetes Care, 12,* 524–529.

Chapter 15

INTELLECTUAL DISABILITY

Jan L. Wallander
Luanne Turrentine

There has been an explosion of interest in the quality of life (QL) of people with intellectual disability, mental retardation, or developmental disabilities (the term intellectual disability will be preferred throughout this chapter for reasons explained below). This is evidenced in part by the numerous volumes published on QL in people with intellectual disability (ID) (e.g., Brown, 1997; Goode, 1994; Renwick, Brown, & Nagler, 1996; Schalock, 1996, 1997), as well as the many journal articles presenting data and discussions on this topic in recent years (see Hughes, Hwang, Kim, Eisenman, & Killian, 1995, for a content analysis of this literature). Schalock (1994) attributed this explosion of interest in QL of people with ID to several phenomena (see also Brown, Renwick, & Nagler, 1997), including: the (a) strong interest in developing and evaluating *quality* in various relevant areas (e.g., service, management); (b) a *paradigm shift* to an emphasis on inclusion, equity, and empowerment in addressing the needs of people with ID; and (c) demonstrable results from successful *habilitation* strategies (e.g., skill training, natural supports). While he notes that the concept of QL is not new to ID, what is new is the belief that QL is an integral part of the service delivery and evaluation of habilitation outcomes for people with ID. Stark and Goldsbury (1990) similarly observed that:

> despite the billions of dollars that have been allocated in implementing policies such as deinstitutionalization, mainstreaming, early intervention, and community integration, we have not yet answered the critical question: "Has it really made a difference in improving the *quality* of life for persons with [intellectual disability]?" (p. 71).

Consequently, QL has emerged as a critical concept in the area of ID. However, as with the other conditions discussed in this volume, the vast majority of the work to date regarding QL and ID has been directed at adults, both explicitly and implicitly. Very few have even discussed issues in applying QL to children and adolescents[1] with ID, much less conducted empirical work with young participants. The overarching goal of this chapter is to stimulate efforts to fill in this gap.

This chapter will commence with a description of ID as a condition and how it may compromise QL in young people. A definition of QL for young people with ID and adoption of an existing model of its content will be proposed. Subsequently, existing quantitative instruments measuring QL in youth with ID will be reviewed, together with a few that have employed alternative qualitative approaches with adults with ID and which may have utility for young people. This is followed by recommendations for future work with the QL concept in the areas of measurement, research, and service relevant to young people with ID.

As a final note in establishing the parameters of this chapter, we will not concern ourselves with the substantial literature regarding defining and measuring personal growth, functional independence, and activities of daily living. These notions have some overlap with QL when applied to people with ID, but are more narrowly defined and have a tradition separate from QL. Measures of these concepts have been reviewed elsewhere (e.g., Leland, 1991; Sattler, 1988).

INTELLECTUAL DISABILITY AS A CONDITION IMPAIRING QUALITY OF LIFE
CORE FEATURES OF INTELLECTUAL DISABILITY

Various terms have been and are being used to refer to what is herein termed ID. We prefer the term ID because of its descriptive nature, highlighting one of the core features of this condition, and its relatively higher international acceptance. For example, it is the preferred term of the International Society for the Study of Intellectual Disability, the largest global association devoted to this condition. Nonetheless, different terms are popular in different countries, such as mental retardation in the US (American Association on Mental Retardation [AAMR], 1992), developmental disability in Ontario, Canada (Woodhill et al., 1994), and learning disability in the UK (e.g., Felce & Perry, 1997).

Further complicating a description of this condition is the fact that different definitions have been used over time (e.g., AAMR, 1959, 1961, 1973, 1983, 1992). Likewise, different definitions are currently being used across countries and cultures as well as in different systems within a country. However at present, most of these definitions include three core features (Hodapp & Dykens, 1996). That is, persons with ID have (a) subnormal intellectual functioning and (b) deficits in adaptive behavior or the ability to perform "daily activities required for personal and social self-sufficiency" (Sparrow, Balla, & Cicchetti, 1984, p. 6), both of which are (c) manifested early in life, generally construed as before age 18 years.

It follows that definitions promulgated by different systems will operationalize these core features in somewhat different ways. For example, the AAMR (1992) currently defines subnormal intellectual functioning as "IQ standard scores of approximately 70 to 75 and below" (p. 5). The American Psychiatric Association (APA, 1994) sets a defining limit in its DSM-IV of "an IQ of approximately 70 or below" (p. 46). The World Health Organization (1992) sets the IQ standard score limit as 69 or less in the ICD-10. While appearing as a slight difference, the more liberal AAMR definition could lead to the diagnosis of twice as many people as having ID purely on statistical grounds (Reschly, 1992). In as much as these definitions vary, there is considerable further variation in definitions applied by different service systems within countries. This can lead to markedly different prevalence rates of ID, for example in school age children in different locations in the United States (Hovinga, 1998).

Of course, no definition of ID applied today relies solely on intellectual deficit. All recognize that adaptive behaviors also need to be deficient to warrant a diagnosis of ID. However, here too differences are apparent between systems. The AAMR holds that a person must show a deficit in two of 10 identified adaptive areas (e.g., communication, self-care, community use), which is similar to the DSM-IV except that it identifies 11 areas. The ICD-10 definition does not list areas, instead it points to diminished social competence as the key feature. This lower specificity is consistent with the ICD-10, being intended to have international relevance and recognition that adaptive behaviors must be culturally referenced. It is conceivable that the defined adaptive behavior areas in the AAMR or DSM-IV definitions are not universally applicable. That is, different adaptive behavior areas could be more important in a technologically advanced, compared to a developing country, or across time in the same country.

Depending on how one defines ID, its prevalence estimates will vary widely. Regardless of the issue of definition, moreover, there have been few solid epidemiological studies of ID using acceptable case-finding procedures. Therefore, discussion of prevalence typically concludes that there is a range of between one and three percent who have ID in the population in developed countries. More males than females are found in developed countries, resulting in part from several sex-linked disorders causing ID. ID is more prevalent among children who are of lower socioeconomic status (SES) and who are from minority groups within each country. However, on closer examination, this over-representation, in relation to population parameters, appears only at the milder levels of ID (Hodapp & Dykens, 1996). Little is known about the prevalence of ID in developing countries.

LEVELS OF FUNCTIONING

ID encompasses individuals with a wide variation in functioning across the core features of intelligence and adaptive behavior. This in turn has numerous implications for QL. Although alternative classifications have been proposed (e.g., AAMR, 1992), most research on ID considers people with ID as functioning at either the mild, moderate, severe, or profound level of disability. Even within these levels, individual differences are quite apparent (cf. Hodapp & Dykens, 1996; AAMR, 1992 for detailed description of levels). Nonetheless, generally the following holds:

Mild ID constitutes the largest group, by far, of people with ID, possibly making up 90% of the total (APA, 1994). Defined typically as having an IQ between 55–70, individuals with mild ID appear similar to those without ID upon initial examination and often blend into the general population in the years before and after formal schooling. Usually there is no co-morbid physical impairment. This level of disability is often not recognized until the child is in school, sometimes not until several years into formal education. In most developed countries, some form of special education is provided for students with ID. Depending on the needs of the student and the prevailing philosophy, this may take any form from attending a segregated school with a specialized curriculum to attending regular classes with age mates where some special services or considerations are given. By the time they reach adulthood, people with mild ID can be described as having a cognitive ability approximately equal to that of average 9–12 year olds without ID. While some will live independently and hold jobs, marry, and raise families, most need help in negotiating problems and tasks in life (Edgerton, Bollinger, & Herr, 1984).

Moderate ID is the second most common level of disability, including people with an IQ typically from 40–54. Children with this level of disability most often are recognized during the preschool years, which may result in them receiving early intervention or at-risk services in an attempt to reduce the impact of the disability. Many individuals with moderate ID have an organic etiology (e.g., chromosomal abnormality, such as Down's Syndrome; significant exposure to teratogens, such as alcohol, during *in utero* development) and co-morbid physical impairment (e.g., seizure activity, motor coordination problems, congenital heart conditions). They typically develop a cognitive capacity by adulthood similar to that of average 6–8 year olds without ID. Most will require supports throughout their lives, such as in the form of employment in a specially designed workshop, living in a group home, and access to a trained person to help deal with both every day and special tasks.

Severe ID includes people with an IQ typically between 25–39. The majority of these individuals have an organic etiology and many show concurrent co-morbid diseases and substantial challenges in activities of daily living. For example, they may need support in completing daily hygiene tasks, feeding, and moving around in the community. Most require special assistance throughout their lives, such as living in completely supervised settings and working in a sheltered workshop or pre-workshop setting. Cognitive development by adulthood can be described to reach that of a 4–6 year old child without ID.

Profound ID is almost always caused by an organic etiology, resulting in an IQ below 25. Because many have severe co-morbid conditions, some die during childhood and early adulthood. All will need substantial supervision, and most will need to reside in facilities with substantial health-care services.

DEFINITIONS AND THE CONTENT OF THE QUALITY OF LIFE CONCEPT

Much effort has gone into establishing specific definitions of QL for people with ID. Samples of these are listed in Table 15.1. Considering there are over 100 definitions (Cummins, 1995), Schalock (1996) proposes rather that QL should not be considered "an entity that one has or does not have to some degree, [but] should be viewed as an organizing concept. [As such, QL] can be used for a number of purposes" (p. 123). Therefore, he argues, it would be reasonable to expect variations in definitions depending on the purpose to which they are applied. Nonetheless, as several have noted (e.g., Borthwick-Duffy, 1997; Cummins, 1997, Felce & Perry, 1995; Schalock, 1996), there are many commonalities in conceptualizing and defining QL evidenced in these many offerings.

Furthermore, QL definitions have included both objective and subjective variables. Generally, four models have been used (Borth-

TABLE 15.1 EXAMPLES OF DEFINITIONS OF QUALITY OF LIFE APPLIED TO PEOPLE WITH INTELLECTUAL DISABILITY

"QUALITY OF LIFE IS BOTH OBJECTIVE AND SUBJECTIVE, EACH AXIS BEING THE AGGREGATE OF SEVEN DOMAINS: MATERIAL WELL-BEING, HEALTH, PRODUCTIVITY, INTIMACY, SAFETY, COMMUNITY AND EMOTIONAL WELL-BEING." (CUMMINS, 1997, P.132)
"QUALITY OF LIFE IS DEFINED AS AN OVERALL GENERAL WELL-BEING WHICH COMPRISES OBJECTIVE DESCRIPTORS AND SUBJECTIVE EVALUATIONS OF PHYSICAL, MATERIAL, SOCIAL, EMOTIONAL, AND PRODUCTIVE WELL-BEING TOGETHER WITH THE EXTENT OF PERSONAL DEVELOPMENT AND PURPOSEFUL ACTIVITY ALL WEIGHTED BY A PERSONAL SET OF VALUES." (FELCE & PERRY, 1993, P. 11)
"THE TIMBRE OF LIFE AS EXPERIENCED SUBJECTIVELY; A PERSON'S FEELINGS ABOUT AND EVALUATIONS OF HIS OR HER OWN LIFE" (GOODE & HOGG, 1994, P. 197)
"THE DISCREPANCY BETWEEN A PERSON'S ACHIEVED AND UNMET NEEDS AND DESIRES." (MATIKKA, 1994, P. 41)
"QUALITY OF LIFE IS DEFINED AS CONCEPT THAT REFLECTS A PERSON'S DESIRED CONDITIONS OF LIVING." (SCHALOCK, 1994, P. 267)
"QUALITY OF LIFE IS THE DEGREE TO WHICH THE PERSON ENJOYS THE IMPORTANT POSSIBILITIES OF HIS OR HER LIFE." (WOODHILL, RENWICK, BROWN, & RAPHAEL, 1994, P. 67)

wick-Duffy, 1992; Felce & Perry, 1995), as discussed in Chapter 2. Thus, QL can be defined as (A) the *objective quality of the conditions* in which the person lives or (B) the person's *subjective satisfaction* with life conditions. However, few contemporary definitions strictly apply to either of these two approaches (Cummins, 1997). Rather, QL is often defined (C) as the *combination* of the objective, life-condition and subjective, satisfaction perspectives. Alternatively, (D) definitions may take into account the *person's values*, aspirations, and expectations while considering both the objective and subjective perspectives. Model D holds that a person's values should moderate the role of life conditions and personal satisfaction in establishing that person's QL (Felce & Perry, 1995). For example, to the extent the conditions of one's residence are not a priority, where one then lives would be weighted less in establishing one's QL than some other domains that are valued more. About 80% of all QL definitions in the ID area apply a combination of objective and subjective perspectives (Cummins, 1997), either as Model C or D.

Regardless of which of these models is applied, there is considerable agreement across definitions that QL is a multidimensional concept. While different approaches have been taken to delineate what are its important dimensions, between five and 15 schemes typically emerge from these efforts, often with hierarchical elements. A sample of these schemes was presented in Chapter 2 (Wallander, this volume),

Table 2.1. There is considerable overlap among the different systems, the differences being due mainly to whether and how much to subdivide. We find Felce and Perry's (1997) delineation of salient domains of QL parsimonious and useful and will use it to organize the discussion of the impact of ID on QL to follow. As shown in Figure 15.1, they suggest consideration for five domains — material, physical, social, emotional, and productive well-being — each of which is further divided.

In summary, we submit that *QL can be defined as well-being in multiple domains of life considered salient in one's culture and time and from both objective and subjective perspectives.* Consistent with the discussion in Chapter 2 (Wallander, this volume), we encourage this definition to be applied generically and do not reserve it for people with ID.

IMPACT OF INTELLECTUAL DISABILITY ON QUALITY OF LIFE

Regardless of associated level of functioning, ID can have a significant impact on the QL experienced by a person. However QL is conceptualized, ID can negatively influence all its salient domains.

Material well-being is typically reduced for children and adolescents with ID. It has been well-documented that children with mild forms of ID more often live in families with reduced financial resources (Hodapp & Dykens, 1996), with many associated consequences for QL. For example, they may reside in substandard housing located in more crowded neighborhoods. Also they may belong to larger families, such that privacy may more often be reduced for young people with ID. Material means would also influence quality and in some cases quantity of food intake, but there may also be differences in food preferences associated with the SES gradient. Dependent on which country they reside in, access to transportation may also be diminished. For example, most locales in the United States have poor public transportation, which disproportionately affects those of low SES, in contrast to, for instance, the Netherlands or Sweden. When transportation is not available, access to many opportunities that could enhance QL in other domains (e.g., training, employment, social and health services, recreational activities) is likely to be limited.

Physical well-being is compromised directly in many people with ID. As noted already, many causes of ID also cause significant physical impairment. For example, the majority (but not all) of the people with cerebral palsy — a condition of an impairment in motor coordination resulting from a brain lesion — also experience some level of ID.

410

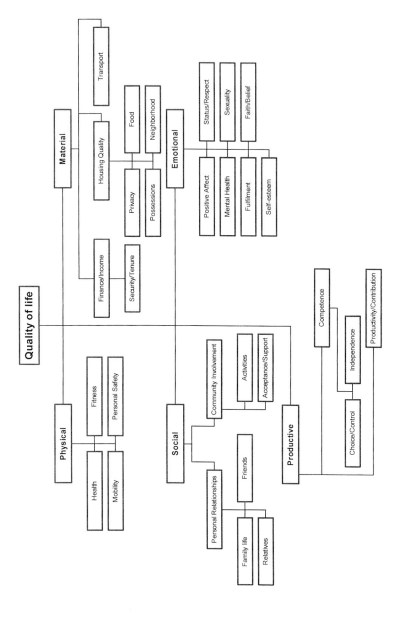

FIGURE 15.1 FELCE AND PERRY'S (1995) ADAPTED SCHEMA OF QUALITY OF LIFE DOMAINS

Beyond this obvious connection between ID and physical well-being due to shared etiology in a portion of this population, the ability of young people with ID to learn and internalize health preventive and promoting behaviors is reduced in many (Raeburn & Rootman, 1997). This may also be aggravated by sub-optimal health behaviors present in lower SES groups. Both immediate and longer-term health consequences may develop as a result.

Limited access to health care may be another influence on the physical well-being of people with ID. This may be especially so in the United States where fewer public resources are devoted to subsidizing health care for people without private or employment-based means to obtain health care (Stark & Faulkner, 1996). Young people with ID here are less likely to have parents employed with full health care benefits. This may be less of a problem in countries with universal health care policies. Also related to more often being members of low SES families, young people with ID may more often live in less safe settings, such as in the inner cities in the United States or suburban apartment housing tracts around major European cities. They are also at higher risk for physical and sexual abuse (Nagler, 1996).

Social well-being has long been observed to be a problem for young people with ID. There are several influences on this. Diminished physical and material well-being likely play a significant role. However, at a more basic level, social development is typically compromised in young people with ID, certainly the many aspects of social relations that are cognitively based (Simeonsson & Rosenthal, 1991). Also being less able to perform age-typical tasks across many areas and typically being programmatically segregated in some way in the school setting, young people with ID are often isolated (Gottlieb, Alter, & Gottlieb, 1991). Same-age peers less often choose them for friendships (Richardson & Koller, 1996). Furthermore, young people with ID have fewer opportunities for community involvement (Landesman, Vietze, & Begab, 1987). Related to the SES covariation, such activities are less available in the settings in which they more often live. In other cases, such activities are often ability-based (e.g., music, sports), for which they are less equipped to compete.

Emotional well-being has been found to be lower in children and adolescents with ID. For example, several studies have shown young people with ID — even at the mild level of disability — to be at increased risk for poorer mental health (e.g., Richardson & Koller, 1996; Wallander, Stankovic, & Brown, 1998). Prevalence estimates suggest a rate of mental health problems that is 2–5 times that observed in the general population of young people. They report or are reported with more mental health symptoms across the range of diagnostic categories. Young people with ID may also be at particularly elevated risk for some specific disorders, such as Pervasive Developmental Disorders or Attention Deficit-Hyperactivity Disorder (Coe & Matson, 1993). The self-esteem of young people with ID is also often described as reduced (e.g., Richardson & Koller, 1996).

Sexuality, as one dimension of emotional well-being, represents a special challenge regarding young people with ID. On the one hand, because being isolated and possibly stigmatized, they may have fewer opportunities to explore their sexuality in an age-typical manner through adolescence. Likewise, people with ID may not receive sex education to the same degree as typical-developing people. Even when it is provided, it may not be well matched to their cognitive development. On the other hand, young people with ID may also be more vulnerable to being used sexually by others as well as subject to frank sexual abuse (Nagler, 1996). Because of their ID, they are less likely to plan for and use contraceptives, causing the prevalence of pregnancy to be elevated in adolescents with ID compared to the general population (Kempton & Stiggall, 1989; Kleinfeld & Young, 1989). The effect on the prevalence of sexually transmitted diseases is not known, but may be elevated as well.

Finally, regarding *productive* well-being, both competence and contribution is severely challenged in young people with ID. The major task of childhood can be argued to be learning. This is certainly the priority in the school environment, where young people in developed countries spend a large portion of their time from about age 5 up to about age 18 years. The defining disability for ID interferes with learning and consequently with the development of competence and sense of contribution. Furthermore, because of a reduced rate of development and the upper limit of that development being lower in people with ID, their choices in life and control over experiences are reduced. Without developmentally appropriate gradual expansion of choice in and control over life, development is arrested and autonomy cannot develop adequately. Consequently, independence is often withheld longer in young people with ID. Indeed, for a significant portion, especially for those with profound or severe ID, independence is withheld indefinitely. While this may be desirable to maintain, for example, physical well-being, it inevitably compromises one's sense of competence and contribution.

In summary, ID can have a substantial impact on QL across all domains and throughout childhood. Although not uniform, because ID presents with considerable individual differences, and people with ID encounter different environmental supports, the vast majority of young people with ID will experience reduced opportunities for well-being across the areas of physical, material, social, emotional, and productive functioning. Even when adulthood is reached, most people with ID will continue to experience a reduced QL in these areas (e.g., Schalock, 1996).

EXISTING MEASURES OF QUALITY OF LIFE FOR PEOPLE WITH INTELLECTUAL DISABILITY

After reviewing over 225 QL instruments, Cummins (1997a) summarized 22 that have direct utility for people with some form of ID. He has furthermore published a detailed review focusing on 13 self-rated QL scales for people with ID (Cummins, 1997b). We can confirm from our own review that none of these were developed specifically for *young people with ID*.

However, two instrument developers have begun to address the need for instruments geared to this age group by constructing *general* adolescent (not specific to adolescents with ID) versions of instruments originally developed for use with adults with and without ID (Cummins et al., 1997; Keith & Schalock, 1994). We will review these instrument "systems" first (both the general adolescent and adult ID versions) and then we will consider a few additional adult ID instruments that are worthy of attention because they introduce alternative assessment approaches.

QUANTITATIVE MEASUREMENT SYSTEMS IN PART ADDRESSING YOUNG PEOPLE

Comprehensive Quality of Life Scale (ComQol)

The Comprehensive Quality of Life Scale (ComQol) consists of three parallel versions intended for use with non-disabled adults (Form A), adults with ID (Form I), and adolescents ages 11–18 attending school (Form S), respectively (Cummins, 1997a, 1997b, 1997c). The same conceptual base and approach supported the development of each form (see Table 15.1 for the relevant QL definition). The ComQol is multidimensional, addressing seven domains: material well-being, health, productivity, intimacy, safety, place in community, and emotional well-being. Moreover, a multi-axial approach is used, taking three separate measurements. Firstly, (a) *objective* and subjective perspectives are collected in each domain. The subjective perspective is then considered separately for its (b) *importance* to the individual as well as (c) perceived *satisfaction*.

There are a total of 35 items, with 21 objective indices to be completed by a proxy, and 7 ratings of importance plus 7 ratings of satisfaction being obtained from the target. Examples (taken from the adolescent version) of objective items are "How many clothes and toys do you have compared with other people of your age?" and "How often do you talk with a close friend?" Subjective items request both importance and satisfaction ratings. Examples of the former are: "How important to you are the things you own?" and "How important to you are close relationships with your family or friends?"; and of the latter: "How satisfied are you with the things you own?" and "How satisfied are you with close relationships with your family?"

On this basis four scores can be calculated in each of the seven domains: the objective, importance, satisfaction, and importance-by-satisfaction product score. The latter product score reflects Cummins argument that subjective QL is a function of both perceived satisfaction with circumstances in a domain and the importance of that domain to the individual. The ComQol takes about 15–20 minutes to complete, with the subjective section alone taking only 5 minutes. Quite well documented manuals are available for each form.

Of particular note is that the form to be used with people with ID (Form I) incorporates a pre-testing protocol to determine whether, and at what level of complexity, respondents are able to use the instrument. The results of this pre-testing inform which response scale should be used for that respondent. For example, if a respondent is only able to manage the choice between two levels of importance, then he or she will be provided with a version of ComQol-I (the other versions are not deemed to require attention to response capability) where Likert scales are presented as a binary choice. If he or she can differentiate three or five levels of responses, then the appropriate version of the instrument would have three or five response choices. In addition, two items are administered to evaluate for acquiescence tendency, which is a concern in the assessment of people with ID (e.g., Sigelman, et al., 1981). Form I takes 45 minutes to complete when this pre-testing phase is added.

Psychometric data are reported from different samples for the different forms. The adolescent form (Form S) was evaluated in two samples of 264 and 524 Australian youngsters ages 12–18 years. Normative data are provided for each sample separately. Cummins has calculated various reliability estimates with considerable sensitivity given the appropriateness of each type for the data at hand and intended uses. Both internal consistency and test-retest reliabilities appear quite reasonable. Validity data for Form S is more scant at this point. However, differences in mean scores between homeless, at risk, and non-homeless community-resident school-attending adolescents, as well as some expected associations with measures of related constructs, provide preliminary validity support.

Psychometric data for Form I, for people with ID, are also available from two samples of 59 and 115 17–63 year old residents in group homes in Australia. They were reported with a Mental Age between 3 and 9 years of age. Reliability estimates appear satisfactory even in a sample with ID, although test-retest suffers quite a bit beyond two weeks. Curiously, no validity data are provided, rather a reference is given to Form A (the general adult version). However, no information could be found in the manual for Form A pertaining to the validity when used with people with ID.

Thus, ComQol has been used with reasonably reliable results with people apparently functioning below the mild level of ID. Taking the results from Form S and Form I together, there is encouragement that ComQol can be used at least with some young people with ID. We expect that youngsters age 14–18 years with mild ID, for example, would be able to respond satisfactorily to this instrument. However, direct applications with young people with ID must be evaluated.

In summary, there is much to commend Cummins for his careful development of the ComQol. In most ways it can stand as a model for QL instrument development. Of course, it also has some outstanding issues. Foremost is the shortage of validity data. Second, the norm samples for Form I are quite small. Finally, the meaning of the four different scores must be elaborated. Widely varying correlations have been reported between the objective and subjective QL scores across the seven domains (r = .09–.41) and between the importance and satisfaction ratings across samples (r = .29–.61). There is little discussion yet about what value may be associated with each. For example, does the added complexity of weighting the subjective satisfaction score by perceived importance truly enhance the information yield or does this represent more of a conceptual distinction?

Quality of Life Questionnaire and Quality of Student Life Questionnaire

The Quality of Life Questionnaire (QOL.Q) and Quality of Student Life Questionnaire (QSL.Q) are parallel versions intended for people with ID (QOL.Q; Schalock & Keith, 1993) and adolescents from the general population attending school (QSL.Q; Keith & Schalock, 1992, 1994, 1995), respectively. To date, the QOL.Q is the most widely used instrument for measuring QL in people with ID (Cummins, 1997b). Each form has 40 items requesting subjective ratings from the respondent on three-point scales. Response scales are tailored to each item. The QSL.Q was modeled after the QOL.Q, with changes mainly in wording to fit adolescents' situations. Both forms represent an entirely subjective perspective on QL and no allowance is made for the objective perspective within these instruments.

The forms take 15–20 minutes to administer. The QSL.Q is administered either as a written questionnaire or in an interview, depending on the ability of the respondent. The QOL.Q should always be administered in an interview. However, if the respondent is not verbal, either form is to be completed by two proxies who know the target well. The proxies are to report how they believe the target would respond. Their scores would then be averaged. In this manner, Schalock and Keith (1993) argue that the QOL.Q can be used with individuals with any level of ID.

In addition to a total score, separate scores are calculated for the four domains of (a) satisfaction, (b) well-being and competence, (c) social belonging, and (d) control and empowerment. These scales have slightly different names in the two versions, largely reflecting the different contexts of adolescents without ID and adults with ID. The subscales represent the authors' theoretical perspective on QL, but were confirmed in factor analyses by the authors as well as others (Rapley & Lobley, 1995). Nonetheless, substantial variance remains in total scores that is not associated with the factor scores, which is an argument for retaining the total score.

Psychometric data for the QSL.Q are based on up to 1,982 students from public schools, colleges, and vocational colleges mainly in Nebraska, but also Oregon (both in the United States) and Japan (Keith & Schalock, 1995). Norms, however, are based on only 340 students in Nebraska, who were overwhelmingly white. Data are also presented for 60 special education students, most with learning disability (by the US definition, having a tested intellectual aptitude basically in the normal range or above, but a significantly reduced educational achievement) and in junior high school (ages 12–15 years). A similar pattern of responding was noted between Nebraska and Oregon samples. College students in the United States, however, scored significantly higher than Japanese college students. Internal consistency and two-week test-retest reliability estimates are more than adequate. Validity support is scant, but preliminary support is provided by data showing that students in special education scored lower on the QSL.Q compared to regular education students as well as scores that increased across age and advancement in education.

Psychometric properties for the QOL.Q, the version for adults with ID, are well established for the most part (Schalock & Keith, 1993). While more validity data exist for this version than the QSL.Q, Cummins (1997b) noted that reliability data were reported only for college students rather than adults with ID. Construct validity is supported through higher scores being achieved by people living in independent rather than supervised settings, which has been independently confirmed in the United Kingdom (Ralley & Beyer, 1996), as well as competitive employment as compared to those in supported employment and sheltered workshops. Moreover, scores have been reported to decrease consistent with the severity of the disabilities of people with ID. Concurrent validity is supported with an association with a general life satisfaction measure. Schalock, Lemanowics, Conroy, and Feinstein (1994) reported that adaptive versus challenging behavior, earnings, integrated activities, and home-type contributed strongly to QOL.Q scores.

QUALITATIVE APPROACHES TO MEASURING QUALITY OF LIFE IN PEOPLE WITH INTELLECTUAL DISABILITY

The above instrument systems appear by far the best currently available for the *quantitative* assessment of QL in people with ID regardless of age. In developing approaches to the assessment of QL in this population, however, there has also been substantial representation of a *qualitative* approach. We feel it is important to consider a diversity of approaches in capturing the heretofore nebulous concept of QL. For this reason we will briefly consider three examples of the qualitative approach. However, to our knowledge no data exist as of yet from their application with young people.

Quality of Life Interview Schedule

The Quality of Life Interview Schedule (QUALIS; Development Consulting Program) has been designed primarily for people who are non-verbal or who have a severe ID (Oulette-Kunts & McCreary, 1995). Consequently, it is completed by trained observers and proxies. The definition of QL serving as the basis for this instrument is cited in

Table 15.1. QUALIS measures 43 indicators grouped into 12 domains (see Wallander, Chapter 2 in this volume, Table 2.1). Notably it omits an evaluation of personal health. Each indicator is rated on four criteria: (a) support availability, (b) access, (c) participation, and (d) contentment. A considerable amount of additional data are collected with both open and closed format items, making it a rather comprehensive assessment of current life situation. Verbal clients are also administered 76 items addressing satisfaction.

This is a complex instrument, requiring assessors to complete a two-day training course to be certified in its use. The actual interview takes about two hours to complete. Some psychometric data are provided (Oulette-Kuntz, 1990; Oulette-Kuntz, McCreary, Minnes, & Stanton, 1994). Although impressive in its depth and breadth, the magnitude of this instrument may be excessive for most purposes for which QL measurement will be used (Cummins, 1997b). However, to the extent that it was designed for individuals at a low level of intellectual development, it may have some aspects worthy of application or modification for developing assessments of QL of younger children with ID.

Rehabilitation Questionnaire

The Rehabilitation Questionnaire (Brown & Bayer, 1992) (also referred to as Quality of Life Questionnaire) employs both qualitative and quantitative items to address a broad range of QL domains, including: home living, activities, health, social life, family life, self-image, leisure, employment, legal aspects, desired support, and life satisfaction. This broad scope is a strength of the instrument, which undoubtedly can provide a wealth of information useful for diagnostic or program planning. Forms are available to be administered to people with ID as well as caregivers. Brown and Bayer state there is generally close agreement between these sources (r = .60–.90). The average time of completion is 1–1.5 hours. It has been used with people with tested IQs from 45–110. Consistent with the authors' assertion that "this is not a test in the formal sense but a means of exploring the 'inner' perceptions of individuals" (Brown & Bayer, 1992, p. vii), there is no standardized scoring system. Each user is encouraged to score items as best fitting their needs. This makes it difficult to use and interpret this instrument reliably. While psychometric data are scant, 12-month test-test correlations were reported in the range of .52–.97, with the majority being cited as "above 0.7". This instrument may inform the development of measures of QL with young people mainly in the richness of information one can obtain with it.

Center for Health Promotion Quality of Life Project

The Center for Health Promotion Quality of Life Project (QLP; Raphael, Brown, Renwick, & Rootman, 1996) measure is the product of an explicit theoretical-philosophical perspective elaborated by, for example, Woodhill and colleagues (1994). Setting out to conceptualize and measure QL for all persons with developmental disabilities, they explicitly state a set of assumptions and a model of QL supporting their measurement approach. Their definition of QL is provided in Table 15.1. As elaborated in Table 2.1 in Chapter 2 (Wallander, this volume), their model of QL is summarized with the terms "being, belonging, and becoming" to reference the key components of QL. Each in turn has three dimensions. Adopting a multi-method approach in addressing these domains, the QLP is really a measurement system encompassing self-report, report-by-others, and independent observations, each using a particular combination of interview, diary, checklist, and observation. Data collection thus requires an on-site visit of at least one day for each client. The organizing theme of these methods is to reflect how important each dimension is to the individual and how satisfied the client is with each. Also, the extent of control that he or she has in each dimension as well as possibilities of enhancement or change in those areas are addressed. Numerous scores can be calculated from these efforts.

Although the authors confess disenchantment with traditional measurement tenets, they have provided some psychometric data (Raphael et al., 1996). Descriptive data are provided only on a small sample of 41. Reliability estimates of various sorts, as appropriate to the scales involved, vary from adequate to unsatisfactory for self-report scores, but are at least adequate for report-by-others and observers. Initial concurrent validity is supported by correlations between self-report and QOL.Q scores. Comparisons of very small groups of people living in different situations that were consistent with expectations provide preliminary construct validity support. These findings are encouraging, but inadequate. The major contribution made by the QLP currently is primarily the care with which the construct of QL was elucidated and assumptions were made explicit. Together with the other two measures discussed in this section, the QLP also points out the possibility that QL for young people with ID needs to be measured through a collection of methods, quantitative and qualitative, especially when people are not highly verbal.

RECOMMENDATIONS
MEASUREMENT

It is clear from our review that considerable effort is needed to establish a QL measurement methodology for *young people with ID*. Basically, it does not yet exist! The most important need is to test the utility of those instruments that have been used with young people (ComQol and QSL.Q) on large samples of different ages and intellectual abilities. These measures appear promising; however, in the absence of additional data, neither measure can be supported currently for use with young people with ID. Further adaptations need to be considered for those instruments which have been developed for the general adolescent population and adults with ID, to make them suitable for younger adolescents and children with ID as well as for young people with severe ID.

Existing adult ID instruments should also be considered as useful models in some respects for the development of new instruments for children and adolescents with ID. We need to have different instruments available to meet the different needs for QL assessment. To this end, the qualitative approaches that have been developed may provide useful directions.

Beyond using one or another specific QL instrument, there are the several general measurement issues that continue to confront both researchers and users of QL information. Schalock (1996) has outlined several issues, which are applicable to young people with ID as well:

(1) What should be measured?

While there is increasing consensus that QL is multi-dimensional, what those dimensions are remains a debate. However, this to us seems largely an issue of semantics and where on a continuum from molar to molecular division one stands. While different purposes may require different dimensional frameworks, there is considerable comparability among models of QL content (see Wallander, Chapter 2, in this volume). We feel that the schema proposed by Felce and Perry (1997) provides a useful compromise among comprehensiveness, applicability across the life span, parsimony, and utility. Likewise, because there are advantages and disadvantages with emphasizing either objective or subjective perspectives on QL (see Wallander, Chapter 2 in this volume, for an elaboration) — and clearly, neither is sufficient by itself — we argue that both are needed when considering young people with ID. When and how to join these perspectives or use them as two equally important, but independent perspectives, requires further research.

(2) How do we measure Quality of Life?

This is a question regarding the method of measurement. Different frameworks have been used to discuss solutions (Schalock, 1996). One tendency is to recommend using three or more sources (e.g., participant observation, others' report, self-report). However, if QL is to be used often to inform decisions about individuals, programs, as well as policies, expedience and ease of use must be a priority. Setting high standards is laudable, but we are afraid that is may result in making QL considerations impractical and therefore uninfluential. We suggest that the two sources of self-report and significant others' report (e.g., parent or teacher) be used to measure QL in young people with ID. Further research is needed, however, to determine when self-report can be reliably used in this population. We strongly recommend Cummins' (1997) pre-testing approach to address this concern in clinical application with individuals. If anything, this approach should be expanded to consider issues beyond response format and acquiescence.

(3) What psychometric standards need to be considered?

There are some tendencies to eschew traditional psychometric standards as not applicable when considering QL in people with ID (e.g., Brown & Bayer, 1992; Woodhill et al., 1994). In contrast, we agree with, for example, Schalock (1996) and Cummins (1997b) that reliability and validity must enter into our considerations. At the same time, we have argued elsewhere for the use of a decision-making model to deal with the dilemma in joining considerations for psychometric standards with considerations of utility (Hubert & Wallander, 1988). This means that psychometric standards are not the exclusive concern, nor are they sufficient standards for using a measure. However, they are necessary initial standards, beyond which we must consider *measurement goals and context*. Measures must be practical given the goals and context of assessing young people with ID.

(4) How do we overcome the unique challenges in measuring Quality of Life in young people with ID?

Among these challenges are risk for acquiescence, tendency toward socially desirable responding, lack of effective communication, and the need to use proxies in some cases. The several recommendations made already may address some of these concerns. Additionally, Schalock (1996) recommends (a) using multiple methods; (b) using simple response scales; (c) correcting statistically for response bias; and (d) resolving differences between self- and proxy-report through discussion and observation. To this we must add that research into these issues is much needed. The details regarding each recommendation need to be filled in.

RESEARCH

Given the paucity of research on QL in young people with ID, it is both easy and difficult to provide recommendations. On the one hand, we could, and should, state that much more research is needed in all directions. On the other hand, which of the many possible directions should be a priority? Several will be recommended (see also Schalock, 1994).

Firstly, the dimensional structure of QL in young people needs further attention. How do prevailing models developed for adults apply to young people, or what modifications are needed? In particular, how do these dimensions play out across development? This question needs to be addressed for both typical-developing children and those with ID.

Secondly, influences on individual differences in QL require investigation. These can be characteristics of the person or the environment. Those associated with reduced QL, which can be termed risk factors, need to be determined as this information can aid in the identification of high-risk groups, to which prevention efforts may be directed. Likewise, factors should be identified that are associated with differential outcomes when the same risk factor(s) is present, which can be termed resilience or protective factors. It is especially important to understand those factors associated with protection against the risk exposure because they can point to targets for intervention in those who experience poor QL. Risk and resilience factors associated with differential QL of course need to be studied within a developmental framework.

Thirdly, the impact of interventions for young people with ID on their QL needs to be investigated. This recommendation encompasses a number of different possibilities. In the area of education alone, this would include, for example, evaluation of the differential impact on QL from different educational placements, degrees of integration or inclusion, types of transition services and/or vocational training, and teaching strategies. Social, family, community, and medical interventions represent other areas where impact on QL should be evaluated. Most generally, public policies for young people with ID need to be evaluated in terms of QL impact.

SERVICES

As Schalock (1994) points out, "once the critical factors associated with [QL] are understood, then the next logical step is to enhance a person's ... [QL] through the application of ... quality enhancement techniques" (p. 274). *Quality enhancement techniques* can be directed at service programs or management techniques. Schalock (1994) for example, lists a variety of programmatic efforts that can be implemented that are believed to enhance QL. These can be focused on the (a) home or community living, (b) education, and (c) health functioning. Just as in the business world, quality management and continuous quality improvement principles can be implemented in the disability service area, with expected positive impact on young people's QL. However, the effectiveness and efficacy of these hypothesized quality enhancement techniques need to be evaluated.

Bringing to the forefront considerations for QL of young people with ID is integral to providing *quality assurance* in service provision. Quality assurance needs to address three dimensions of a service program (Schalock, 1994): (a) structure, (b) process, and (c) outcomes. QL, as discussed herein, plays a large role in measuring the quality process and outcomes within such a schema. Quality assurance is dependent on a well-developed definition and process for indexing quality. Even though we can acknowledge that this has not yet taken place for young people with ID, quality assurance processes are rarely discussed in reference to service programs for them, such as special education or transition services.

CONCLUSION

There clearly remains much work to be done to advance our study, understanding, and use of the QL concept in attending to the needs of young people with ID. This represents a significant challenge. The importance of taking on this challenge, however, was well put by Schalock (1994):

> How [the QL] concept unfolds — and the use we make of it — is both challenging and frightening. Challenging because it can result in significantly enhanced conditions of living for persons with disabilities; but at the same

time frightening because we can let the concept be diluted and/or bastardized. The [QL] concept thus represents potentially either our best or worst. (p. 281).

NOTE

[1]   We will use the terms "young people", "children and adolescents," and "youth" interchangeably to refer to those in the age range from birth to about 20 years in this chapter. When more specificity is desired, the term "adolescents" will be used to refer approximately to those aged from 12 to 20 years and "younger children" to those aged 11 years and less.

References

American Association on Mental Retardation. (1992). *Mental Retardation: Definition, classification, and systems of supports.* Washington, DC: American Association on Mental Retardation.

American Psychological Association. (1994). *Publication manual of the American Psychological Association* (4th ed.). Washington, DC: Author.

Borthwick-Duffy, S.A. (1992). Quality of life and quality of care in mental retardation. In L. Rowitz (Ed.), *Mental retardation in the year 2000* (pp. 52–66). Berlin: Springer-Verlag.

Borthwick-Duffy, S.A. (1996). Evaluation and measurement of quality of life: Special considerations for persons with mental retardation. In R.L. Schalock (Ed.), *Quality of life* (Vol. 1) (pp. 105–119). Washington, DC: American Association on Mental Retardation.

Brown, I., Renwick, R., & Nagler, M. (1996). The centrality of quality of life in health promotion and rehabilitation. In R. Renwick, I. Brown, & M. Nagler (Eds.), *Quality of life in health promotion and rehabilitation: Conceptual approaches, issues, and applications* (pp. 3–13). Thousand Oaks, CA: Sage Publications.

Brown, R.I. (1997). *Quality of life for people with disabilities.* London: Stanley Thornes Ltd.

Brown, R.I., & Bayer, M.B. (1992). *Rehabilitation questionnaire and manual: A personal guide to the individual's quality of life.* Toronto: Captus University Publications.

Coe, D.A., & Matson, J.L. (1993). Hyperactivity and disorders of impulse control. In J.L. Matson, R.P. Barrett et al. (Eds.), *Psychopathology in the mentally retarded* (2nd. ed., pp. 253–271). Boston, MA: Allyn & Bacon.

Cummins, R.A. (1995). *Directory of instruments to measure quality of life and cognate areas.* Melbourne, Australia: Deakin University.

Cummins, R.A. (1997a). Assessing quality of life. In R.I. Brown (Ed.), *Quality of life for people with disabilities* (2nd ed., pp. 116–150). London: Stanley Thornes Ltd.

Cummins, R.A. (1997b). Self-rated quality of life scales for people with an intellectual disability: A review. *Journal of Applied Research in Intellectual Disabilities, 10,* 199–216.

Cummins, R.A., McCabe, M.P., Romeo, Y., Reid, S., & Waters, L. (1997). An evaluation of the comprehensive quality of life scale — intellectual disability. *International Journal of Disability, Development and Education, 44,* 7–20.

Edgerton, R.B., Bollinger, M., & Herr, B. (1984). The cloak of competence: After two decades. *American Journal of Mental Deficiency, 88,* 345–351.

Felce, D., & Perry, J. (1993). *Quality of life: A contribution to its definition and measurement.* Cardiff, Wales, UK: Mental Handicap in Wales Applied Research Unit.

Felce, D., & Perry, J. (1995). Quality of life: Its definition and measurement. *Research in Developmental Disabilities, 16,* 51–74.

Felce, D., & Perry, J. (1997). Quality of life: The scope of the term and its breadth of measurement. In R.I. Brown (Ed.), *Quality of life for people with disabilities* (2nd ed., pp. 56–71). London: Stanley Thornes Ltd.

Goode, D.A. (1994). *Quality of life for persons with disabilities: International perspectives and issues.* Boston: Brookline Books.

Goode, D.A., & Hogg, J. (1994). Towards an understanding of holistic quality of life in persons with profound intellectual and multiple disabilities. In D.A. Goode (Ed.), *Quality of life for persons with disabilities: International perspectives and issues* (pp. 197–207). Cambridge, MA: Brookline.

Gottlieb, J., Alter, M., Gottlieb, B.W. (1991). Mainstreaming mentally retarded children. In J.L. Matson, J.A. Mulick, et al. (Eds.), *Handbook of mental retardation* (2nd ed., pp. 63–73). New York, NY: Pergamon Press.

Hodapp, R.A., & Dykens, E.M. (1996). Mental retardation. In E.J. Mash, R.A. Barkley, et al. (Eds.), *Child psychopathology* (pp. 362–389). New York, NY: Guilford Press.

Hubert, N.C., & Wallander, J.L. (1988). Instrument selection. In T.D. Wachs, & R. Sheehan (Eds.), *Assessment of young developmentally disabled children* (pp. 43–60). New York: Plenum.

Hughes, C., Hwang, R., Kim, J.H., Eisenman, L.T., & Killian, D.J. (1995). Quality of life in applied research: A review and analysis of empirical measures. *American Journal on Mental Retardation, 99,* 623–641.

Keith, K.D., & Schalock, R.L. (1993). Assessing the quality of student life. *Issues in Special Education and Rehabilitation, 7,* 87–97.

Keith, K.D., & Schalock, R.L. (1994). The measurement of quality of life in adolescence: The quality of student life questionnaire. *The American Journal of Family Therapy, 22,* 83–87.

Keith, K.D., & Schalock, R.L. (1995). *Quality of student life questionnaire.* Worthington, OH: IDS Publishing Co.

Kleinfeld, L.A., & Young, R.L. (1989). Risk of pregnancy and dropping out of school among special education adolescents. *Journal of School Health, 59,* 359–361.

Landesman, S., Vietze, P.M., & Begab, M.J. (Eds.) (1987). *Living environments and mental retardation.* Washington, DC: AAMR.

Leland, H. (1991). Adaptive behavior scales. In J.L. Matson, J.A. Mulick, et al. (Eds.), *Handbook of mental retardation* (2nd ed., pp. 211–221). New York, NY: Pergamon Press.

Matikka, L. (1994). The quality of life of adults with developmental disabilities in Finland. In D. Goode (Ed.), *Quality of life for persons with disabilities: International perspectives and issues* (pp. 22–38). Cambridge, MA: Brookline.

Nagler, M. (1996). Quality of life of people with disabilities who have experienced sexual abuse. In R. Renwick, I. Brown, & M. Nagler (Eds.), *Quality of life in health promotion and rehabilitation: Conceptual approaches, issues, and applications* (pp. 190–203). Thousand Oaks, CA: Sage Publications.

Oullette-Kuntz, H. (1990). A pilot study in the use of the quality of life interview schedule. *Social Indicators Research, 23,* 283–298.

Oullette-Kuntz, H., & McCreary, B.D. (1995). Quality of life assessment for persons with severe developmental disabilities. In R. Renwick, I. Brown, & M. Nagler (Eds.), *Quality of life in health promotion and rehabilitation: Conceptual approaches, issues, and applications* (pp. 268–278). Thousand Oaks, CA: Sage Publications.

Oullette-Kuntz, H., McCreary, B.D., Minnes, P., & Stanton, B. (1994). Evaluating quality of life: The development of the quality of life interview schedule (QUOLIS). *Journal on Developmental Disabilities, 3,* 17–31.

Raeburn, J.M., & Rootman, I. (1996). Quality of life and health promotion. In R. Renwick, I. Brown, & M. Nagler (Eds.), *Quality of life in health promotion and rehabilitation: Conceptual approaches, issues, and applications* (pp. 14–25). Thousand Oaks, CA: Sage Publications.

Raphael, D., Brown, I., Renwick, R., & Rootman, I. (1996). Assessing the quality of life of persons with disabilities: Description of a new model, measuring instruments, and initial findings. *International Journal of Disability, Development, and Education, 43,* 25–42.

Rapley, M., & Beyer, S. (1996). Daily activity, community participation and quality of life in an ordinary housing network. *Journal of Applied Research in Intellectual Disabilities, 9,* 31–39.

Rapley, M., & Lobley, J. (1995). Factor analysis of the Schalock and Keith (1994) quality of life questionnaire: A replication. *Mental Handicap Research, 8,* 194–202.

Renwick, R., Brown, I., & Nagler, M. (1996). *Quality of life in health promotion and rehabilitation: Conceptual approaches, issues, and applications.* Thousand Oaks, CA: Sage Publications.

Reschley, D.J. (1992). Mental retardation: Conceptual foundations, definitional criteria, and diagnostic operations. In S.R. Hooper, G.W. Hynd, et al. (Eds.), *Developmental disorders: Diagnostic criteria and clinical assessment* (pp. 23–67). Hillsdale, NJ: Erlbaum.

Richardson, S.A., & Koller, H. (1996). *Twenty-two years: Causes and consequences of mental retardation.* Cambridge, MA: Harvard University Press.

Sattler, J.M. (1988). *Assessment of children* (3rd ed.). San Diego, CA: Author.

Schalock, R.L. (1994). The concept of quality of life and its current applications in the field of mental retardation/developmental disabilities. In D. Goode (Ed.), *Quality of life for persons with disabilities: International perspectives and issues* (pp. 57–74). Cambridge, MA: Brookline Books.

Schalock, R.L. (1996). *Quality of Life Volume I: Conceptualization and measurement.* Washington, DC: American Association on Mental Retardation.

Schalock, R.L. (1997). *Quality of life Volume II: Application to persons with disabilities.* Washington, DC: American Association on Mental Retardation.

Schalock, R.L., & Keith, K.D. (1993). *Quality of life questionnaire.* Worthington, OH: IDS.

Schalock, R.L., Lemanowicz, J.A., Conroy, J.W., & Feinstein, C.S. (1994). A multivariate investigative study of the correlates of quality of life. *Journal on Developmental Disabilities, 3*, 59–73.

Sigelman, C.K., Schoenrock, C.J., Winer, J.L., Spanhel, C.L., Hromas, S.G., Martin, P.W., Budd, C., & Bensberg, G.J. (1981). Issues in interviewing mentally retarded persons: An empirical study. In R.H. Brunininks, C.E. Meyers, B.B. Sigford, & K.C. Lakin (Eds.), *Deinstitutionalization and community adjustment of mentally retarded persons* (pp. 114–129). Washington, DC: American Association on Mental Deficiency.

Simeonson, R.J., & Rosenthal, S.L. (1991). Qualitative-developmental processes. In J.L. Matson, J.A. Mulick, et al. (Eds.), *Handbook of mental retardation* (2nd ed., pp. 529–538). New York, NY: Pergamon Press.

Sparrow, S.S., Balla, D.A., & Cicchetti, D.V. (1984). *Vineland Adaptive Behavior Scale.* Circle Pines, MN: American Guidance Service.

Stark, J.A., & Goldsbury, T. (1990). Quality of life from childhood to adulthood. In R. Schalock (Ed.), *Quality of life: Perspectives and issues.* Washington, DC: American Association on Mental Retardation.

Stark, J., & Faulkner, E. (1996). Quality of life across the life span. In R.L. Schalock (Ed.), *Quality of life, Volume I* (pp. 23–32). Washington, DC: American Association on Mental Retardation.

Wallander, J.L., Stankovic, S., & Brown, D. (1997). *Mental health in special education adolescents: Mental health problems in African American adolescents in EMR special education reported by multiple sources.* Paper submitted for publication. University of Alabama at Birmingham, Birmingham, AL.

Woodhill, G., Renwick, R., Brown, I., & Raphael, D. (1994). Being, belonging, becoming: An approach to the quality of life of persons with developmental disabilities. In D. Goode (Ed.), *Quality of life for persons with disabilities: International perspectives and issues* (pp. 57–74). Cambridge, MA: Brookline.

World Health Organization. (1992). *Mental disorders: Glossary and guide to their classification in accordance with the Tenth Revision of the International Classification of Diseases* (10th ed.). Geneva: Author.

CONCLUSIONS AND FUTURE DIRECTIONS

Chapter 16

CHALLENGES IN CHILD AND ADOLESCENT QUALITY OF LIFE RESEARCH

Hans M. Koot
Jan L. Wallander

The quality of life (QL) of children and adolescents has only recently received the attention it rightfully deserves. Of course, the psychosocial development of people younger than the adult age has been the focus of a great deal of attention, in terms of research, care and policy. However, QL as an overarching concept for this age group has only recently received broader attention, mainly in the context of health care. Not surprisingly, being a relatively young endeavor, there is considerable diversity in conceptualization of and operational approach to QL. Despite the relatively advanced status of QL research in adults with health problems or intellectual disabilities, it has not as yet become mainstream in the field. The diversity of approaches described in the chapters of this book attest to that fact.

The aim of this concluding chapter is to summarize the findings and issues discussed in the other chapters in this book, and to identify unresolved conceptual and practical issues. To this end, we summarize QL related consequences of different childhood chronic conditions, as well as existing generic and condition-specific QL measures for this age group. Further, the chapter identifies needs and underdeveloped areas regarding childhood QL research and measurement, and possible applications of the concept in research, services, and care.

This book is a reflection of the short history of QL research with children and adolescents, with most findings and products springing from research on so-called health-related quality of life. This summary partly reflects that history. However, it should be noted that QL is an overarching concept applicable across all young people, regardless of their condition. This view is maintained throughout this chapter.

QUALITY OF LIFE AS AN ORGANIZING CONCEPT
IMPACT OF CONDITIONS

This book includes reviews of the impact of a number of the most common chronic childhood conditions: abdominal disorders, asthma, cancer, cardiovascular disease, cystic fibrosis, headaches, insulin-dependent diabetes mellitus, and intellectual disabilities. These reviews illustrate an enormous diversity, which makes it hard to compare QL work with different conditions and/or draw firm conclusions regarding impact and associated needs. It is immediately obvious, then, that a common framework for the evaluation of effects of chronic conditions is lacking across these chapters. Earlier attempts to summarize the impact of childhood chronic conditions perforce relied primarily on standardized questionnaires for behavioral/emotional problems, completed by parents and child self-esteem ratings (e.g., Lavigne & Faier-Routman, 1992, 1993; Wallander & Thompson, 1995; Wallander & Varni, 1998), thus covering only a portion of what we consider as QL.

The foremost advantage of the QL concept is that it is an organizing concept that can be used for "evaluating core dimensions associated with a life of quality, providing direction and guidance in providing appropriate services" (Schalock, 1996, p. 124). To immediately take advantage of QL as an organizing framework, we summarize the findings from these reviews using the core QL dimensions described by Felce and Perry (1995) as the organizing framework. These include material, physical, social, emotional, and productive well-being (Table 16.1).

Although Table 16.1 summarizes the impact of chronic conditions on QL dimensions, the entries are overwhelmingly based on health care professional and parental reports of physical limitations and psycho-social adjustment; the traditional topics of outcome research. Notable exceptions are the child self-reports of pain, anxiety, depression, and self-esteem mentioned in many reviews. Apart from a description of physical and treatment-related limitations, the emphasis in most reviews is on psychiatric and behavioral/emotional problems. Very little appears to be known about social functioning, as LaGreca (1990) has repeatedly pointed out, although impact on school functioning and participation in clubs and organizations are mentioned. This is probably largely influenced by the inclusion of several items on the Achenbach instruments, the most widely used outcome measure for children. The data on productivity mostly refer to reduced intelligence and other aspects of cognitive functioning. Information on material conditions are lacking for virtually all of the conditions. On the other hand, most chapters mention serious impact on family functioning and relations with and between other family members.

It should be noted that these summary statements are necessarily only estimates. However, the entries in Table 16.1 show an enormous

TABLE 16.1   QUALITY OF LIFE IMPACT OF CHRONIC CONDITIONS BASED ON REVIEWS IN THIS VOLUME

	MATERIAL	PHYSICAL	SOCIAL	EMOTIONAL	PRODUCTIVE
ABDOMINAL DISORDERS	?	***	**	***	?
ASTHMA	?	***	***	***	*
CANCER	?	***	***	***	*
CARDIOVASCULAR DISEASE	?	*	*	*	*
CYSTIC FIBROSIS	?	***	?	***	?
HEADACHES	?	***	**	**	+
DIABETES MELLITUS	?	*	+	*	*
INTELLECTUAL DISABILITY	**	*	***	***	***

NOTE: QL IMPACT IS ORDERED ALONG THE CORE QL DIMENSIONS DELINEATED BY FELCE AND PERRY (1995).
* MINOR OR NONE, ** MODERATE, *** SUBSTANTIAL, ? = NO DATA

variation of impact across conditions. While serious effects on virtually all dimensions appear for some conditions (e.g., cancer, intellectual disabilities), for other conditions relatively small effects or even above average functioning are mentioned (e.g., cardiovascular disease, IDDM). However, variation within conditions is likely as large as variation between conditions, which is mainly due to the significant variation in severity and type of treatment.

As a summary table, Table 16.1 yields two firm conclusions: First, a fair comparison across conditions cannot be made given the variety of instruments used and type of data available on each condition. Second, virtually nothing is known about the *quality of life* of these young people; that is when defined as "the combination of objectively and subjectively indicated well-being in multiple domains of life considered salient in one's culture and time, while adhering to universal standards of human rights" (cf. Wallander, Chapter 2).

CRITIQUE OF PREVIOUS WORK

The reviews in this volume point out several shortcomings in the collective work conducted thus far. We will highlight four that in our opinion are paramount.

First, we need to make a compelling argument for the use of information obtained from youth themselves. For example, a nation-wide US study among parents of youth in the general population (Newacheck & Taylor, 1992) showed that the amount of bother produced by chronic childhood conditions cannot be predicted from the type of condition nor the amount of associated functional limitations. As a case in point, while 58% of those affected by epilepsy seem to encounter limitations in their usual activities, only 19% of them seem to experience a great deal of bother. By contrast, while only 17% of those with chronic headache encounter functional limitations, 57% of them are bothered a great deal (Newacheck & Taylor, 1992). Thus, based on epidemiological data, we may expect only a limited association between the functional and psychological impact for each chronic condition.

In addition, average correlations between biomedical tests of disease parameters and patient reports of well-being are fairly low, especially in children (e.g. Guyatt, Juniper, Feeny, & Griffith, 1997). Therefore, it is not surprising that the ability of physicians and nurses to accurately rate their patients' QL is limited. Both under- and over-estimations of limitations, pain, and psychological impact occur (see Sprangers & Aaronson, 1992). Moreover, in medical treatment in particular we frequently see a discrepancy between efficacy of a treatment from the provider's and patient's point of view. Similarly, ratings of behavioral and emotional functioning by youths themselves tend to have a low correlation with ratings by parents, teachers, or mental health workers (Achenbach, McConaughy, & Howell, 1987; Verhulst & Koot, 1992). Insights such as these have led to the reasoning that QL is best understood from the perspective of the individual (e.g., Joyce, McGee, & O'Boyle, 1999; Schalock, 1996; Spilker, 1996). While this is well acknowledged in the field of adult QL research, methods to obtain children's and adolescents' views on their QL are only beginning to be developed (e.g., Varni, Seid, & Rode, 1999).

Second, there is poor agreement on the core quality of life dimensions. While many specific schemas have been proposed, they do in fact overlap considerably (see Wallander, Chapter 2). Most approaches reviewed herein, which were based in the healthcare system, have included in some form or another the physical, emotional, and social dimensions. However, broader conceptualizations of QL in individuals across the life span consistently identify additional dimensions targeting material and productive well-being. As argued elsewhere (Wallander, Chapter 2), we find Felce and Perry's particular conceptualization of QL dimensions useful and would urge adoption of this hierarchical system as the base for identification of core QL dimensions.

Third, the modus operandi has been to develop setting or condition specific QL instruments, almost for each separate research project or clinic. This approach has made it virtually impossible to develop a knowledge base on the impact of chronic conditions on children or what are effective and efficacious interventions or policies for improving their QL. We need to move towards the adoption of a select few QL instruments that can be applied generically to summarize information from children and adolescents as well as their parents, caretakers, and health providers. These generic instruments need to be construed broadly enough to be applicable to all children, whether or not they have a health-threatening condition. This is the only way we will acquire the necessary knowledge to make informed decisions regarding the effects on children's QL. We find the notion of disease-specific QL misleading. QL is by its nature a holistic concept; an attempt to describe how well or poorly life works at a particular point in time. How can one's life be separated into that which is influenced by a disease and that which is influenced by all current and past experiences. Of course, we may at times be interested in learning about disease impact. Presumably, this becomes an issue of what specific known symptoms and consequences of a disease are present. These may in turn may be correlates of QL. However, QL and disease impact are theoretically distinct concepts and need to be measured separately.

Finally, the work thus far to understand QL in children and adolescents has lacked a broad theoretical framework to organize questions and findings. Once the conceptual base has been established and a few instruments have been identified to operationalize QL, studies on differences and similarities between conditions regarding their impact and explanatory factors, as well as subsequent efforts to improve them, may begin. A valuable framework for the study of explanatory factors is the disability-stress-coping model proposed by Wallander and Varni (1998) which identifies risk and resilience factors for QL. Included in the former are disease/disability parameters, functional limitations, and psychosocial stress, and the latter, stress processing, intrapersonal factors, and social-ecological factors.

EVALUATION OF QUALITY OF LIFE INSTRUMENTS FOR YOUNG PEOPLE
DESIDERATA

Many instruments have been developed in a relatively short period of time to measure QL in young people. This reflects the rapidly growing interest shown over the past decade or so in the broad impact of health conditions and interventions on young people's lives and mirrors, albeit in the typically delayed fashion, what has transpired with adult populations. There are several dozen instruments reviewed in this volume that purport to measure QL in young people and more are published every year. This interest is of course satisfying for those of us who believe that QL can be a very useful notion for improving the lives of children and adolescents.

The outcome of these efforts to date is, however, less satisfying. That is, *as a whole, the instruments available to measure QL in young people at this point in time are lacking on many counts*. While there is considerable diversity in the measurement methodology available today, the quality of the resulting products is generally poor. No one instrument can be recommended without limitations. The chapters so charged in this volume review many QL instruments, either in a general context (e.g., Hanson, Chapter 7; Spieth, Chapter 3) or relevant to a specific condition (see Part 4), generally coming to the same conclusion.

On the one hand, the negative evaluation of the available instruments should not be surprising. Measuring QL in young people is a relatively new endeavor, explaining in part the current state. There are many measurement issues to address, which take time. These issues have been discussed in detail in many chapters and we summarize our recommendations for how to address them in a following section.

It is necessary to highlight here that some specific issues have not been well handled, by and large, in this collective body of work thus far. Foremost is the lack of conceptual development, discussion, and consensus seeking specifically applied to young people. QL measures will be hard pressed to improve without adequate attention being paid to this foundational development. The QL notion will simply flounder and possibly die out as a useful construct without adequate conceptual undergirding. A particular obstacle against conceptual development, in our opinion, has been the bifurcation of efforts to construe QL as a generic or disease-specific construct. This and other more specific issues in the conceptual domain were discussed earlier in this chapter as well as in the chapters in Part 2.

High on the list of important issues to be addressed are those issues that can generally be described as developmental in nature. In addition, more attention needs to be paid to psychometric development and evaluation to produce better instruments. Most efforts have been lacking in one or both of these respects. We will summarize recommendations regarding these two sets of issues in a later section of this chapter and further detailed discussion can be found in Chapter 2 (Wallander).

Although the QL measurement methodology is not where we would like it to be today, there is reason to be optimistic about its development. Given the many different efforts and the increased attention, and given the many challenges in developing high quality instruments to measure QL, we expect considerable improvements will be evident in the near future. Some of the instruments available today indeed appear promising and these will be highlighted below. Those few instruments should emerge as the most worthy of our use during the next phase of this work, which should result in those instruments being further improved. Not only is this a natural evolution in a developing area of inquiry, but this will also serve to improve the knowledge base about QL of young people with health and developmental conditions. When a select set of instruments is used to operationalize QL, then we will be much better able to compare findings from different studies and across populations and contexts.

GENERIC INSTRUMENTS

We believe that much will be gained if efforts from this point forward are devoted primarily to considering QL as a construct that is applicable across all young people. No differentiation should be made between those who have *specific* health or developmental conditions, *any* health or developmental conditions, or *no* health or developmental conditions. That is, standards for a life of quality cannot depend on the challenges a young person experiences. Those standards must be universal. Therefore, the body of generic QL measures should provide the most useful pool from which to develop the next generation of QL measures for young people.

Spieth (Chapter 3) reviews some 17 generic QL instruments in detail. However, it is hard to select a few specific instruments from this pool worthy of further consideration. They were clearly developed for different purposes, such as epidemiological surveys, policy and program evaluation, and patient assessment. Those labeled by Spieth as health profiles and multidimensional instruments come closest to the conceptualization of QL that we emphasize. Each instrument within these two categories, however, has shortcomings, such as being overly long, targeting only adolescents, requesting only self- or parent-report, or focusing on a "health-related" perspective on QL.

Nonetheless, from among these instruments we recommend that further consideration be given the RAND Health Status Measure of Children (Eisen et al., 1979), Child Health Rating Inventories (Kaplan et al., 1995), How Are You? (Bruil et al., 1997), and Quality of Life Profile (Raphael et al., 1996). None of these are completely satisfactory at present, but they contain elements that will serve as a good base for future work. To this set we would like to add two instruments for further consideration.

One is the Comprehensive Quality of Life Scale (Cummins, 1997). Although this instrument was reviewed in the context of measures of QL in young people with intellectual disability (Wallander & Turrentine, Chapter 15), one of its forms is intended for all adolescents. We appreciate its clear conceptual basis, broad multidimensional construction of QL, use of objective and subjective indicators, brevity, and careful psychometric attention. One of its limitations is its exclusive use thus far by Cummins in Australia.

The other instrument that should be considered further is the PedsQL, a generic measurement system developed by Varni and colleagues (Varni, Seid, & Rode, 1999) and published after Spieth's review for this volume. While the initial goal was to measure QL in children with cancer (Varni et al., 1998a, 1998b), it is now available in a fourth generic edition. It consists of a 15-item core, addressing the physical, mental, and social health domains. These scales provide an overall QL score. To this can be added disease-specific modules, of which several are available or currently being tested (e.g., cancer, diabetes, cystic fibrosis). Non-English versions are also being developed. This is a reasonable way of avoiding confusion between generic QL and what others term health-related and disease-specific QL. Versions are available for ages 8–12 and 13–18 years which differ in wording only to match the ability of each age range, as confirmed by formal assessment of reading levels. There are parallel forms for self- and parent proxy-report and a pictorial response format version for ages 5–7 years is currently being tested. Internal consistency reliability estimates for a total score as well as for domain scores were found to be adequate. Discriminant validity, using the known-groups approach, was demonstrated for young patients with cancer on- and off-treatment. Construct validity has received initial support from confirming the expected correlation patterns with standardized psychosocial questionnaires. The PedsQL appears promising — it is clearly a second generation instrument — but is in need of further, and especially independent, use and testing.

DISEASE-SPECIFIC INSTRUMENTS

As discussed previously, we find the disease-specific approach quite limited, if not misguided. It is hard for us to understand the idea of disease-specific QL, or even health-related QL. It seems impossible to differentiate what conditions or circumstances influence what aspect of one's life. Moreover, it makes little sense to us to measure the impact of a disease by limiting a priori what could be due to the disease, as is typically done in the disease-specific or health-related approaches. Rather, QL must be viewed as having universal standards (see earlier proposed definition), and the impact of any disease is then best learned by comparing the QL, broadly construed, of people with and without the disease (either through a between- or within-groups study). Given our premise, we can therefore not recommend any specific disease-specific QL measures.

Many colleagues, however, have not shared our premise. The chapters in Part 4 of this volume show that there are numerous disease-specific instruments available purported to measure QL. Certainly, one theme to be observed in the development of instruments to measure QL in young people with health or developmental conditions has been the plethora of disease-specific instruments. Even within distinct diseases, especially for asthma, diabetes, and cancer, there have been many different instruments developed. Unfortunately, most studies of the QL of children with a diagnosis have relied on its own measure of QL and therefore comparisons based on different approaches and measures are near impossible. Rarely have comparison groups been used to provide any type of standard and consequently, the body of knowledge about each condition or about health and developmental conditions overall has suffered.

In our view, those instruments purported to be disease-specific QL measures may be useful for measurement of the more limited construct of *perceived disease impact*. The utility of the construct must be evaluated first, of course. We certainly would not advocate the substitution of this construct in studies to learn of the impact of a condition, treatment, or care policy on young people. These must be evaluated in terms of QL broadly construed. In many cases, this may be supplemented, at least in theory, with consideration for perceived disease impact.

Furthermore some of the instruments used to measure QL in young people with specific diseases have been developed after considerable thought and effort. Several contain elements that should inform the generic efforts we advocate. For example, we are impressed with the developmental approach used by French et al. (1994) in developing different forms to be useful for young people with asthma at different ages. Also, Eiser et al.'s (1995) child centered approach in developing the Perceived Illness Experience measure is another nice example of this.

Some of the disease-specific instruments may also provide a good basis for the development of a generic QL measure, as was illustrated above with the PedsQL. This would require editing items and evaluating their use with a broader sample of children. Likewise, some of these instruments provide nice examples for how some of the specific measurement issues can be addressed. We draw examples from these instruments in providing recommendations below.

MEASUREMENT ISSUES AND RECOMMENDATIONS
ACCOUNTING FOR DEVELOPMENT

As discussed by Wallander (Chapter 2) development is a pervasive challenge for the study of QL in youth. Development does and should affect our choices of: which QL dimensions to tap, item content, instrument format, the use of proxy information, and the feasibility of certain approaches, such as the utility approach. Development and associated child and adolescent competencies should be of concern for anyone involved in the study of QL.

DIMENSIONS AND DOMAINS

Although there is general agreement that QL measures should tap multiple dimensions, hardly anything is known about the relative importance of accepted QL dimensions for children and adolescents. This is unlike the knowledge base of psychosocial adjustment, where we are guided by our knowledge on the importance of certain themes such as the development of attachment to parents, language, peer relations, school competence, sexual roles, and identity. However we do not know how important specific QL domains are in the eyes of the typical youngster. Surveys and focus group discussions involving youth of different ages and conditions can give us the necessary detailed information on desirable content of QL measures for youth. The challenge is to cover the life of young people and at the same time choose dimensions and domains that are relevant across ages and sociocultural contents. One approach would be to develop modules that may be used depending on the developmental age of the child, and then compute average domain scores.

INSTRUMENT FORMATS

As with adults, most QL instruments for children and adolescents use a questionnaire format. Provided that a child can understand simple questions about his or her own experience and that acquiescense tendencies are ruled out, for example by using the pretesting protocol developed by Cummins (1997; see Chapter 2 by Wallander), a large variety of formats is now available. Starting with the preschool age we may use simple questions and pictorial scales. Recently, computer simulations have also been developed for the youngest age group (e.g. Buller, 1999). Starting with age six, more comprehensive items and response formats may be used such as those in the three different versions of the Childhood Asthma Questionnaires (see French, Chapter 9). In addition to subjective experience or satisfaction ratings, importance ratings may be used (e.g., Juniper, Guyatt, Feeny, Ferrie, Griffith, & Townsend, 1996). However it is as yet unclear what added value importance ratings have over and above satisfaction ratings. It is important to note that utility ratings such as used with adults (e.g., Kaplan, see Chapter 4) are far too complex for use with children under age 15 years (Juniper, Guyatt, Feeny, Griffith, & Ferrie, 1997).

OBJECTIVE AND SUBJECTIVE MEASURES

Although QL has most often been defined in terms of subjective well-being, there are at least two reasons to also include objective measures. First, it may simply be impossible to obtain reliable subjective information from youths themselves, when for example they are too young, have cognitive limitations, or are severely ill. The limited capacity of some people to judge their own QL necessitates the collection of information on objective living circumstances. This approach of having available methods to obtain both subjective and objective information has served our study of psychological adjustment well (e.g., Achenbach, 1991a, 1991b). A second reason lies in the fact that subjective QL ratings may be heavily influenced by personal frames of reference that run counter to generally accepted standards. People may lower their standards to unacceptable levels as a form of adaptation to conditions. This is exemplified when changes occur in QL ratings without objective changes in conditions such as in QL ratings by terminally ill or psychiatric patients (e.g., Bury, 1991).

SELF-REPORT AND PROXY REPORT

Given the lack of congruence between self- and proxy reports and the simultaneous necessity to obtain proxy reports in many cases, it is imperative to find ways to increase the validity of proxy reports and develop useful strategies for how to combine these sources of information. One of the first questions to answer is from what age onward reliable child reports can be obtained. Children may have difficulty with any of the following: reporting about the period beyond the immediate present; using standard response formats; adapting to changes between positive and negative questions; answering pain-related questions; and answering private or intrusive questions.

Second, should we use child or parent proxy reports or both? The validity of both reports may vary across domains and development. Parents may be more sensitive to impairments than children themselves. However, parents may have limited sensitivity to the child's experiences and changes therein. Therefore, we need to assess the reliability and validity of both types of reports using repeated measures and external validation criteria. Further, we should test the typical degree of congruence between informants across different domains to assess how much confidence we can have in each. Finally, we should test algorithms to combine or integrate self-ratings and ratings from multiple proxies to obtain optimal information on the child's QL.

GENERIC AND CONDITION-SPECIFIC MEASURES

As outlined above and argued by Spieth (Chapter 3) there are several advantages to the use of generic QL instruments. First, since generic measures are designed to assess all relevant QL domains that are likely to be affected by the condition, they are more comprehensive than condition-specific ones. Second, the rater is dismissed from the difficult, if not impossible, task of judging QL only in regard to when it is solely "health-related". Third, it enables the comparison of QL outcomes across conditions as well as the value of allocation of resources to different service systems (e.g., health care vs. social services vs. education).

However, generic instruments are unlikely to be sensitive to all detectable changes in the condition. We might argue that changes that do not affect QL as tapped by generic QL measures are not really important. However, there might be important effects that are only detectable in the long run. For example, reduction of diarrhea in youth with certain bowel disorders may increase mobility, which may subsequently increase social participation. Therefore, short-term effects of specific treatments may be more easily tapped by condition-specific instruments. However, to avoid confusion, these should be referred to as disease-impact measures.

Reliability and validity

As argued in several chapters (e.g. Wallander, Chapter 2, and Spieth, Chapter 3) QL measurements need to meet universal standards of reliability and validity. Most QL instruments for youth do not meet even basic criteria of validity, and in most cases the study of critical characteristics such as the power to discriminate between known groups, or sensitivity to change, have just started. Consequently, a lot of effort has to be devoted to the psychometric evaluation of QL measures. However, the following are examples of issues which may challenge these efforts: (a) limited internal consistency may be expected given the heterogeneity of domains covered by QL measures; (b) the limited value of test-retest reliability given the changeable nature of QL; (c) the lack of sensitivity to differences between groups with different conditions and between children with chronic conditions and the general population; (d) the uncertain clinical importance of differences in QL scores between groups or across time; and (e) the clinical relevance of instruments developed for research.

Sensitivity to change

The important issues in regard to sensitivity to change include: statistical sensitivity of QL measurements to change; the clinical significance of statistically significant changes; the importance of individual change scores; and the comparison with clinically relevant changes in health status (e.g., use of medication; absent days). Many QL instruments (including those developed for adults) have only been validated in relation to sensitivity to group differences. However, an important application of QL is to evaluate treatment, services, and policies. This broad use requires that the instrument is sensitive to group mean change. Using repeated measures in a case-control design, changes in groups can be tested using paired t-tests or repeated measures analysis of variance. When more than two measurements are available on large samples, individual differences in growth curves can be tested. However, in clinical practice, reliable assessment of intraindividual change is difficult. Individual's ratings of change are subject to response shift; that is, people tend to adjust the criteria of their judgments across time. For example, Mathijssen et al. (in press) asked parents of children referred for mental health services to indicate after one year whether the problem for which the child had been referred had improved. Differences in ratings were mostly related to the present level of problem behavior, independent of the level of problem behavior at intake. Goal Attainment Scaling may be a better option, if both objective and subjective measures are included. Another question is — how much of the measured change is clinically significant? Individual clinical decision making requires high-quality instruments that produce very low standard errors of measurement. This in turn is dependent on internal consistency and test-retest reliability, both of which benefit from a large number of items.

Scoring and interpretation

For QL measurements to be useful, scores are necessary that are sensitive to both statistically and clinically relevant differences. Relatively little attention has been paid to the presentation and interpretation of QL scores. Several suggestions can be made as to how to present information regarding QL measurement in manuals as well as scientific publications: scores and changes in scores may be presented as the population attributable risk for obtaining a certain score. Effects of clinical trials may be illustrated by presenting the percentage of scores indicating reliable improvement or deterioration, or by relating the amount of change to known measures of consumption of care (e.g. hospital days) or clinically significant differences in health status. Another way is to relate scores to known population distributions of QL scores, for example, by indicating how much scores have shifted from the mean of the dysfunctional group to the population mean; by transforming raw QL-scores to percentile scores; by indicating the percentage of the group whose scores shifted from the deviant range to the normal range in the population; or by indicating the p-value for a specific amount of change (see also Lydick & Epstein, 1996).

RESEARCH APPLICATIONS

Apart from research on measurement issues, two main areas of research are expected to receive a lot of attention in the near future. To get a better idea of the meaning of QL in children and adolescents we need to study the determinants of QL. This information should lead to interventions to improve QL in a wide variety of settings, which in turn need to be evaluated. Such research on QL will be enhanced by taking into account the following recommendations.

RESEARCH DESIGNS

Three study designs are most commonly applied in QL research (Testa & Simonson, 1996). The first one is the *cross-sectional or nonrando-*

mized longitudinal study that is focused on predictors of QL by comparing different patient groups or analyzing predictive power of the condition, person, or environmental characteristics. For example, a recent secondary analysis of SF-36 data on more than 10,000 patients in the Netherlands compared the QL of adult patients with a range of chronic diseases (De Haes et al., 1997). QL was lower for almost all patients than for individuals from the general population. In general lower QL was associated with higher age, being female, lower education, living alone, and more severe disease and comorbidity. Further, differences between patient groups were larger for physical than for mental functioning. However, the balance between physical and mental burden differed greatly among diseases. Mental functioning was most taxed for people with psychiatric, cerebral-vascular and neurological diseases, while physical functioning was most limited for patients with musculoskeletal problems.

Similar comparisons can be made for childhood conditions if the same generic instrument is used for all. This can be illustrated by results from a meta-analysis of studies on behavioral/emotional problems in children with chronic physical conditions in which the same outcome instrument was used, that is the parent-completed Child Behavior Checklist (Koot & Hoogerheide, 1999). Based on 103 empirical studies it could be shown that the average level of problem behavior for children with chronic conditions was 1 SD above the general population mean and 0.5 SD below the mean of a population referred to mental health services. Effect sizes ranged from 2.58 for neurologic disorders to 0.01 for juvenile rheumatoid arthritis. Effect sizes were stronger for disorders with an intermittent course, neurologic disorders, diseases with acute onset and acquired (vs. congenital) conditions. Unfortunately, these data are based on proxy reports and therefore cannot be readily interpreted to reflect children's QL. A broadly accepted generic QL instrument is clearly needed.

A second common design is the *randomized clinical intervention*. This design requires measures that reflect the nature of the condition, are responsive to clinically meaningful changes and are sensitive to changes within the domains that are to be affected by the intervention. This type of application is still very scarce in childhood QL research (see Ravens-Sieberer & Bullinger, Chapter 6). However, it is encouraging to know that self-report instruments can be developed that reliably assess QL in children in a large age range (7–17 years), and are valid for both discriminative (survey) and evaluative (clinical trial/practice) use, as is the case with the Paediatric Asthma Quality of Life Questionnaire (Juniper et al., 1996).

A third design is the *cost-effectiveness and cost–benefit analysis*. Several examples based on health outcomes expressed in Quality-Adjusted Life Years are elaborated by Kaplan (Chapter 4). However, the use of QL ratings for the purpose of managed health care evaluation is not without dispute. Measurement of QL in order to evaluate the human and financial costs and benefits, and determine whether expenditures for health care are justified, cannot replace decisions based primarily on the individual patients' preferences.

DEFINITION OF QUALITY OF LIFE

If we cannot agree upon the concept of QL, it will be very difficult to advance the field. Study questions, methods, and results will then be too divergent to be comparable. Wallander's definition of QL as "the combination of objectively and subjectively indicated well-being in multiple domains of life considered salient in one's culture and time, while adhering to universal standards of human rights" (Chapter 2) is attractive. It summarizes all important aspects that are covered in the literature, it is broad, and at the same time it is precise enough to allow operational definitions and empirical testing. Furthermore, by allowing individual and cultural variation in content it avoids premature closure, and enables further conceptual and empirical development. To advance the field, it is important to allow multiple domains to be included as well as multiple perspectives.

IDENTIFICATION OF QUALITY OF LIFE DOMAINS

The type and number of domains and subdomains to be included in the study of QL is undetermined. As indicated in Chapter 1, the purpose of studying QL is of importance, not only in determining the level of analysis or measurement, but also the type and amount of domains to be covered. Broadly defined core domains such as material, physical, social, emotional, and productive well-being (cf. Felce & Perry, 1995) should provide the common framework. However, these core domains may well be more precisely and specifically defined in any particular study. For example, if we want to change the QL of people with both intellectual and hearing disabilities, intervention may include the application of a hearing aid as well as training for its use, acoustic environmental improvements, caregiver instruction, and communication training. QL improvements may then be expected with regard to hearing function, communication, self-help, social involvement, emotional well-being, and level of problem behavior. Thus, both specific and general, broadband domains of functioning are involved. This does not mean that domains are independent, but improvement of the functional hearing level may have implications for psychological and social functioning, and thus for overall QL.

A definition of QL that includes both subjective and objective indicators implies that we should include both children and adults, professionals, and laymen in the identification of relevant domains. Children, and for that matter all participants in a study who are dependent on adults, are seldom asked to participate in the construction of domains, items, or instruments. However, for both the content and wording of generic and domain-specific instruments and items, target groups should be interviewed or addressed through focus groups of people who are all familiar with the condition at hand. For example, Griffiths (1999) asked youths with Crohn's disease or ulcerative colitis to produce functional, social, and emotional issues related to their physical condition and to rank them according to importance. It appeared that both the prevalence and rank order of similar complaints were very different across conditions. Thus, this type of finding underscores the utility of including target groups in the development of instruments to obtain valid information on content and importance.

QL may be culture-dependent. Although a number of domains and values are considered universal, as documented in the Universal Declaration of Human Rights, their valuation may differ across cultures or according to local circumstances. For example, while it seems important for most adults in the US to be able to drive a car, this is definitely less so in Papua New Guinea. Thus, a material domain of QL would need to be operationalized differently in these cultures. Cross-cultural comparisons may make clear to what extent cultural differences in values and local conditions, such as standard of living, may influence the relative importance and rating of several aspects of QL.

NORMATIVE STANDARDS

An unaddressed issue related to QL assessment in children regards the normative basis against which to compare QL data. QL standards may vary considerably both between and within cultures. For example, Weisz, Suwanlert, Chayasit, Weiss, Walter, and Anderson (1988) asked parents in Thailand and the US to respond to case vignettes of internalizing and externalizing child problems. Thai parents, compared to American parents, rated the children's problems as less serious, less unusual, less likely to worry them if they were the child's parent or teacher, and more likely to improve over time without intervention. These findings suggest that the same child behavior may lead to quite different levels of adult concern. Similar problems may be encountered when searching for adequate norms for children's QL. Even within nations, norms for QL may vary across subcultures.

APPLICATIONS IN SERVICES AND CARE

To determine quality of care as indicated by Ravens-Sieberer and Bullinger (Chapter 6), the common denominator of most of the applications of the QL notion (except the purely individual) is that QL is viewed from a patient group perspective. That is, the main focus has been on how a specific patient group can be described in terms of needs and effects to enable recommendations for clinical care in that patient population. This use of QL should be helpful to evidence-based medicine, in which systematized knowledge is collected about effects of treatment regimens. Likewise, QL considerations should inform managed care plans, by providing information about economical yet effective use of services. Below we suggest some possible applications, illustrated with examples on specific, mostly physical conditions. Similar applications may be developed to improve the QL of youths with psychosocial problems or living in otherwise unfavorable situations.

TO DETERMINE QUALITY OF LIFE DIFFERENCES BETWEEN DIFFERENT GROUPS

If the same standardized, generic measure of QL is used in different groups, the resulting quantitative expression may be used to indicate the relative impact of a specific condition on the invidual's QL. This can be expressed in relation to the average QL of children with other chronic conditions as well as in reference to norms for the general population. However, comparisons across conditions are only possible if a generic instrument or a utility index is used. If differential impact on different aspects of QL are to be detected, an instrument yielding a profile will be necessary.

TO DETERMINE HOW COMPLICATIONS UNRELATED TO DISEASE ACTIVITY AFFECT QUALITY OF LIFE

Several complications of conditions are not directly caused by disease activity, but may have a considerable impact on QL of the child. For example, incontinence, strictures, obstruction, pain, and physical deformity, but also growth retardation, delayed sexual development, and enteric fistulas, may be present in Crohn's disease and all potentially affect QL. Knowledge about the adverse effects of this type of complication can provide a valuable focus of care.

TO DETERMINE WHETHER CONDITION-RELATED DIFFERENCES EXIST BETWEEN DIFFERENT SUBGROUPS

For example, although Crohn's disease and ulcerative colitis present with some similar symptoms, patients within each group may be distinguished in terms of symptom characteristics, location of the affected gastrointestinal section, symptom specificity, course, treatment, complications, and psychological impact. QL studies on broadly defined groups could account for these distinctions.

TO USE IN INTERVENTION TRIALS

Evaluating intervention effects is complex, requiring measurement of potential effects at multiple levels. QL measurement should be one important level. As an illustration, consider the study by Feagan et al. (1995), who reported a randomized trial of treatment with methotrexate in 141 adult patients with chronically active Crohn's disease despite at least 3 months of prednisone therapy. The treatment was effective in that patients who received methotrexate were twice as likely to be in clinical remission following 16 weeks of treatment than those who received placebo, and actively treated patients received less prednisone and showed less disease activity. However, the decision to give methotrexate depends on the weighing of benefits and risks against the increase in well-being as experienced by the patient. Therefore, in this study patients completed the Inflammatory Bowel Disease Questionnaire, a 32-item disease impact instrument that addresses bowel function, emotional function, systemic symptoms, and social function. The authors chose a disease impact instrument because it includes problems that are deemed to reflect patients' primary symptoms, and may be more powerful than generic instruments in detecting treatment effects. However, although the effect of the methotrexate was statistically significant, the study was inconclusive in three important ways. First, the QL measure used in this study did not measure adverse effects of methotrexate treatment, such as nausea, lethargy, rash, or mouth ulcers, nor effects on QL more broadly. Second, it was not clear from the report how clinically significant the difference in disease impact between the study group and control group was. Finally, effects of the intervention on QL more broadly could not be assessed. Thus, although disease impact was carefully evaluated, QL assessment was notably lacking.

TO DETERMINE THE ASSOCIATION BETWEEN CHILDHOOD QUALITY OF LIFE AND OTHER PROGNOSTIC FACTORS AND OUTCOME IN PROSPECTIVE STUDIES

Collection of QL measures over time can help to track both changes and rates of changes in outcomes as they relate to disease activity, medical treatment, and other life changes. For example, independent of disease activity or treatment, social and emotional aspects of QL in children with inflammatory bowel disease may decline when they reach puberty. This is because they experience difficulties in achieving an age-appropriate position in their peer group due to disease-related physical problems. Nothing is known about these children's differential reactions to their condition depending on disease characteristics and related stress, personal make-up, developmental status, and available environmental support. However, several models have been developed to identify factors relevant for the adjustment of children with chronic conditions (e.g. Wallander & Varni, 1998). These models may be applicable to illuminate both between and within group differences in QL.

TO ASSESS THE RELATIONSHIP BETWEEN SUPPORT AND QUALITY OF LIFE OUTCOMES

This is a general topic, which may be well illustrated by an ongoing study on adolescent insuline dependent diabetes. In puberty, both psychological and physiological changes cause a deterioration of diabetes control, while the need to improve and stabilize metabolic control is increased. The enormous demands of daily management of diabetes are associated with symptoms of depression and anxiety, particularly in adolescents. Numerous investigators have found adolescents with diabetes to have poorer treatment adherence than younger children. Furthermore, cases of serious noncompliance commonly seem to emerge in mid-adolescence and to be protracted. In view of these findings, efforts to better understand factors that may promote or enhance treatment adherence among adolescents with diabetes is a critical area for pediatric research. Preliminary evidence (La Greca et al., 1995; La Greca & Thompson, 1998; Thompson et al., 1997, submitted) shows that both family members and friends are important and complementary sources of tangible and emotional support for adolescents with diabetes, and that support from friends is associated with improved adherence and glycemic control. Of course, a crucial question is whether these improvements lead to simultaneous improvements in overall QL.

TO ASSIST IN THE ALLOCATION OF RESOURCES AND PUBLIC POLICY DECISION MAKING

One of the advocated goals of QL assessment is to provide data regarding the true costs of a disease, taking into account the number of life-years saved after adjustment for quality of these years, the so-called quality-of-life-adjusted years. Although hypothetically this type of data can be useful to reach decisions regarding the allocation of limited human and financial resources, it will prove very difficult to obtain the required children's preferences to reach utility weightings. Issues involve the methods by which preferences are derived, the sample from which they are derived, and the interpretation of the weightings. Similar issues have been raised against using this approach with persons with intellectual disability (see Wallander and Turrentine, Chapter 15).

ACCEPTANCE IN THE FIELD OF CARE

Some authors maintain that QL research "will be fully accepted by [health care] practitioners only when it answers questions directly related to clinical programs and therapeutic choices" (Testa & Simonson, 1996, p. 839). This quote reflects the limited focus of QL research in one of its major fields of application. Many, especially in the medical field, would feel that separate attention to QL issues would be outside their circle of influence and competence. Many consider it unnecessary and not useful to address QL as an outcome of medical treatment beyond disease impact. Several reasons underlie this view-point. Most health care providers are still unfamiliar with QL concepts and its measurement. It is certainly very different from biomedical measures. In addition, there is considerable disagreement as to whether QL is an appropriate goal for health care. The lack of familiarity with QL concepts and psychosocial measurement as a whole is expressed as skepticism against "subjective" data. There is also resistance against the use of structured or standardized formats to assess QL as well as toward posing "private" questions. Admittedly, before health care providers will spend time and money on QL there are numerous issues to solve.

TABLE 16.2 NEEDS FOR CONNECTING RESEARCH AND HEALTH CARE PRACTICE FOCUSED ON QUALITY OF LIFE

1. ATTITUDE FORMATION AND SCHOOLING IN THE PRINCIPLES AND METHODS OF QL ASSESSMENT
2. FURTHER DEVELOPMENT AND REFINEMENT OF GENERIC AND CONDITION-SPECIFIC INSTRUMENTS THAT ARE RELEVANT FOR CARE AND SENSITIVE TO CHANGES IN TREATMENT AND CARE
3. PRACTICALLY ORIENTED RESEARCH INTO THE BEST PRESENTATION OF QL METHODS AND DATA
4. COLLECTION OF NORMATIVE QL DATA FOR REPRESENTATIVE POPULATIONS
5. DEVELOPMENT OF MODELS FOR THE EVALUATION OF CARE
6. FURTHER DEVELOPMENT OF QL DATA MANAGEMENT, SCORING, AND INTERPRETATION
7. FURTHER DEVELOPMENT OF VERSIONS OF QL INSTRUMENTS THAT CAN BE USED IN DIFFERENT AGE AND ABILITY GROUPS
8. RESEARCH ON TIMING, METHODS AND CONTRIBUTION OF FOLLOW-UP ASSESSMENTS
9. DEVELOPMENT OF GUIDELINES AND PROCEDURES TO USE QL DATA IN THE PRACTICE OF CARE
10. DEVELOPMENT OF QL BASED PROTOCOLS FOR FOLLOW-UP AND SUBSIDIARY CARE

These include better definition of the QL domain and its relevance for the practice of care, as well as the very limited guidelines for care that can as yet be derived from our current state of knowledge based on QL. To this end, combined research and practical efforts need to address issues such as summarized in Table 16.2.

CONCLUSION

As maintained throughout this chapter, many issues have to be solved in the study and application of QL measurements in youth. To set up really useful studies addressing aspects of QL in children and youths, we need to adhere as much as possible to methodological principles of large-scale and, possibly, cross-cultural research. Expanding on some guidelines formulated by Huerny et al. (1992) and summarized by Ravens-Sieberer & Bullinger in this volume (Chapter 6), the following list has been composed of requirements for an effective implementation of QL measurement in studies on children and adolescents that are easily overlooked (see Table 16.3). Regard for these recommendations in QL studies involving children and adolescents is very likely to enhance the validity and interpretability of their results.

Although, the use of the QL notion and its empirical knowledge base is in its infancy, we feel the contributions in this volume suggest that furthering their development will be worthwhile. We further believe that the QL notion has the potential to represent the ultimate standard against which to judge the impact on children from whatever conditions they encounter — health-related and otherwise — and the efforts of

TABLE 16.3   BASIC QUESTIONS IN THE IMPLEMENTATION OF QUALITY OF LIFE MEASUREMENTS IN MULTI-CENTRE STUDIES

STUDY DESIGN
- IS THE QL ASSESSMENT AN INTEGRAL PART OF THE STUDY? ARE OBJECTIVES, METHODS AND GUIDELINES EXPLICITLY STATED IN THE PROTOCOL?
- ARE ALL STUDY PARTICIPANTS, INCLUDING CHILDREN AND PARENTS/CARETAKERS CONSULTED DURING THE DESIGN AND DEVELOPMENT OF THE PROTOCOL?

INSTRUMENT
- ARE ITEMS INCLUDED THAT ARE LABELED BY STUDY PARTICIPANTS AS THE MOST IMPORTANT IN THEIR DAILY LIVES?
- IS THE INSTRUMENT SENSITIVE TO ADVERSE EFFECTS OF INTERVENTION OR TREATMENT?
- IS THE INSTRUMENT'S FORMAT APPROPRIATE FOR THIS AGE GROUP?
- CAN PROXY REPORT BE CONSIDERED VALID, IF NEEDED?
- IS THE INSTRUMENT RELIABLE AND VALID?
- IS THE INSTRUMENT CROSS-CULTURALLY ADAPTED?
- IS THE INSTRUMENT SHORT ENOUGH TO BE FILLED OUT REPEATEDLY, E.G. DURING THE COURSE OF AN INTERVENTION?
- DOES THE INSTRUMENT DISCRIMINATE BETWEEN GROUPS WITH DIFFERENT CONDITIONS OR WITH DIFFERENT TREATMENTS/INTERVENTIONS WITHIN ONE CONDITION GROUP?
- IS THE INSTRUMENT SENSITIVE TO CHANGES OVER TIME IN HOW PARTICIPANTS FEEL?

DATA COLLECTION AND MANAGEMENT
- IS A CENTRAL STUDY COORDINATOR AVAILABLE, WHO HAS ONGOING CONTACT WITH LOCAL COORDINATORS AND PROVIDES BOTH INDIVIDUALIZED AND STANDARDIZED FEEDBACK TO ALL INSTITIUTIONS, ALSO INCLUDING GROUP MEETINGS ON THE EXPERIENCE WITH AND EVOLUTION OF THE STUDY?
- IS MANAGEMENT OF QL DATA AND OTHER BIOPSYCHOSOCIAL DATA JOINTLY ORGANIZED AND CARED FOR BY ONE RESPONSIBLE AND TRAINED LOCAL DATA MANAGER PER INSTITUTION?
- IS THE STUDY SUPPORTED BY THE RESPONSIBLE HEAD OF THE INSTITUTION OR DEPARTMENT BY PROVIDING TIME AND SPACE FOR THE STUDY?
- IS SELECTIVE INCLUSION FOR QL ASSESSMENT AVOIDED? ARE PARTICIPANTS FULLY INFORMED ABOUT STUDY GOALS AND REQUESTS? IS ASSISTANCE OF THE PARTICIPANTS IN QUESTIONAIRE COMPLETION AVAILABLE?

DATA ANALYSIS
- WHAT STATISTICALLY SIGNIFICANT EFFECT ON QL WILL BE CONSIDERED PRACTICALLY AND CLINICALLY SIGNIFICANT?
- WHAT METHOD WILL BE USED TO EXPRESS THE EFFECT SIZE?
- WILL THE RESULTS HAVE AN IMPACT ON THE WAY CHILDREN AND PARENTS/CARETAKERS WILL BE INFORMED, TREATED, SUPPORTED, OR CARED FOR, NOW OR IN THE FUTURE?

---

society to enhance their development. Certainly, all who work with or are otherwise concerned with children would hold as one of their most important goals that of ensuring that children experience a life of quality.

References

Achenbach, T.M. (1991a). *Manual for the Child Behavior Checklist and 1991 Profile*. Burlington, VT: University of Vermont Department of Psychiatry.

Achenbach, T.M. (1991b). *Manual for the Youth Self-Report and 1991 Profile*. Burlington, VT: University of Vermont Department of Psychiatry.

Achenbach, T.M., McConaughy, S.H., & Howell, C.T. (1987). Child/adolescent behavioral and emotional problems: Implications for cross-informant correlations. *Psychological Bulletin, 101,* 213–232.

Bruil, J., Maes, S., Le Coq, E., & Boeke, A. (April, 1997). *Assessing quality of life among children with a chronic illness: The development of a questionnaire*. Paper presented at the Sixth Florida Conference on Child Health Psychology, Gainesville, FL.

Büller, H. (1999). Assessment of quality of life in the younger child: The use of an animated computer program. *Journal of Paediatric Gastroenterology and Nutrition, 28,* S53–55.

Bury, M. (1991). The sociology of chronic illness. *Social Health Illness, 13,* 451–468.

Cummins, R.A. (1997). *Comprehensive Quality of Life Scale — Student (Grades 7–12): ComQoL-S5.* (5th ed.). Melbourne: School of Psychology, Deakin University.

Cummins, R.A. (1997). Assessing quality of life. In R.I. Brown (Ed.), *Quality of life for people with disabilities* (2nd ed., pp. 116–150). London: Stanley Thornes Publishers, Ltd.

De Haes, J.C.J.M., Sprangers, M.A.G. et al. (1997). *Adaptieve opgaven bij chronische ziekte.* [Adaptive tasks of chronic disease]. Report. The Hague: NWO.

Eisen, M., Ware, J., & Donald, C. (1979). Measuring components of children's health status. *Medical Care, 17,* 902–921.

Eiser, C., Havermans, T., Craft, A., & Kernahan, J. (1995). Development of a measure to assess the perceived illness experience after treatment for cancer. *Archives of Disease in Childhood, 72,* 302–307.

Feagan, B.G., Rochon, J., Fedorak, R.N., Irvine, E.J., Wild, G., Sutherland, L., et al. (1995). Methotrexate for the treatment of Crohn's disease. The North American Crohn's Study Group Investigators. *New England Journal of Medicine, 332,* 292–297.

Felce, D., & Perry, J. (1995). Quality of life: Its definition and measurement. *Research in Developmental Disabilities, 16,* 51–74.

French, D.J., Christie, M.J., & Sowden, A.J. (1994). The reproducibility of the Childhood Asthma Questionnaires: Measures of quality of life for children with asthma aged 4–16 years. *Quality of Life Research, 3,* 215–224.

Griffiths, A.M., Nicholas, D., Smith, C., Munk, M., Durno, C., & Sherman, P.M. (1999). Development of a quality of life index for paediatric inflammatory bowel disease: Dealing with differences related to age and IBD type. *Journal of Paediatric Gastroenterology and Nutrition, 28,* S46–52.

Guyatt, G.H., Juniper, E.F., Feeny, D.H., & Griffith, L.E. (1997). Children and adult perceptions of childhood asthma. *Pediatrics, 99,* 165–168.

Huerny, C., Bernhard, J., Joss, R., Willems, Y., Cavalli, F., Kiser, J., Brunner, K., Favre, S., Alberto, P., Glaus, A. et al. (1992). Feasibility of quality of life assessment in a randomized phase III trial of small cell lung cancer — a lesson from the real world — The Swiss Group for Clinical Cancer Research SAKK. *Annals of Oncology, 3,* 825–831.

Johnson, S.B. (1995). Insulin-dependent diabetes mellitus in childhood. In M.C. Roberts (Ed.), *Handbook of pediatric psychology* (pp. 263–285). New York: Guilford Press.

Joyce, C.R.B., McGee, H.M., & O'Boyle, C.A. (1999). *Individual quality of life: Approaches to conceptualisation and assessment.* Amsterdam: Harwood Academic Publishers.

Juniper, E.F., Guyatt, G.H., Feeny, D.H., Ferrie, P.J., Griffith, L.E., & Townsend, M. (1996). Measuring quality of life in children with asthma. *Quality of Life Research, 5,* 35–46.

Juniper, E.F., Guyatt, G.H., Feeny, D.H., Griffith, L.E., & Ferrie, P.J. (1997). Minimum skills required by children to complete health-related quality of life instruments for asthma: comparison of measurement properties. *European Respiratory Journal, 10,* 2285–2294.

Kaplan, S.H., Barlow, S., Spetter, D., Sullivan, L., Khan, A., & Grand, R. (1995). Assessing functional status and health-related quality of life among school-aged children: Reliability and validity of a new self-reported measure [Abstract]. *Quality of Life Research, 4,* 444.

Koot, H.M., & Hoogerheide, K. (1999). Behavioral/emotional problems in children with chronic conditions: A meta-analytic review. Unpublished paper.

LaGreca, A.M. (1990). Social consequences of pediatric conditions: Fertile area for future investigation and intervention. *Journal of Pediatric Psychology, 15,* 285–307.

LaGreca, A.M. (1992). Peer influences in pediatric chronic illness: An update. *Journal of Pediatric Psychology, 17,* 773–784.

La Greca, A.M., Auslander, W.F., Greco, P., Spetter, D., Fisher, E.B., Jr., & Santiago, J.V. (1995). I get by with a little help from my family and friends: Adolescents' support for diabetes care. *Journal of Pediatric Psychology, 20,* 449–476.

La Greca, A.M. & Thompson, K. (1998). Family and friend support for adolescents with diabetes. *Analise Psicologica, 1,* 101–113.

Lavigne, J.V., & Faier-Routman, J. (1992). Psychological adjustment to pediatric physical disorders: A meta-analytic review. *Journal of Pediatric Psychology, 17,* 133–157.

Lavigne, J.V., & Faier-Routman, J. (1993). Correlates of psychological adjustment to pediatric physical disorders: A meta-analytic review and comparison of existing models. *Journal of Pediatric Psychology, 17,* 133–157.

Lydick, E.G., & Epstein, R.S. (1996). Clinical significance of quality of life data. In B. Spilker (Ed.), *Quality of life and pharmacoeconomics in clinical trials* (pp. 461–466). Philadelphia: Lippincott-Raven.

Mathijssen, J.J.J.P., Koot, H.M., & Verhulst, F.C. (Submitted). One-year outcome of referred children and adolescents: Perceived changes, need for help, and dropping out.

Maes, S., & Bruil, J. (1995). Assessing quality of life of children with a chronic illness. *Health psychology and quality of life research, proceedings of the 18th annual conference of the European Health Psychology Society* (pp. 637–652). Alicante: Health Psychology Department, University of Alicante.

Newachek, P.W., & Taylor, W.R. (1992). Childhood chronic illness: Prevalence, severity, and impact. *American Journal of Public Health, 82,* 364–371.

Raphael, D., Rukholm, E., Brown, I., Hill-Bailey, P. & Donato, E. (1996). The Quality of Life Profile-Adolescent version: Background, description and initial validation. *Journal of Adolescent Health, 19,* 366–375.

Schalock, R.L. (1996). Reconsidering the conceptualization and measurement of quality of life. In R.L. Schalock (Ed.), *Quality of life, Volume I: Conceptualization and measurement* (pp. 23–32). Washington: American Association on Mental Retardation.

Spilker, B. (1996). Introduction. In B. Spilker (Ed.), *Quality of life and pharmacoeconomics in clinical trials* (2nd ed.) (pp. 1–10). Philadelphia: Lippincott-Raven.

Sprangers, M.A.G., & Aaronson, N.K. (1992). The role of health care providers and significant others in evaluating the quality of life of patients with chronic disease: A review. *Journal of Clinical Epidemiology, 45,* 743–760.

Testa, M.A., & Simonson, D.C. (1996). Assessment of quality-of-life outcomes. *New England Journal of Medicine, 334,* 835–840.

Thompson, K.M., La Greca, A.M., & Shaw, K.H. (submitted). Family and peer support for diabetes care among African-American and Hispanic adolescents. Manuscript submitted for publication.

Varni, J.W., Katz, E.R., Seid, M., Quiggins, D.J.L., Friedman-Bender, A., & Castro, C.M. (1998a). The Pediatric Cancer Quality of Life Inventory (PCQL): I, Instrument development, descriptive statistics, and cross-informant variance. *Journal of Behavioral Medicine, 21,* 179.

Varni, J.W., Katz, E.R., Seid, M., Quiggins, D.J.L., & Friedman-Bender, A. (1998b). The Pediatric Cancer Quality of Life Inventory-32 (PCQL-32): I. Reliability and validity. *Cancer, 82,* 1184.

Varni, J.W., Seid, M., & Rode, C.A. (1999). The PedsQL™: Measurement Model for the Pediatric Quality of Life Inventory. *Medical Care, 37,* 126–139.

Verhulst, F.C., & Koot, H.M. (1992). *Child psychiatric epidemiology: Concepts, methods and findings.* Newbury Park: Sage Publications.

Wallander, J.L., & Thompson, R.J. Jr. (1995). Psychosocial adjustment of children with chronic physical conditions. In M.C. Roberts (Ed.), *Handbook of pediatric psychology* (2nd ed., pp. 124–141). New York: Guilford Press.

Wallander, J.L., & Varni, J.W. (1998). Effects of pediatric chronic physical disorders on child and family adjustment. *Journal of Child Psychology and Psychiatry, 39,* 29–46.

Weisz, J.R., Suwanlert, S., Chayasit, W., Weiss, B., Walter, B.A., & Anderson, W.W. (1988). Thai and American perspectives on over- and undercontrolled child behavior problems: Exploring the threshold model among parents, teachers, and psychologists. *Journal of Consulting and Clinical Psychology, 56,* 601–609.

(ECMO) 224, 225, 314, 320, 322; and cognitive function 322, 325

face validity 64
FACT 158
factor analysis 14
family: adjustment 187–93, 195, 198, 202; assessing 136; beliefs/attitudes 193–5, 197; buffering role 189, 191, 195, 201, 341, 350; climate 186, 192, 203; cohesion 190, 191, 198, 199, 200; coping styles 195–7, 201, 203; effect on child 189–91; flexibility 190, 191; functioning 6, 11, 185, 188, 190, 191, 432; miscarried helping 199; resources 150, 196, 203; role restriction 364; support 189, 196, 197–200, 201, 204, 350, 351
Family Environment Scale 345
family impact 11, 15, 126; cancer 289; chronic illnesses 11, 15, 126, 188–93; Crohn's disease 222; CVD 308, 309, 311; cystic fibrosis 125, 340–42, 345, 350; headaches 363–4; IDDM 380, 392, 394; RAP 217
family QL perspective 181, 182, 186, 187, 202, 203; and child development 189; concepts 185–8, 202; conceptual models 184–5; definitions 185–7; and disease course 189, 190, 192, 193, 200; disease-specific 188; functional 188; gender differences 187; parental behavior 186; sibling effects 192–3, 203; stress 188, 189, 193, 195, 198, 199, 200, 201, 203, 308, 309, 311, 364
feeding difficulties 307, 313, 324, 329
Feeling Thermometer 12
FLIC questionnaire 158
freedom, and QL 5
French, D.J. 241–61, 439
functional approach, chronic childhood illness 124, 125–9, 188
Functional Disability Inventory 215
functional effects 5, 154, 435; asthma 242, 258; in CF 351–2; in IDDM 377–8; measures 8, 11, 53, 54, 67–72, 134–7
Functional Status-II-R 54, 69–70, 135, 136, 253, 256; Measure (FSI) 69; psychometric characteristics 135
Functional Status Measure II (FS-II) 386
functionality, conceptions of 137

gastrointestinal disorders see abdominal disorders
gender: and cognitive function 327; and QL issues 138, 159, 187
General Health Policy Model (GHPM) 89, 97, 98–100, 102, 104; duration of symptoms 99, 101; morbidity 98, 101;

mortality 98, 101; prognosis 98, 99–100; utility 98, 99, 103
generic health-related QL 49–83, 155, 163; advantages 82–3; clinical practice 49; clinical research trials (intermediate level 50) 49, 50; definitions 49; developmental framework 80–82; disadvantages 83; health care policy (macro level) 49, 50; individual assessment approach (micro level) 51; physical functioning 49, 154; population surveys 50; psychological functioning 49; social functioning 49
generic instruments 11, 49, 51, 52–5, 155, 435, 437–8, 440, 442; clinical outcome measures 53, 67–77; epidemiological 11, 52; evaluations 59–77, 442; functional status 11, 53, 54, 67–72; health profiles 11, 52, 62–7; interpretation 78; use in IBD 223; multi-dimensional 11, 54, 72–7, 116; psychometric standards 51–9, 159; selection 77; staff burden 78; taxonomy of instruments 51, 52–5; utility measures 11, 52, 60–62, 440
genetic screening, cystic fibrosis 106–8
Goal Attainment Scaling 444
goal orientated approach 274, 275–6
goldstandard see normative standards
growth abnormalities 11, 94, 167, 168, 222, 227; and CF 335, 336; and chemotherapy 272; and CHD 307, 313, 324; IBD 218, 222

Handicap-Related Problems for Parents Inventory 11, 12
Hanson, C.L. 181–204
headaches 11, 357–68; adult QL studies 364–3; causality 361; child QL studies 365–7; cluster 358; and cognitive function 363; diagnosis 358; duration 359; and family life 363–4; migraine 358–9, 365; and physical functioning 361–2; prevalence 360–61; and psychological functioning 362–3, 366; and psycho-social problems 359; and QL domains 357, 361–2, 366; and schooling 363, 367; and social functioning 363–4; subjective nature of 357; support 368; tension 358, 360, 364, 365; treatment selection 357–8, 368
health care policy perspective 5, 6, 8, 9, 14, 49, 50, 89–116
health care, special 126, 128; for at-risk groups 128, 129
health: definition of 6, 27, 29, 181, 183; goals 90, 93; perceptions 5; profiles 11, 52, 62–7; promotion 90
health-related QL 5, 27, 36, 181; generic 49–83; specific 49

item selection strategy 30; criterion-based 30; internal consistency 30; item-response theory 30

Johnson, S.B. 373–94
Journal of Developmental and Behavioural Pediatrics 7
Journal of Pediatric Psychology 7
Juvenile Arthritis Functional Assessment Report for Children 136, 137
juvenile chronic arthritis (JCA) 129; and gender 138

Kant, I. 24
Kaplan, R. 89–116
Karlish, L. 335–52
Kawasaki disease 301
KINDL 170
Koot, H.M. ix–xi, 3–17, 431–53

Langveld, J.H. 357–68
latent traits 24, 30
learning disability *see* intellectual disability
leukemia 134, 142, 164, 271, 286, 302; *see also* cancer
Life Activities Questionnaire for Childhood Asthma 250–51; parental assistance with 251; psychometric features 251
life satisfaction 7, 27, 29, 36; and control 37
Life Situation Scale for Parents 12
list-based *see* condition-specific approach
longitudinal studies 153, 155, 161, 167, 168, 171, 203, 223, 444–5
low birth weight 168
lung cancer 158
lung transplantation 103

magnetic resonance imaging (MRI) 321
managed care organizations (MCOs) 125
Marfan's syndrome 300–301
material well-being 40, 409
matrix approach to evaluation 95, 96
Medical Outcomes Study Short Form Health Survey (SF-20) 364, 385
medication *see* treatment
Mental Development Index 321, 323
mental health *see* psychological functioning
mental retardation *see* intellectual disability
miscarried helping 199
Missouri Child Behavior CheckList (MCBC) 344
mortality 3, 8, 98, 101
Multi-attribute health status classification system 277–9; domains 278; standard gamble 278
myocardial disease 301–2
myocarditis 301

National Association of Children's Hospitals and Related Institutions (NACHRI) 132
National Health Interview Survey (NHIS) 52, 59–60, 125; Disability Supplement 148–50
National Longitudinal Study of Adolescent Health 105
nephrology 160
neurology 159–60, 167
neuromuscular disorders 11
nomological net 26
non-categorical approach *see* functional approach
non-insulin dependent diabetes mellitus (NIDDM) 373
normative standards 10, 36, 44, 45, 64, 72, 78, 80, 155, 169, 283, 416, 447–8
Nottingham Health Profile 155, 159
NYHA classification 159

objective measures *see* quantitative approaches
obsessive-compulsive disorder 159, 220, 221
oncology *see* cancer
Ontario Child Health Study (OCHS) 52, 60
otitis media 11
outcomes: importance of 99; non disease 105–15
outcome measures 94; QL as 6–7, 53, 67–77, 152, 260
outcomes model 90–94; approach to health care 91; cost–benefit 91–2; life-expectancy 93; patient-centered 91; patient reports 90, 92, 93; and prevention 90, 92, 93, 94; and QL 93, 450
overprotection 314, 328

Paediatric Asthma Caregiver's Quality of Life Questionnaire (PACQLQ) 12, 255–6; psychometric properties 256
Paediatric Asthma Quality of Life Questionnaire (PAQLQ) 253–4, 259; psychometric properties 254, 446
Paediatric Cancer Quality of Life Inventory (PCQL) 280–81
Paediatric Oncology Quality of Life Scale (POQL) 279–80, 286; psychometric characteristics 280
pain 167, 432; control 286; and psychological well-being 363; underrating 15, 434
parental: behavior 186, 196; overprotection 314, 328
parental QL: assessment 11, 12; asthma 246, 255–6, 257; cancer 268